Imaging Atlas of the Pelvic Floor and Anorectal Diseases

Mario Pescatori • F. Sérgio P. Regadas • Sthela M. Murad Regadas •
Andrew P. Zbar

Imaging Atlas of the Pelvic Floor and Anorectal Diseases

Forewords by
Clive I. Bartram
Robert D. Madoff

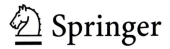 Springer

MARIO PESCATORI, MD, FRCS, EBSQ
Chairman, Coloproctology Unit
Ars Medica Hospital
Rome, Italy

F. SÉRGIO P. REGADAS, MD, PhD
Professor of Surgery and Coordinator
Digestive Surgery Course
School of Medicine
Federal University of Ceara
Head of the Department of Surgery
Clinic Hospital
Federal University of Ceara
Fortaleza, Brazil

STHELA M. MURAD REGADAS, MD, PhD
Adjunct Professor of Digestive Surgery
School of Medicine
Federal University of Ceara
Head of the Anorectal Physiology Unit
Clinic Hospital
Federal University of Ceara
Fortaleza, Brazil

ANDREW P. ZBAR, MD (Lond) MBBS, FRCS
(Edin), FRCS (Gen), FRACS, FSICCR
Conjoint Associate Professor
Universities of New England
and Newcastle
Tamworth Regional Referral Centre
New South Wales, Australia

Library of Congress Control Number: 2008926120

ISBN 978-88-470-0808-3 Springer Milan Berlin Heidelberg New York
e-ISBN 978-88-470-0809-0

Springer is a part of Springer Science+Business Media
springer.com
© Springer-Verlag Italia 2008

Typesetting: C & G di Cerri e Galassi, Cremona, Italy
Printing and binding: Printer Trento S.r.l., Trento, Italy

Printed in Italy
Springer-Verlag Italia S.r.l., Via Decembrio 28, I-20137 Milan, Italy

To our parents for their permanent dedication and love during our entire lives, and to our children, for the patience during the times we have been out of their convivial company

F.S.P. Regadas and S.M. Murad Regadas

To my parents who instilled in me the desire for knowledge through its articulation, dedication to its pursuit and in its recapitulation

A.P. Zbar

To my daughter Camilla and my son Lorenzo Carlo

M. Pescatori

Foreword

Imaging is now central to the investigation and management of anorectal and pelvic floor disorders. This has been brought about by technical developments in imaging, notably, three-dimensional ultrasound and magnetic resonance imaging (MRI), which allow high anatomical resolution and tissue differentiation to be presented in a most usable fashion. Three-dimensional endosonography in anorectal conditions and MRI in anal fistula are two obvious developments, but there are others, with dynamic studies of the pelvic floor using both ultrasound and MRI coming to the fore.

This atlas provides an easy way to gain a detailed understanding of imaging in this field. The atlas is divided into four sections covering the basic anatomy, anal/perianal disease, rectal/perirectal disease and functional assessment.

One of the difficulties with developing an atlas is to strike the right balance between text and images. Too much text and it is not an atlas; too little text and the images may not be understood. The editors of this atlas are to be congratulated on achieving an appropriate balance. The images are all that one expects from an atlas, and the diagrams are excellent. The commentaries at the end of invited chapters are a valuable addition, placing what are relatively short, focussed chapters into context. They add balance and depth to the work and are well worth reading.

The range covered in this atlas is extensive and includes all the coloproctologist would expect to encounter. Anorectal cancer is included, as are other primary pelvic tumours and metastatic diseases. Again, this increases the breadth of the work, as when working in this field it is important to know about tumours in other related systems. I am pleased that colonic transit time is included, as this is such an integral part of the investigation of constipation and pelvic floor disorders. The chapters on ultrasound, which more directly address clinicians, are detailed, practical and well illustrated.

This is a well-laid-out atlas, with several imaginative innovations. It is readily accessible and will be most helpful to all health care providers in this field of expertise.

London, June 2008   *Professor Clive I. Bartram, FRCS, FRCP, FRCR*
Consultant Radiologist
Princess Grace Hospital
London, UK

Foreword

The field of coloproctology is an increasingly complex one. Knowledge of both benign and malignant anorectal diseases has expanded dramatically, and with this growth, a new array of available treatment options has emerged. In addition, continued steady progress in the study of pelvic floor disorders has led to an ever-broadening range of available therapies. Moreover, treatment of anorectal and pelvic floor disorders, be they organic or functional, is increasingly informed by the anticipated functional consequences of the proposed therapy. Gone are the days when every fissure was treated by sphincterotomy, fistula by fistulotomy, or cancer by radical surgery (or radical surgery alone).

In order to optimally treat these difficult problems, the surgeon must have the most accurate possible preoperative information, including – especially – imaging. Fortunately, the increasing availability of new imaging techniques, coupled with a dramatic improvement in image quality, is now positioned to provide exactly this information. However, as with many opportunities, this one comes with a challenge. Colorectal surgeons need to know which test to perform when, and how to interpret the results. Radiologists need to understand the fine points of functional anatomy and the clinical relevance of specific findings. Much is written advocating a "team approach" to complex clinical problems, and the concept applies particularly well to disorders of the anorectum and pelvic floor. *Imaging Atlas of the Pelvic Floor and Anorectal Diseases* fills an important void at the interdisciplinary juncture.

There is much to recommend this book. The authors are internationally recognized authorities, many of them pioneers in their specific subspecialty fields. The book is practical, logically organized, and clearly written. The illustrations and diagrams are sharp, well labeled, and easy to understand. At the end of several chapters, the editors provide helpful commentaries that emphasize key issues and provide the appropriate clinical context.

I congratulate Drs. Pescatori, Regadas, Murad Regadas, and Zbar on this outstanding work, which can only serve to advance the dialog between specialties and care of affected patients.

Minneapolis, June 2008

Robert D. Madoff, MD
Stanley M. Goldberg, MD Professor of Surgery
Chief, Division of Colon and Rectal Surgery
University of Minnesota
Minneapolis, MN, USA

Table of Contents

**SECTION IV   Large Bowel and Pelvic Floor Functional Assessment:
Imaging Indications and Technical Principles**

List of Contributors

HERAND ABCARIAN
Department of Surgery
University of Illinois
Chicago, IL, USA

FELIX AIGNER
Department of General and
Transplant Surgery
Innsbruck Medical University
Innsbruck, Austria

BRENDA AVALOS
Colorectal Gold Surgery Service
LAC+USC Medical Center
Los Angeles, CA, USA

ROSILMA GORETE LIMA BARRETO
Medical School of the Federal
University of Ceara
São Luis, Maranhão, Brazil

PEDRO C. BASILIO
Section of Colégio Brasileiro de
Cirurgiões – CBC, and
Colorectal Surgery
Hospital Samaritano
Rio de Janeiro, RJ, Brazil

MARC BEER-GABEL
Pelvic Floor Unit
Chaim Sheba Tel-Hashomer
Medical Center
Tel-Aviv, Israel

ANA KARINA NASCIMENTO BORGES
Department of Diagnostic Imaging
Cancer Hospital of Barretos
Barretos, SP, Brazil

ALICE BRANDÃO
Clínica Radiológica
Luiz Felippe Mattoso
Rio de Janeiro, RJ, Brazil

ALEXANDRE CECIN
Department of Diagnostic Imaging
Cancer Hospital of Barretos
Barretos, São Paulo, Brazil

GERALDO MAGELA G. CRUZ
Colorectal Department
Santa Casa de Belo Horizonte
Belo Horizonte, MG, Brazil

RAFAEL DARAHEM
Department of Diagnostic Imaging
Cancer Hospital of Barretos
Barretos, SP, Brazil

ALBERTO DIAZ-CARRANZA
Keck School of Medicine at USC
Los Angeles, CA, USA

HANNES GRUBER
Department of Radiodiagnostics
Innsbruck Medical University
Innsbruck, Austria

JOSE J. GUILLEM
Department of Surgery
Memorial Sloan-Kettering Cancer Center
New York, NY, USA

ANGELITA HABR-GAMA
School of Medicine
University of Sao Paulo
Sao Paulo, SP, Brazil

José Marcio Neves Jorge
School of Medicine
University of Sao Paulo
Sao Paulo, SP, Brazil

Howard S. Kaufman
Division of Pelvic Floor and
Colorectal Surgery
Keck School of Medicine at USC
and General Surgery Service
USC University Hospital
Los Angeles, CA, USA

Harry Kleinübing Jr.
Department of Surgery
Hospital Municipal São José
University of Região de Joinville
Joinville, Santa Catarina, Brazil

Hector Lugo-Colon
Keck School of Medicine at USC
Los Angeles, CA, USA

Armando Melani
Department of Surgery
Cancer Hospital of Barretos
Barretos, SP, Brazil

Roberto Misici
Pelvic Floor Functional Disorders Unit
"Faculdade Integrada do Ceara (FIC)"
Aldeota, Fortaleza, Ceará, Brazil

Caio Sergio R. Nahas
Department of Gastroenterology
Surgical Division
University of Sao Paulo
Sao Paulo, SP, Brazil

Sergio Carlos Nahas
Department of Gastroenterology
Surgical Division
University of Sao Paulo
Sao Paulo, SP, Brazil

Adrian E. Ortega
Keck School of Medicine at USC
and Colorectal Gold Surgery Service
LAC+USC Medical Center
Los Angeles, CA, USA

Frida R. Pena
Department of Surgery
Keck School of Medicine at USC
Los Angeles, CA, USA

Vittorio Piloni
Diagnostic Imaging Centre
Private Clinic "Villa Silvia"
Senigallia, Ancona, Italy

Mauro S.L. Pinho
Department of Surgery
Hospital Municipal São José
University of Região de Joinville
Joinville, Santa Catarina, Brazil

Manoel de Souza Rocha
Department of Radiology
University of Sao Paulo
Sao Paulo, SP, Brazil

Lusmar Veras Rodrigues
Colorectal Department
Clinic Hospital of the Federal
University of Ceara
Fortaleza, Ceara, Brazil

Bianca Santoni
Department of Colorectal Surgery
Cleveland Clinic Florida
Weston, FL, USA

Liana Spazzafumo
Center of Statistics
Department of Ageing Geriatric Research
Institute I.N.R.C.A.
Ancona, Italy

Jaap Stoker
Department of Radiology
University of Amsterdam
Amsterdam, The Netherlands

Steven D. Wexner
Department of Surgery
Division of General Surgery
University of South Florida
College of Medicine
Tampa, FL, USA, and
Department of Colorectal Surgery
Division of Research and Education
Cleveland Clinic Florida
Weston, FL, USA

SECTION I
Normal Anal Canal and Rectum Anatomy

CHAPTER 1

Two-dimensional Ultrasonography of Pelvic Floor and Anorectal Anatomy

Felix Aigner, Hannes Gruber

Abstract

This chapter should help to clarify the anatomical relationships and complex anorectal topography that can be clearly visualized by modern ultrasound techniques and should be recognized by the pelvic surgeon. The pelvic floor forms the supportive and caudal border of the abdominal cavity. Previous anatomical studies have demonstrated that the pelvic connective tissue can be divided into three compartments: anterior, middle, and posterior. This chapter is dedicated to the posterior compartment and reflects the supportive function of the pelvic floor muscle systems as well as its impact on continence function and defecation.

Introduction

Diagnosis of pelvic-floor and complex anorectal disorders has been revolutionized by the introduction of endosonography over the last 20 years. Additional applications of ultrasound to the perineum, such as noninvasive transperineal ultrasound (NITUS) or three-dimensional (3-D) endoanal ultrasound extend the spectrum of imaging this complex anatomical region with regard to the longitudinal extent of normal anal structures and of perianal pathologies. Techniques such as endorectal (ERUS) or endoanal (EAUS) ultrasound gained popularity among physicians mainly because of their minimally invasive, painless, and inexpensive modality compared with other imaging techniques such as computed tomography (CT) scan or magnetic resonance imaging (MRI). Moreover, improvements in the technology of ultrasound transducers, such as high-resolution 3-D machines, also increased the accuracy of ERUS and EAUS for local staging of malignant lesions in the anorectal region. However, history and physical examination remain essential cornerstones of diagnosis, especially concerning the pelvic floor, and should inevitably precede any imaging technique in proctological practice.

Main indications for ERUS and EAUS are local staging of rectal and anal carcinomas, on the one hand, and evaluation of fecal incontinence, on the other hand. The accuracy of endosonography in staging primary rectal cancer varies from 69% to 93% [1], which is stage dependent and thus high in T1 and T2 tumors and low in locally advanced rectal cancer (T3 and T4) with regard to tumor depth and perirectal lymph node involvement. Several other conditions can be evaluated by endosonography or transperineal ultrasound, such as inflammatory disorders and fistulas in ano. This is especially so in areas marginally accessible for MRI or CT scan, such the intersphincteric or rectogenital compartments. By consequence, NITUS techniques – using "conventional" curved array ultrasound probes – improved over recent years as first-line ultrasound modalities for assessing the perirectal and perianal soft tissues – even with the possibility of including color-Doppler ultrasound (CDUS) techniques.

To summarize, high-resolution endosonography represents a useful tool for evaluating anorectal anatomy and its topographical relationships. The information they provide is indispensable for clinical routine to improve and optimize surgical treatment for both benign and malignant conditions.

M. Pescatori, F.S.P. Regadas, S.M. Murad Regadas, A.P. Zbar (eds.), *Imaging Atlas of the Pelvic Floor and Anorectal Diseases*. ISBN 978-88-470-0808-3. © Springer-Verlag Italia 2008

Techniques

We recommend cleaning the rectum from feces for both ERUS and EAUS, even though the anal canal is usually devoid of stool. This is attained by using a cleansing enema of sodium phosphate 1 h prior to the examination. Patients are then positioned in the left lateral position with their knees and hips flexed. Digital examination should precede the endosonography procedure. This allows the examiner to assess the anal canal width as well as the anal sphincter apparatus for morphological disorders and for functional analysis (i.e., anal resting tone and squeeze pressure). Proctoscopy/anoscopy should be performed prior to ERUS to exclude any obstruction of the distal rectum, which cannot be reached by digital examination. The ultrasound probe is then inserted through the proctoscope, which is pulled back as far as possible to obtain reliable ultrasound imaging. For EAUS the proctoscope is not necessary, as the probe is inserted into the anal canal blindly after thorough digital examination.

For ERUS a 5-10 MHz transducer is used with a balloon filled with degassed water placed over the transducer. Air bubbles should be completely removed from the balloon to produce high-quality images. After insertion into the rectum, the balloon is further filled with 40-60 ml of water, which should be adjusted according to the rectal diameter. For EAUS a hard plastic cone is used to cover the 5-10 MHz transducer, which is rotated mechanically so that the beam is emitted at right angles for a 360° radial-swept image [2]. A condom containing ultrasonic gel is placed over the transducer and lubricated on its exterior. Recently, a 3-D ultrasound system using computerized software with data interpolation to create 3-D images of the anal canal (Pro Focus 2202, B-K Medical, Herlev, Denmark) with a 6-16 MHz 360° rotating endoprobe was introduced into proctological practice. Thus, it seems a promising strategy to define constitutive gender and age differences in the normal anal canal [3]. For NITUS we use a normal curved-array ultrasound probe. In this context, our standard iU22 ultrasound device (ATL Philips, Washington, DC, USA) with use of a 9-4 MHz broadband curved-array transducer shows sufficient resolution power versus penetration combined with the depiction of all necessary topographic landmarks [4]. For transperineal ultrasound, the probe must be covered by a lubricant-filled plastic sac. Thereby, the handling of the probe is not hampered. Patients are positioned in the left lateral position with their knees and hips flexed. The probe

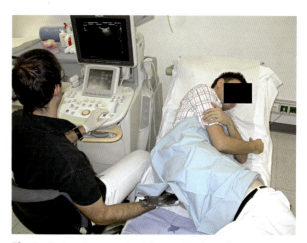

Fig. 1. Noninvasive transperineal ultrasound with use of a 9-4 MHz broadband curved-array transducer. The patient is positioned in the left lateral position with the knees and hips flexed. The probe is attached to the perineum sagittally

is attached to the perineum sagittally (Fig. 1). Thus, all perineal structures can be assessed to an acceptable extent in real time, and CDUS assessments can be easily performed. This procedure is performed very quickly without patient preparation in a relatively convenient manner.

Normal Anatomy

Pelvic floor connective tissue is divided into three compartments: anterior, middle, and posterior. Each one contains the respective pelvic organs as well as different kinds of connective tissue. The posterior compartment can be subdivided into the presacral subcompartment with the presacral vessels and the perirectal subcompartment or mesorectum, which develops along the rectal vessels, nerves, and lymphatics and is enveloped by the mesorectal or rectal fascia. The latter is crucial for rectal resection techniques and a powerful predictor for oncological outcome and local recurrence rate following treatment of rectal cancer. The anterior and middle compartments contain the urogenital organs, with the middle compartment existing only in the female individual.

The Rectum

In ERUS the rectal wall can be divided into concentric rings of hypo- and hyperechoic regions (Fig. 2). According to Beynon et al. [5], the series of rings starts with an inner hyperechoic ring representing the interface of the balloon with the rectal mucosa. The inner hypoechoic ring indicates the muscularis mu-

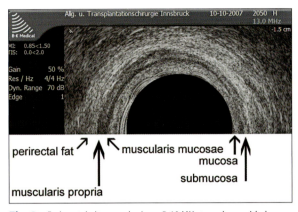

Fig. 2. Endorectal ultrasound using a 5-10 MHz transducer with demonstration of the typical concentric rings of hypo- and hyperechoic regions [5]. *Mucosa* inner hyperechoic ring, *muscularis mucosae* inner hypoechoic ring, *submucosa* middle hyperechoic ring, *muscularis propria* outer hypoechoic ring, *perirectal tissue* outer hyperechoic ring

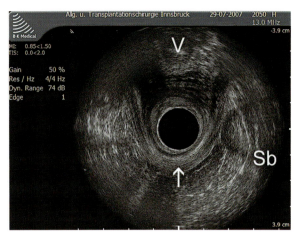

Fig. 3. Endorectal ultrasound of the anorectal junction demonstrating the puborectalis muscle sling (*arrow*) and adjacent structures to the rectal wall, such as the vagina (*V*) and small bowel (*Sb*) in a female individual

cosae and is surrounded by the next hyperechoic layer, which represents the submucosa. The outermost hypoechoic ring corresponds to the muscularis propria and is bordered by the outer hyperechoic ring, which represents the interface between the muscular coat of the rectum and the perirectal fat. Adjacent structures or organs to the rectal wall, such as the prostate and the seminal vesicles in the male and the vagina and uterus in the female individual are detected even with lower resolution (Fig. 3). Blood vessels and lymph nodes are visualized as hypoechoic structures. The rectum is surrounded by the perirectal subcompartment or mesorectum, which develops along the superior rectal vessels and therefore is broad in dorsolateral position and thin in ventral position. The rectal fascia constitutes the external border of the mesorectum, which is directly attached to the inferior hypogastric plexus at the lateral pelvic wall in the male and the uterosacral ligament, which lies between the rectal fascia and the autonomic nerve plexus, in the female individual.

The Anal Canal

The anal canal length can be defined either from a functional or an anatomical point of view. The functional anal canal extends from the intersphincteric groove at the anal verge to the anorectal junction (approximately 4 cm). The latter corresponds with the level of the striated puborectalis muscle sling, which is part of the pelvic diaphragm (levator ani muscle). The anatomical anal canal extends between the anal verge and the dentate line and therefore is roughly half the distance of the functional anal canal. In

EAUS the anal canal can be divided into three levels: the *upper anal canal* is the level midway between the inferior margin of the puborectalis muscle sling and the complete formation of the deep portion of the external anal sphincter (EAS) muscle anteriorly (Fig. 4a). At this level, the inner hypoechoic ring corresponds with the circular layer of the muscular coat of the rectum. Three-dimensional reconstructions of histological sections of the pelvis demonstrated that the deep portion of the EAS is not a completely circular muscle in ventral position at the anorectal level (Fig. 4b) [6]. However, the muscular components of the pelvic diaphragm (puborectalis, pubococcygeus, and iliococcygeus) are usually depicted as hypoechoic linear structures. They are separated by their respective fascias, which are depicted as shiny hyperechoic linear bands orientated to the course of the respective muscle.

The *middle anal canal* is defined by the completion of the EAS anteriorly in combination with the maximum thickness of the internal anal sphincter (IAS) muscle [7] (Fig. 5), which forms a direct continuation of the circular layer of the muscular coat of the rectum and is uniformly hypoechoic. This area also corresponds with the high-pressure zone of the anal canal, which can be assessed by anal manometry. The IAS is sharply demarcated from the anal subepithelial tissue medially (inner hyperechoic ring) and the intersphincteric longitudinal anal muscle laterally, which forms a direct continuation of the longitudinal layer of the muscular coat of the rectum and is of heterogeneously hyperechoic appearance (Fig. 5). The IAS thickness positively correlates with age and body mass index [7], in contrast to EAS width, which decreases with age.

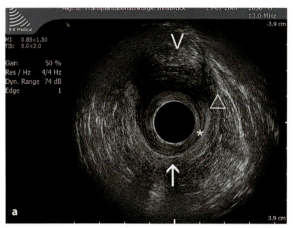

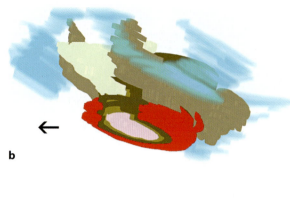

Fig. 4 a, b. Endoanal ultrasound using a 5-10 MHz transducer. **a** Upper anal canal with the puborectalis muscle sling (*arrow*) and the muscular coat of the distal rectum (*asterisk*). At this level, the deep portion of the external anal sphincter muscle (*arrowhead*) is attached to the puborectalis and is not completely circular in ventral position. *V* vagina. **b** Three-dimensional reconstruction of histological sections of the pelvis demonstrating that the deep portion of the external anal sphincter muscle (*red*) is not a completely circular muscle in ventral position (*arrow*) at the anorectal level. Puborectalis (*light brown*), muscular coat of the distal rectum (*dark brown*). Reprinted from [6]

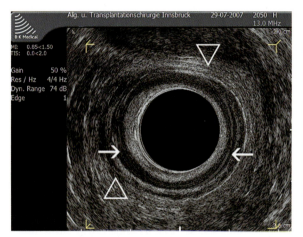

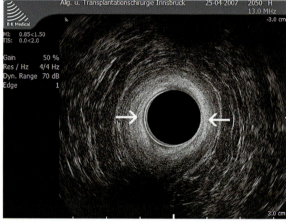

Fig. 5. Endoanal ultrasound of the middle anal canal showing the external (*arrowheads*) and internal (*arrows*) anal sphincter muscles in the high-pressure zone

Fig. 6. Endoanal ultrasound of the lower anal canal showing the subcutaneous portion of the external anal sphincter muscle (*arrows*)

The *low anal canal* is defined as the level below the inferior margin of the IAS and comprises the subcutaneous portion of the EAS, which is complete ventrally (Fig. 6). In dorsal position, the EAS turns inward and forms a muscular continuum with the smooth IAS and the longitudinal muscles. According to Gold et al. [8], the EAS is generally longer in the male than in the female individual (32.6 ± 5.3 mm vs. 15.3 ± 2.8 mm; $p < 0.001$) and thinner anteriorly in the female than in the male individual.

The EAS remains an anatomical structure difficult to visualize at its outermost layers and to discriminate them from surrounding structures, such as the perianal and/or ischioanal adipose tissue. For better visualization of the perianal and perirectal region, NITUS is a promising strategy for detection of perianal abscesses, fistula tracks, or simply variations in the anorectal vascularization status.

The Perineal Body

The perineal body can be visualized by EAUS and its thickness measured by inserting a finger, held gently against the posterior vaginal wall, into the vagina and measuring the distance between the inner surface of the IAS and the ultrasonographic reflection of the finger (Fig. 7) [9]. Studies confirmed that perineal body thickness < 10 mm was more commonly associated with fecal incontinence [10]. The perineal body consists of dense connective tissue and separates the urogenital hiatus from the anal hiatus.

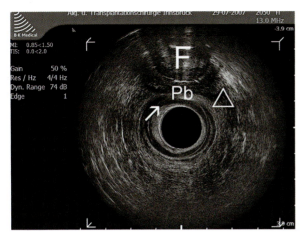

Fig. 7. Perineal body measurement using a finger (*F*), held gently against the posterior vaginal wall, into the vagina and measuring the distance between the inner surface of the internal sphincter (*arrow*) and the ultrasonographic reflection of the finger. Fibers of the subcutaneous portion of the external anal sphincter muscle (*arrowhead*) intermingle with the perineal body (*Pb*)

Fig. 8. Noninvasive transperineal ultrasound showing the rectogenital septum (*S*) cephalad to the perineal body (*Pb*), which constitutes an incomplete partition ventrocranial between the rectum (*R*) and the urogenital organs. Anal canal (*A*), internal anal sphincter (*double arrow*), subcutaneous portion of the external anal sphincter muscle (***), puborectalis muscle sling (****), anorectal flexure of the rectum (*arrow*); male individual

It is intermingled with numerous originating and inserting muscles (subcutaneous portion of the EAS, longitudinal anal muscle, bulbospongiosus and superficial transverse perineal muscle), along with the longitudinal smooth muscle fibers of the rectogenital septum. It must be considered a tendinous center for muscles without bony origin or attachment.

Cephalad to the perineal body, the rectogenital septum (Denonvilliers fascia) constitutes an incomplete partition to the ventrocranial segment between the rectum and the urogenital organs (Fig. 8). It is formed by local condensation of mesenchymal connective tissue during the early fetal period and intermingled by longitudinal smooth muscle fibers, which can be traced back to the longitudinal layer of the rectal wall. The rectogenital septum serves as a guiding structure for the cavernous nerves arising from the autonomic inferior hypogastric plexus at the lateral pelvic wall. It forms a borderline for limiting the spread of malignancy and inflammation and a functional gliding sheath between urogenital organs and rectum, enabling shortening and opening of the anal canal during defecation. It is crucial for stabilizing the ventral rectal wall as well as in rectal filling and asymmetric rectal distension [11], which is also visualized in dynamic transperineal ultrasound.

Anorectal Blood Supply

Blood supply to the rectum and the transitional zone comprising the corpus cavernosum recti (CCR), an arteriovenous cavernous network without interposition of a capillary system, is provided by the superior rec-

tal artery. The anal canal and the anal sphincter muscles receive branches from the variable middle and the inferior rectal arteries. The CCR is located within the rectal submucosa above the dentate line at about 3–5 cm from the anal verge. Its filling and drainage partly depends on the contraction status of the IAS and forms a gas-tight seal of the anal canal at anal resting tone, thus sustaining fecal continence. The CCR is drained through transsphincteric veins during IAS relaxation at defecation. The CCR supplying arterial vessels courses downward in the rectal submucosa, on the one hand, and continues the course of extramural terminal branches by perforating the rectal wall in an axial plane close to the levator ani muscle, on the other hand. These afferent vessels as well as CCR drainage can be detected and even assessed by NITUS, especially for assessing the vascularization status in hemorrhoidal disease (Fig. 9). Arterial and venous drainage signals can be clearly analyzed at this depth by performing spectral wave analyses, which could be groundbreaking concerning the differentiation of several different functional forms of hemorrhoidal disease presently under definition [12]. Changes of arterial and venous spectra – all found in extensive grades of hemorrhoidal disease – may resemble shunt-flow patterns detected usually also in, e.g., arteriovenous fistulas (e.g., intrahepatic vascular malformations).

It was demonstrated that NITUS is a relatively sensitive procedure for assessing perianal inflammatory conditions [13]. Resembling the previous descriptions, the rectal and anal walls are layered hyper- and hypoechoically but are depicted linearly. The entire extent of the anorectum is usually shown in its course distally from the distal sacral flexure. When

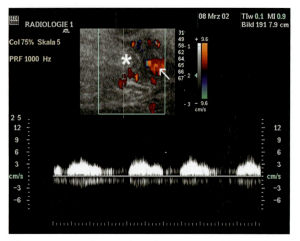

Fig. 9. Detection of anorectal vascularization in a healthy male individual by noninvasive transperineal ultrasound. The corpus cavernosum recti is shown (*arrow*) with the supplying arterial vessels and the respective flow spectrum. Some vessels perforate the rectal wall close to the anal sphincter complex (*asterisk*)

tilting the probe, the levator ani is shown encompassing the anorectal junction. Combined gray-scale and CD ultrasonography have a high detectability rate and comprehensive characterization of perianal abscesses and fistulas. Compared with the walls of the anal canal or rectum, respectively, they usually present hypoechoic nodular to globular structures, where pus can often be detected by compression and decompression of the probe.

Conclusion

In conclusion, 2-D and 3-D endosonography and NI-TUS represent innovative tools for diagnosing complex anorectal disorders. Knowledge of the normal anorectal anatomy and its topographical relationships is necessary for deciding upon the appropriate treatment of anorectal diseases.

References

1. Arumugam PJ, Patel B, Beynon J (2005) Ultrasound in coloproctologic practice: endorectal/endoanal ultrasound. In: Wexner SD, Zbar AP, Pescatori M (eds) Complex anorectal disorders. Investigation and management. Springer, London, pp 217–245
2. Sultan AH, Nicholls RJ, Kamm MA et al (1993) Anal endosonography and correlation with in vitro and in vivo anatomy. Br J Surg 80:508–511
3. Zbar AP, Frudinger A (2005) Three-dimensional endoanal ultrasound in proctological practice. In: Wexner SD, Zbar AP, Pescatori M (eds) Complex anorectal disorders. Investigation and management. Springer, London, pp 263–274
4. Bonatti H, Lugger P, Hechenleitner P et al (2004) Transperineal sonography in anorectal disorders. Ultraschall Med 25(2):111–115
5. Beynon J, Foy DMA, Channer JL et al (1986) The endoscopic appearances of normal colon and rectum. Dis Colon Rectum 29:810–813
6. Fritsch H, Brenner E, Lienemann A, Ludwikowski B (2002) Anal sphincter complex. Dis Colon Rectum 45:188–194
7. Frudinger A, Halligan S, Bartram CI et al (2002) Female anal sphincter: age-related differences in asymptomatic volunteers with high-frequency endoanal US. Radiology 224:417–423
8. Gold DM, Bartram CI, Halligan S et al (1999) 3-D endoanal sonography in assessing anal canal injury. Br J Surg 86:365–370
9. Zetterström JP, Mellgren A, Madoff RD et al (1998) Perineal body measurement improves evaluation of anterior sphincter lesions during endoanal ultrasonography. Dis Colon Rectum 41(6):705–713
10. Oberwalder M, Thaler K, Baig MK et al (2004) Anal ultrasound and endosonographic measurement of perineal body thickness: a new evaluation for fecal incontinence in females. Surg Endos 18(4):650–654
11. Aigner F, Zbar AP, Ludwikowski B et al (2004) The rectogenital septum: morphology, function and clinical relevance. Dis Colon Rectum 47:131–140
12. Aigner F, Bodner G, Gruber H et al (2006) The vascular nature of hemorrhoids. J Gastrointest Surg 10(7):1044–1050
13. Mallouhi A, Bonatti H, Peer S et al (2004) Detection and characterization of perianal inflammatory disease: accuracy of transperineal combined grayscale and color-Doppler sonography. J Ultrasound Med 23(1):19–27

CHAPTER 2

Three-Dimensional Ultrasonography of Pelvic Floor and Anorectal Anatomy

F. Sérgio P. Regadas, Sthela M. Murad Regadas, Rosilma Gorete Lima Barreto

Abstract

Here we discuss precisely the anatomic configuration of the anal canal and the length and thickness of the anal sphincters using 3D anorectal ultrasonography in both genders, demonstrating the anal canal's asymmetrical configuration. The rectum and all adjacent pelvic organs are shown in multiple anatomic planes.

Anatomic Planes: Ultrasound View

Advances in ultrasound scanning technology over the past few years includes the development of the 360° rotating anorectal transducers featuring high frequency and between 6-16 MHz, focal distance between 2.8 and 6.2-cm, and automatic image acquisition without manual movement of the transducer. Images up to 6.0-cm long are captured along the proximal-distal axis during up to 55 s by moving two crystals on the extremity of the transducer. The examination involves a series of transaxial microsections up to 0.20-mm thick producing a high-resolution digitalized volumetric image (cube) (Fig. 1). This image is highly mobile and allows for real-time evaluation in all planes, multiview (4–6 simultaneous images) (Fig. 2), and volume-rendered (VR) 3D imaging with low-brightness and high-contrast adjustment for semitransparent dark cavities (Fig. 3). The several anatomic planes are in accord with the planimetric display suggested by Santoro and Fortling [1] (Figs. 4–8).

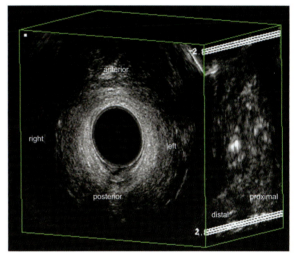

Fig. 1. Digital volume image

Anal Canal Configuration

In a recent study using 3D anorectal ultrasonography, Regadas et al. [2] demonstrated the asymmetrical shape of the anal canal and compared positions and sizes of anal sphincters between genders (Fig. 9). The anterior anal canal starts and ends more distally and it is formed by the external anal sphincter (EAS) and the internal anal sphincter (IAS). The distance between the anterior anorectal junction and the EAS is called the gap. It corresponds to the upper anal canal and is formed by normal rectal wall proximally and by the IAS distally (Fig. 10). The lateral EAS and puborectalis (PR) muscle were significantly longer than

M. Pescatori, F.S.P. Regadas, S.M. Murad Regadas, A.P. Zbar (eds.), *Imaging Atlas of the Pelvic Floor and Anorectal Diseases*. ISBN 978-88-470-0808-3. © Springer-Verlag Italia 2008

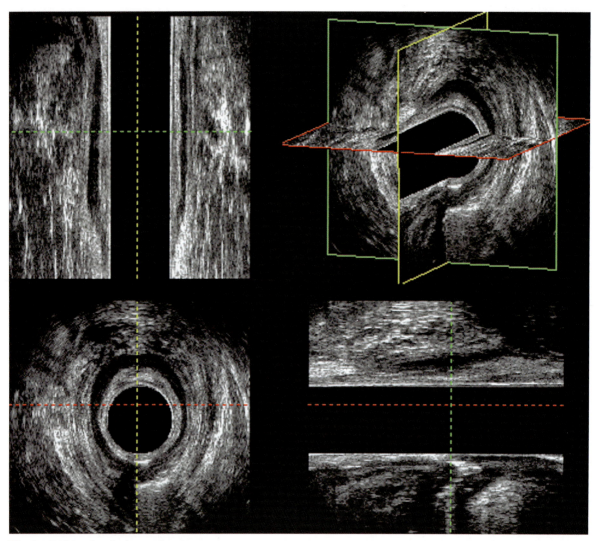

Fig. 2. Multiview: four simultaneous images

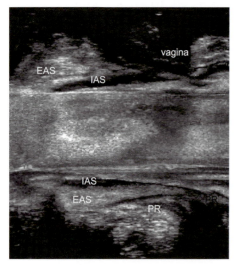

Fig. 3. Female anal canal: midsagittal plane, render mode, enhanced image. *EAS* external anal sphincter, *IAS* internal anal sphincter, *PR* puborectalis muscle

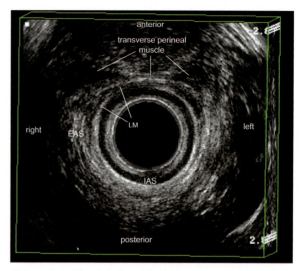

Fig. 4. Normal female anal canal; longitudinal muscle: axial plane (transverse). *EAS* external anal sphincter, *LM* longitudinal muscle, *IAS* internal anal sphincter

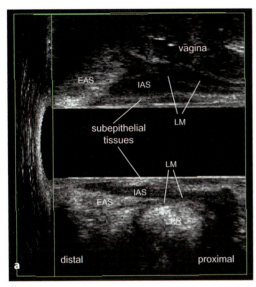
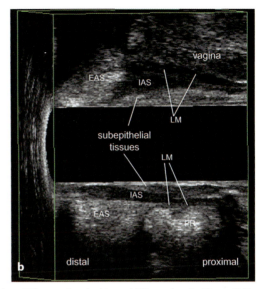

Fig. 5 a, b. Normal female anal canal: **a** sagittal plane; **b** midsagittal plane. *EAS* external anal sphincter, *IAS* internal anal sphincter, *LM* longitudinal muscle, *PR* puborectalis muscle

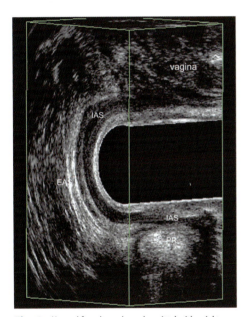

Fig. 6. Normal female anal canal: sagittal with axial transverse planes. *EAS* external anal sphincter, *IAS* internal anal sphincter, *PR* puborectalis muscle

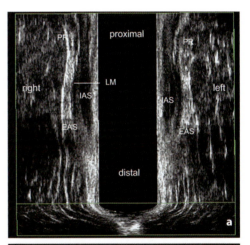
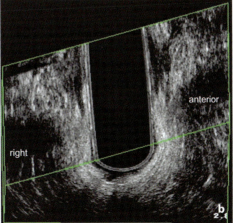

the posterior part of the muscles in men (3.9 cm vs. 3.6 cm, respectively) than in women (3.6 cm vs. 3.2 cm, respectively). They form at the same level but the lateral part of the EAS-PR ends more distally (Fig. 10). The anterior IAS was significantly shorter than the posterior and lateral parts of the muscle in men (2.7 cm vs. 3.5 cm vs. 3.5 cm, respectively) than in women (2.0 cm vs. 3.0 cm vs. 3.3 cm, respectively)

Fig. 7 a, b. Normal female anal canal: **a** coronal plane; **b** coronal with diagonal planes. *EAS* external anal sphincter, *IAS* internal anal sphincter, *LM* longitudinal muscle, *PR* puborectalis muscle

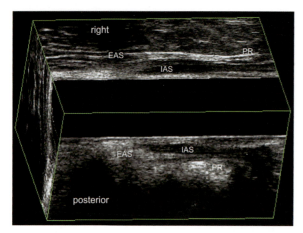

Fig. 8. Normal female anal canal: midsagittal with coronal planes. *EAS* external anal sphincter, *IAS* internal anal sphincter, *PR* puborectalis muscle

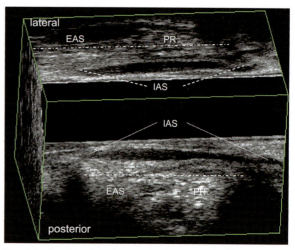

Fig. 10. Female anal canal: transverse and midsagittal planes. Lateral anal canal is longer than the posterior anal canal. Internal anal sphincter (*IAS*) is formed before the puborectalis (*PR*) muscles in both quadrants. *EAS* external anal sphincter

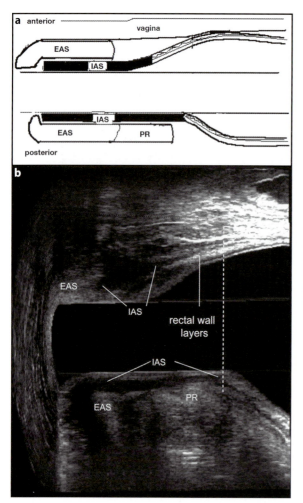

Fig. 9 a, b. Female anal canal and anorectal junction: **a** schematic representation [2]; **b** 3D ultrasound image, midsagittal plane. *EAS* external anal sphincter, *IAS* internal anal sphincter, *PR* puborectalis muscle

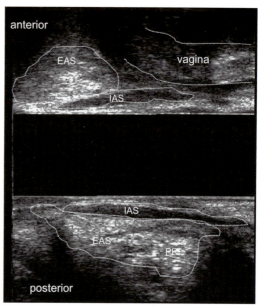

Fig. 11. Female anal canal: midsagittal plane. *EAS* external anal sphincter, *IAS* internal anal sphincter, *PR* puborectalis muscle

(Fig. 11). However, no statistically significant difference was identified in the length of the posterior and lateral quadrants between genders. Comparing the posterior IAS with the EAS-PR, no significant difference in length was determined between men (3.5 cm vs. 3.6 cm) and women (3.0 cm vs. 3.2 cm). However, the posterior IAS is formed proximally but the EAS-PR ends more distally in both genders (Fig. 12). The anterior IAS was significantly thinner than the posterior IAS in women (0.12 cm vs. 0.18 cm).

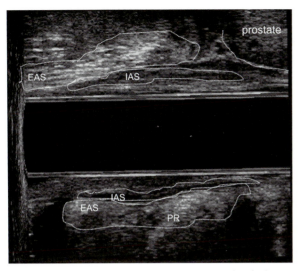

Fig. 12. Male anal canal: midsagittal plane. *EAS* external anal sphincter, *IAS* internal anal sphincter, *PR* puborectalis muscle

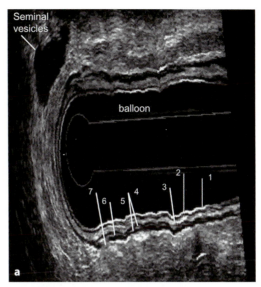

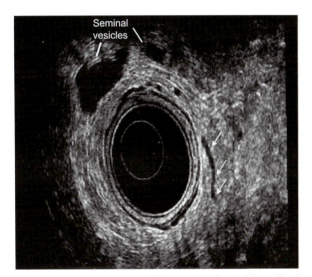

Fig. 14. Normal male rectum: axial (transverse) and sagittal planes. Blood vessel (*arrows*)

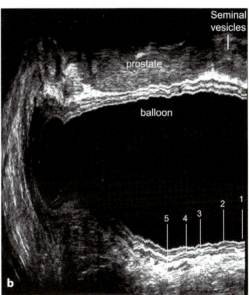

Fig. 13 a, b. Normal male rectum: sagittal plane. **a** Rectal wall is formed by seven layers: *1* mucosa (hyperechoic); *2* muscularis mucosa (hypoechoic); *3* submucosa (hyperechoic); *4* muscularis propria (circular; hypoechoic); *5* muscularis propria (longitudinal; hypoechoic); *6* white line separating both muscular layers; *7* perirectal fat (hyperechoic). **b** Five layers: *1* mucosa; *2* muscularis mucosa; *3* submucosa; *4* muscularis propria; *5* perirectal fat

Comparison between Genders

Comparing muscle distribution between genders, it was identified that the anterior EAS (2.2 cm) was significantly shorter and the gap (1.2 cm) significantly longer in women than in men (3.4 cm and 0.7 cm, respectively) (Fig. 12). The posterior EAS-PR was significantly longer in men (3.6 cm) than in women (3.2 cm) (Fig. 12). The anterior and posterior IAS were significant shorter in women than in

men, whereas the anterior IAS was thicker in men (0.19 cm) than in women (0.12 cm) but without significant difference in the posterior muscle.

Rectal Anatomy: Three-dimensional View

All pelvic organs adjacent to the rectum are clearly visualized, identifying its relation with the rectal wall layers (between 5 and 7 layers) in multiple anatomic planes (Figs. 13–16).

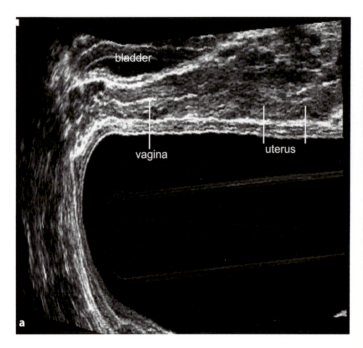

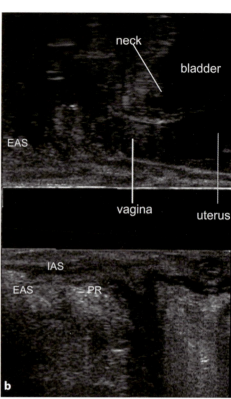

Fig. 15 a, b. Normal female rectum: sagittal plane. **a** With balloon, vagina, uterus, and bladder; **b** without balloon (focal distance 6.0 cm). *EAS* external anal sphincter, *IAS* internal anal sphincter, *PR* puborectalis muscle

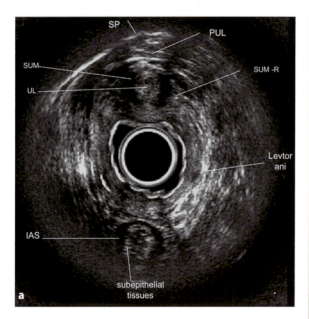

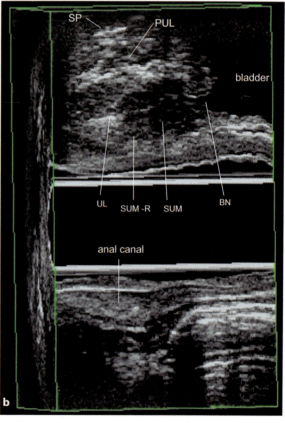

Fig. 16 a, b. Three-dimensional transvaginal ultrasound. All anatomic structures of the pelvic floor are clearly visible. **a** Axial (transverse) plane, **b** sagittal plane. *BN* bladder neck, *IAS* internal anal sphincter, *PUL* puborectal ligament, *SP* symphysis pubis, *SUM* smooth urethral muscle, *SUM-R* striated urethral muscle rhabdosphincter, *UL* urethra lumen

References

1. Santoro GA, Fortling B (2006) New technical developments in endoanal and endorectal ultrasonography. In: Santoro GA, Di Falco G, eds. Benign anorectal diseases. Springer-Verlag Italia, p 23

2. Regadas FSP, Murad-Regadas SM, Lima DMR et al (2007) Anal canal anatomy showed by three-dimensional anorectal ultrasonography Surg Endoscopy 21(12):2207–2211

Commentary

Mario Pescatori

The ultrasonography (US) finding of a shorter muscle in the anterior aspect of the anal canal may have clinical implications when dealing with anterior anal fistulae, especially in female patients, who are likely to have a thin external and internal sphincter stretched by vaginal deliveries. Therefore, a conservative policy may be preferable in such cases, i.e., fistulectomy and rectal advanced flap may achieve better postoperative continence than either fistulotomy or fistulectomy and cutting seton.

In case of rectocele, an anterior smooth muscle defect at the level of both the rectovaginal septum and the lower rectum may also occur, requiring a muscle plication. A new-onset fecal incontinence may occur after transanal manual rectocele repair and the stapled transanal rectal resection (STARR) procedure, ranging between 5% and 12%, respectively. Therefore, either sphincter reconstruction or

pelvic floor rehabilitation may be required more frequently in women, as the above-mentioned US studies showed that the muscle component is weaker in women.

Interestingly, the anatomical muscle differences found at US studies between anterior, lateral, and posterior aspects of the anal canal have also been found at anal manometry, as recently reported by Bove et al [1]. The different resting tone may play a role in the pathogenesis of anal fissure.

Recently, Shafik and coworkers [2] investigated the functional role of the transverse perineal muscle in eliciting the rectoperineal reflexes, which are involved in the continence and defecation mechanisms. Anal US studies on this muscle component are expected to give further contribution to the knowledge of the complex physiology of the pelvic floor and to its influence on surgical policy.

References

1. Bove A, Balzano A, Perotti P et al (2004) Different anal pressure profiles in patients with anal fissure. Tech Coloproctol 8(3):151–156

2. Shafik A, Sibai OE, Shafid AA (2007) A novel concept for the surgical anatomy of the perineal body. Dis Colon Rectum 50(12):2120–2125

CHAPTER 3

Transperineal Ultrasonography of Pelvic Floor and Anorectal Anatomy: Technique and Images

Harry Kleinübing Jr., Mauro S.L. Pinho

Abstract

Transperineal ultrasonography performed with conventional equipment and probes can be used as an important diagnostic tool in the assessment of anorectal disorders to demonstrate the anatomy of the perianal region. Advantages of this procedure include low costs and high availability, and extensive perineal scanning provides combined images including transverse, longitudinal, and oblique ultrasonographic sections. Also, it is a minimally invasive procedure without anal introduction but with particular advantages with regard to painful anorectal conditions. The aim of this chapter is to describe the technique of transperineal ultrasonography and to show normal images of the anal region.

Introduction

Transperineal ultrasonography performed with conventional equipment and probes was introduced in 1997 [1, 2]. It has been used to demonstrate the anatomy of the perianal region as an important diagnostic tool in the assessment of anorectal disorders, providing similar images to anal endosonography [1–6]. Advantages of this procedure include:

- Low cost and high availability
- Extensive perineal scanning providing combined images, including transverse, longitudinal, and oblique ultrasonographic sections
- Less invasive procedure without anal introduction and with particular advantage in painful anorectal conditions.

Transperineal ultrasonography is performed with conventional ultrasonography equipment (Fig. 1) using linear (Fig. 2a), endocavitary (Fig. 2b), and trapezoid 5 to 10 MHz probes. Higher-capacity probes may produce a better definition image, but lower-capacity probes may be useful to assess deeper structures and, consequently, obese patients.

Examinations are undertaken without bowel preparation with the patient in a supine position with

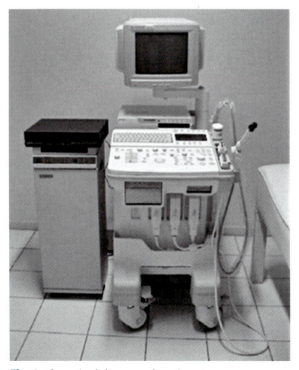

Fig. 1. Conventional ultrasonography equipment

M. Pescatori, F.S.P. Regadas, S.M. Murad Regadas, A.P. Zbar (eds.), *Imaging Atlas of the Pelvic Floor and Anorectal Diseases*. ISBN 978-88-470-0808-3. © Springer-Verlag Italia 2008

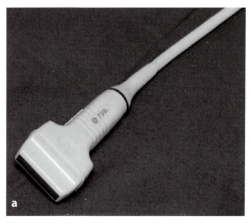
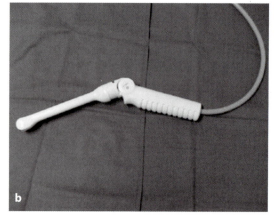

Fig. 2 a, b. Linear (**a**) and endocavitary (**b**) probes

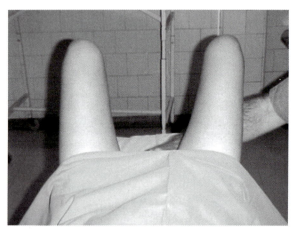

Fig. 3. Patient positioning for the examination

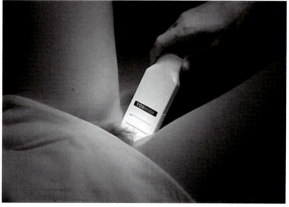

Fig. 4. Probe in transverse position for transverse cross-sectional view of the anal canal

partially opened and semiflexed legs (Fig. 3). Ultrasonography examination is performed by positioning the probe, covered with a condom and lubricated, at the midportion of the perineum in backward orientation at a 45° angle to obtain transverse images of anal sphincters (Fig. 4). Sequential cross-section images of the anal canal are obtained by slight movements of the perineal probe (Fig. 5).

Internal anal sphincter is observed as a dark (hypoechoic) circular layer 2- to 3-mm thick and may be used as reference to identify other surrounding structures, such as the inner, folded submucosal and mucosal layers characterized by a mixture of hypoechoic and hyperechoic images. External to the hypoechoic internal anal sphincter circle the external anal sphincter is demonstrated as a mixed but predominantly hyperechoic and thicker (4–7 mm) layer (Fig. 6). In the deep anal canal, the puborectalis muscle can be identified as a "V" shape (Fig. 7).

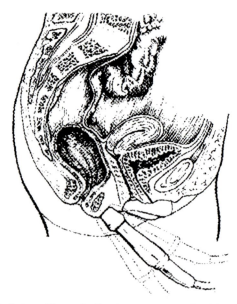

Fig. 5. Probe position required for a transverse cross-sectional view of the anal canal

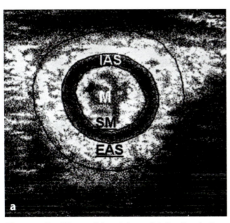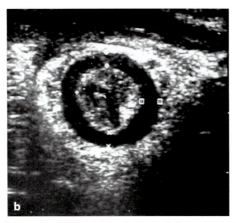

Fig. 6 a, b. Diagram (**a**) and picture (**b**) showing the layers of the anal canal. *EAS* external anal sphincter, *IAS* internal anal sphincter, *SM* submucosa, *M* mucosa

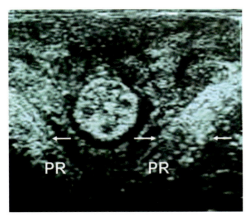

Fig. 7. Transverse section image. The puborectalis (*PR*) muscle is identified as a "V" shape in the deep anal canal

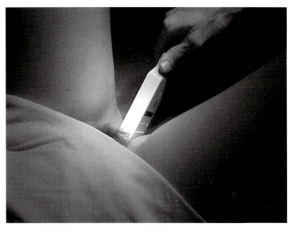

Fig. 8. Probe in a longitudinal position for a sagittal image of the anal canal

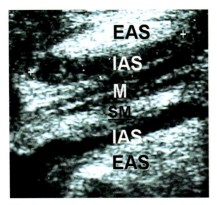

Fig. 9. Longitudinal layers of the anal canal. *EAS* external anal sphincter, *IAS* internal anal sphincter, *M* mucosa, *SM* submucosa

Sagittal images of the anal canal are obtained by longitudinal perineal positioning of the probe (Fig. 8). Similar to transverse sections, slight anterior-posterior movements are required to obtain the ideal angle for structure identification. In this sagittal approach, the internal anal sphincter is demonstrated as two longitudinal, parallel, dark (hypoechoic), thick lines separated by two layers of mixed echogenic submucosal and two hypoechoic mucosal layers (Fig. 9). The external anal sphincter can also be seen as a thicker, clear hyperechoic layer external to the internal sphincter. The anorectal angle (ARA) can be identified at the end of anal canal (Fig. 10).

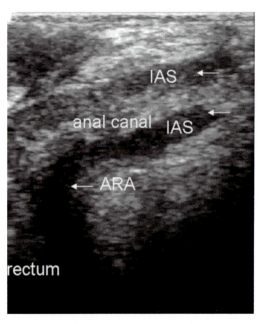

Fig. 10. Sagittal section showing the internal anal sphincter (*IAS*), anal canal, anorectal angle (*ARA*), and rectum

References

1. Peschers UM, Delancey JOL, Schaer GN, Schuessler B (1997) Exoanal ultrasound of the anal sphincter: normal anatomy and sphincter defects. B J Obstet Gynaecol 104:999–1003
2. Kleinübing H Jr, Jannini JF, Malafaia O et al (1997) Ultra-sonografia transperineal: novo método de imagem da região anorretal. Presented at 1° Encontro Catarinense de Colo-Proctologia
3. Rubens DJ, Strang JG, Bogineni-Misra S, Wexler IE (1998) Transperineal sonography of the rectum: anatomy and pathology revealed by sonography compared with CT and MR imaging. AJR Am J Roentgenol 170:637–642
4. Kleinübing H Jr, Jannini JF, Malafaia O et al (2000) Transperineal ultrasonography: new method to image the anorectal region. Dis Colon Rectum 43:1572–1574
5. Roche B, Deléaval J, Fransioli A, Marti M-C (2001) Comparison of transanal and external perineal ultrasonography. Eur Radiol 11:1165–1170
6. Beer-Gabel M, Teshler M, Barzilai N et al (2002) Dynamic ultrasound in the diagnosis of pelvic floor disorders. A pilot study. Dis Colon Rectum 45:239–248

CHAPTER 4

Computed Tomography and Magnetic Resonance Imaging of Pelviperineal Anatomy

Adrian E. Ortega, Frida R. Pena, Brenda Avalos, Howard S. Kaufman

Abstract

Magnetic resonance imaging (MRI) and computed tomography (CT) scan are essential in the practice of pelvic-floor and colorectal surgery. This chapter discusses the conceptual anatomic constructs essential for understanding pelviperineal anatomy. Selected CT scan and MRI of normal anatomy are presented, highlighting the important osseous and myofascial landmarks.

Introduction

Pelviperineal anatomy can confound surgical students as well as masters. It represents a unique challenge to surgical educators and medical illustrators. In its present state of the art, surgical anatomy is represented in two-dimensional media. Medical illustration of the complex three-dimensional human pelviperineal anatomy is challenging. Nonetheless, understanding two-dimensional conceptual constructs is essential for integrating information provided by CT scan and MRI. The following figures provide the necessary nomenclature and theoretic constructs required for correct interpretation of CT scan and MRI. (Figs. 1 and 2).

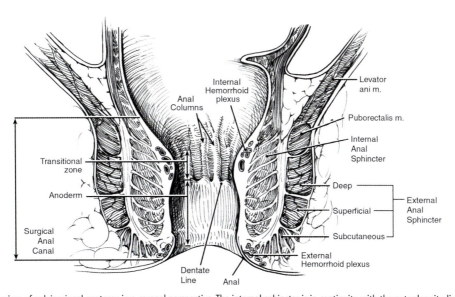

Fig. 1. Classic view of pelviperineal anatomy in a coronal perspective. The internal sphincter is in continuity with the outer longitudinal muscle of the rectum. It is encased by the external sphincter, which is supported posterolaterally at its proximal base by the most medial of the levator ani – the puborectalis muscle

M. Pescatori, F.S.P. Regadas, S.M. Murad Regadas, A.P. Zbar (eds.), *Imaging Atlas of the Pelvic Floor and Anorectal Diseases*. ISBN 978-88-470-0808-3. © Springer-Verlag Italia 2008

Axial Anatomy

Evaluating complex abscesses should include the lower abdomen, pelvis, and extrapelvic regions at least down to the gluteal folds and superior aspect of the femur. Important anatomic landmarks include the ischial spines covered by the fascia of the obturator internus muscle, the anococcygeal ligament, and the tip of the coccyx. A natural route for extension of pelvic infections to extrapelvic sites (bilateral ischioanal fossae) exists in Alcock's canal. Because the pubococcygeus and ileococcygeus muscles insert on the sides of the coccyx, any fluid collection above the tip of the coccyx is supralevator by definition. The bulbocavernosus muscle is another useful landmark because of its continuity with the external sphincter. Conceptually, the bulbocavernosus forms a figure-eight configuration, with the external sphincter divided at its waist by the superficial transverse perineal muscles in the axial plane (Figs. 3 and 4). The puborectalis muscle appears as a U-shaped sling around the sphincter complex (Fig. 5). Three important structures insert at the coccyx: the pubococcygeus, the ileococcygeus, and the anococcygeal ligament (Fig. 6).

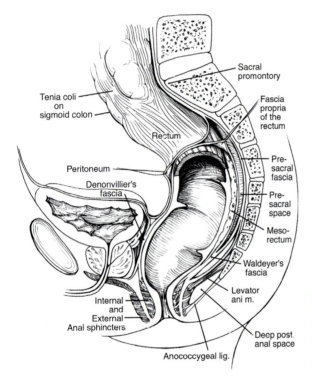

Fig. 2. Classic sagittal view of male pelviperineal anatomy. The important osseous structures include the pubis and coccyx. Significant myofascial landmarks include the anococcygeal ligament, the insertions of the levator ani onto the sides of the coccyx, the presacral and fascia propria of the rectum, and Waldeyer's fascia formed at their point of fusion. Reproduced from [1], with permission from Elsevier

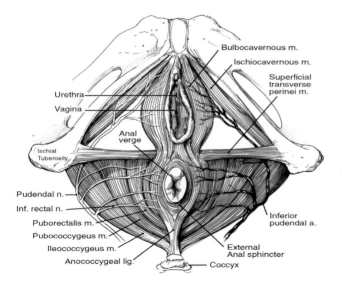

Fig. 3. The female pelvic diaphragm: axial perspective. It is useful to conceive the pelvic floor as divided into anterior and posterior compartments separated by transverse perinei muscles. The anococcygeal ligament attaches the superficial component of the external sphincter to the coccyx. The bulbocavernosus muscle forms a figure-eight configuration, with the external sphincter anchored at the waist of the figure eight by the superficial transverse perinei muscles. Reproduced from [1], with permission from Elsevier

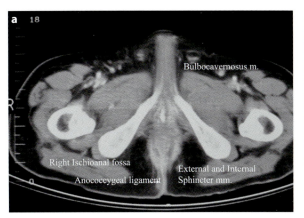
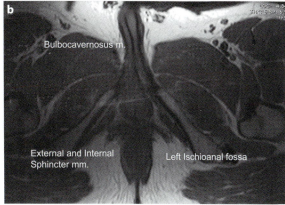

Fig. 4 a, b. Computed tomography (**a**) and magnetic resonance (**b**) images of the lower male pelvis, illustrating the near-contiguous relationship of the bulbocavernosus and external sphincter muscles

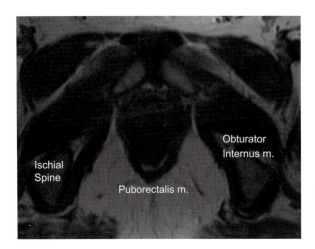

Fig. 5. Magnetic resonance imaging, axial view, of the ischial spines covered medially by obturator internus and its fascia defining the vortex of the ischioanal space. The U-shaped sling around the sphincter complex is the puborectalis muscle clearly evident in this image

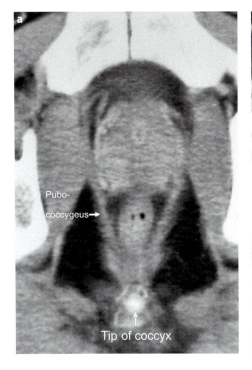
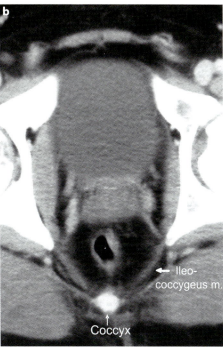

Fig. 6 a, b. **a** Pubococcygeus, **b** ileococcygeus, **c** anococcygeal ligament (see Figs. 4a and 9)

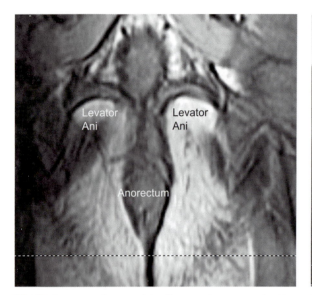

Fig. 7. Levator muscles: coronal view. These muscles appear as shoulders on each side of the rectum, separating pelvic organs from the extrapelvic region

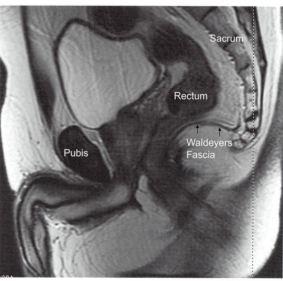

Fig. 8. Pelvis: sagittal view. Demonstrates Waldeyer's fascia (*arrows*) formed at the point of fusion of the fascia propria of the rectum and the presacral fascia

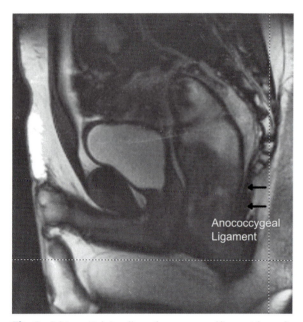

Fig. 9. Pelvis: sagittal view. Shows the anococcygeal ligament (*arrows*)

Coronal and Sagittal Anatomy

MRI offers three views of the pelvic anatomy: (1) axial, (2) coronal, and (3) sagittal. Important anatomic landmarks in both the coronal and sagittal planes include the levator muscles (Figs. 7-9).

Reference

1. Kaiser AM, Ortega AE (2003) Anorectal Anatomy. Surg Clin N Am 82(6):1125

SECTION II

Anal and Perianal Diseases

Two- and Three-dimensional Ultrasonography of Anatomic Defects in Fecal Incontinence

F. Sérgio P. Regadas, Sthela M. Murad Regadas, Lusmar Veras Rodrigues

Abstract

Here we discuss the role of endoanal ultrasound (US) scanning in fecal incontinence. Two-dimensional (2-D) US demonstrates precisely the type and extent of muscle injuries in relation to the anal circumference, whereas 3-D scanning shows it in relation to anal canal length. Interpretation of 3-D imaging is simpler, as muscle length can also be measured longitudinally. The exact identification of the injured muscles is important in deciding upon the best therapeutic option. Anal US can also be useful in evaluating the results of surgical repair, identifying adjacent or overlapping muscles, and documenting persisting muscle injury.

Introduction

Whereas 2-D endoanal ultrasound (US) scanning identifies injured muscles and the extent of the injury in relation to the anal circumference, 3-D scanning shows it in relation to anal canal length [1–3]. The lesion angle is measured by drawing two lines tangentially to the injured muscle and making them converge at the center of the circumference. On US scans, muscle injuries appear as interruptions (or changes) in the echogenicity of the original musculature. Internal anal sphincter (IAS) injuries appear as lighter-colored single or multiple disruptions of the normal hypoechoic circumferential image, whereas external anal sphincter (EAS) injuries are characterized as areas of reduced hyperechogenicity, depending on the amount of fibrous tissue formed. The "septum maneuver," used routinely in measuring the perineal body, is helpful in identi-

fying sphincter injuries of the anterior quadrant, as it helps view the extremities of damaged muscles. It consists of measuring the distance between the internal border of the IAS and the finger of the examiner held against the posterior vaginal wall (normal > 10.0 mm) [4] (Fig. 1). However, this technique cannot be used clinically with patients previously submitted to perineoplasty with sphincteroplasty, as the size of the perineal body in these patients exceeds 10 mm, even before muscle repair (Fig. 2).

The absence of the EAS from the anterior quadrant of the proximal part of the mid-anal canal in women (the EAS becomes completely circular only in the distal part of the mid-anal canal) has led to interexaminer differences in US interpretation or even to false-positive diagnosis. This is due to the difficulty in differentiating the natural gap (absence of EAS) from muscle injury, especially in the 2-D scanning mode, although the diagnosis may be facilitated by other findings. The borders of injured muscles are irregular, separated by fibrosis, and located up to 1.5–2.0 cm from the anal margin (distal part of the mid-anal canal) and/or associated with IAS injuries [5] (Fig. 3). In the 3-D scanning mode, the interpretation is simpler, as the sagittal view makes it possible to measure the length of the muscle. Injury should be suspected in muscles shorter than 1.7 cm [6] (see Chap. 2). Muscle injury caused by obstetric trauma may lead to a number of complications. These can range from severe perineal tears, as indicated by complete damage of the IAS and EAS in the anterior hemiquadrant along the entire anal canal (Fig. 4), to lesions located in the distal part of the mid-anal canal involving the IAS and/or EAS and occasionally extending to the inferior anal canal. Such cases are better diagnosed in the 3-D scanning mode when

M. Pescatori, F.S.P. Regadas, S.M. Murad Regadas, A.P. Zbar (eds.), *Imaging Atlas of the Pelvic Floor and Anorectal Diseases*. ISBN 978-88-470-0808-3. © Springer-Verlag Italia 2008

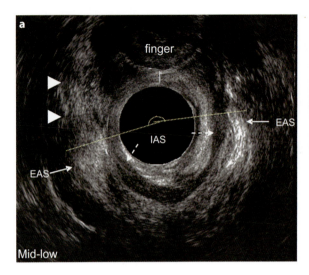

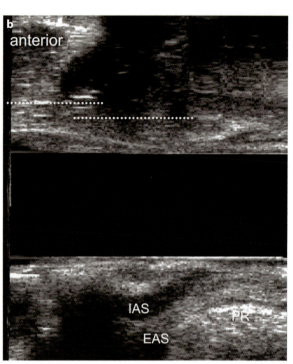

Fig. 1 a, b. Sphincteric muscle injury after a complicated vaginal delivery. **a** Axial plane: external anal sphincter (*EAS*) and internal anal sphincter (*IAS*) injuries 8-2 o'clock (*white arrows*) with scar tissue substituting the EAS (*white arrowheads*). Defect angle 188°. Perineal body thickness < 10.0 mm. **b** Mid-sagittal plane: anterior EAS and IAS are injured in their entire length

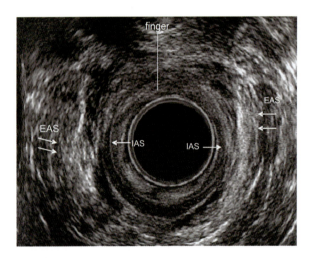

Fig. 2. Sphincteric muscle injury after vaginal delivery, subsequently submitted to a perineoplasty procedure. Complete external anal (*EAS*) and internal anal (*IAS*) sphincter injury 3-9 o'clock. Perineal body measurement > 10 mm

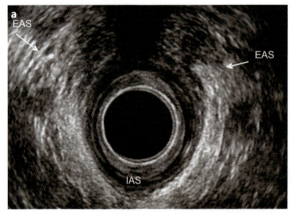

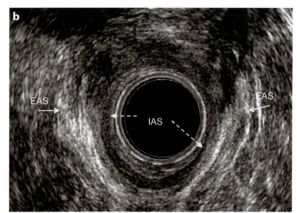

Fig. 3 a, b. **a** Proximal mid-anal canal; natural gap. External anal sphincter (*EAS*) with regular edges (*white arrows*). **b** Distal mid-anal canal. EAS defect with scar tissue 9-3 o'clock (*arrows*). Internal anal sphincter (*IAS*) injury 9-5 o'clock (*arrows*)

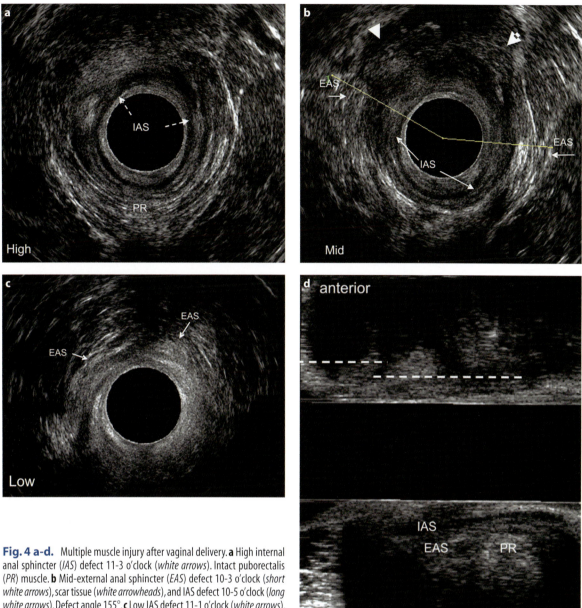

Fig. 4 a-d. Multiple muscle injury after vaginal delivery. **a** High internal anal sphincter (*IAS*) defect 11-3 o'clock (*white arrows*). Intact puborectalis (*PR*) muscle. **b** Mid-external anal sphincter (*EAS*) defect 10-3 o'clock (*short white arrows*), scar tissue (*white arrowheads*), and IAS defect 10-5 o'clock (*long white arrows*). Defect angle 155°. **c** Low IAS defect 11-1 o'clock (*white arrows*). **d** Mid-sagittal EAS and IAS injury in their entire longitudinal length

the injured muscle is viewed sagittally, thus showing the importance of possessing information on muscle length in healthy individuals (Figs. 5 and 6). Injuries from surgical procedures may be simple, single, or multiple and may involve one or more quadrants, depending on the surgical approach (Figs. 7 and 8). However, injury produced by anal dilatation appears as multiple lesions (fragmentation type) in the IAS (Fig. 9).

Anal US is also particularly useful in evaluating results of surgical repair of the anterior and posterior anal sphincter, identifying adjacent or overlapping muscles (Fig. 10), or documenting persisting muscle injury [7, 8].

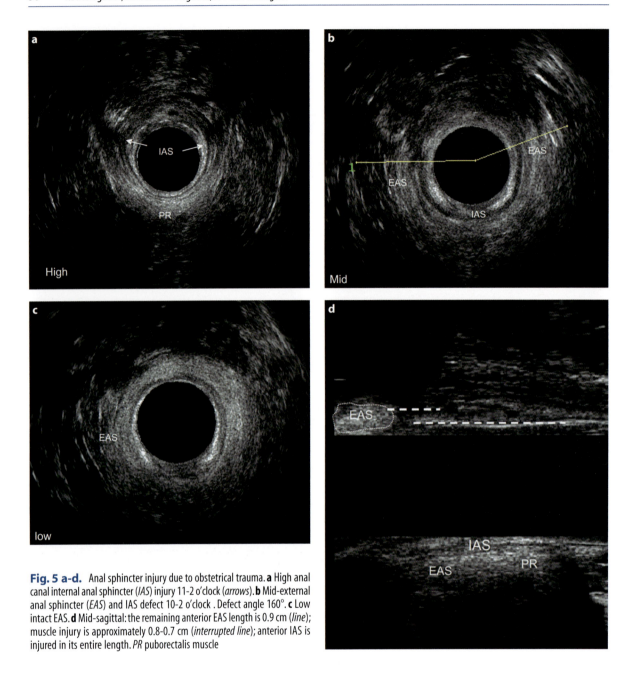

Fig. 5 a-d. Anal sphincter injury due to obstetrical trauma. **a** High anal canal internal anal sphincter (*IAS*) injury 11-2 o'clock (*arrows*). **b** Mid-external anal sphincter (*EAS*) and IAS defect 10-2 o'clock . Defect angle 160°. **c** Low intact EAS. **d** Mid-sagittal: the remaining anterior EAS length is 0.9 cm (*line*); muscle injury is approximately 0.8-0.7 cm (*interrupted line*); anterior IAS is injured in its entire length. *PR* puborectalis muscle

Changes in muscle thickness may correlate with symptoms of fecal incontinence and are easier to measure in the lateral quadrants between the 3 and 9 o'clock position. Reduced muscle thickness may be observed in incontinent patients, in primary degeneration of the EAS, and following ileoanal anastomosis [9]. The muscle may not be well defined in the anterior quadrant where it joins the longitudinal muscle and the EAS forming the perineal body.

EAS atrophy may result from damage to the pudendal nerve during vaginal delivery and should be identified in patients with indication for surgical repair due to sphincter injuries, since the prognosis may be poor with regard to postoperative function [10].

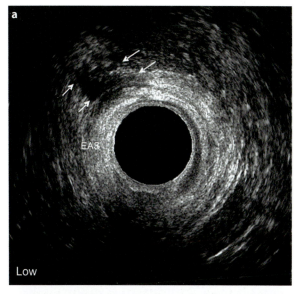

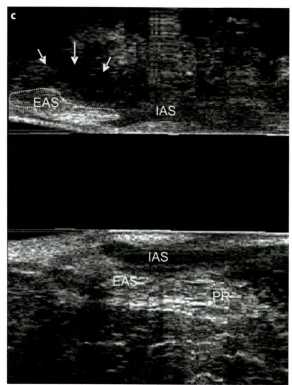

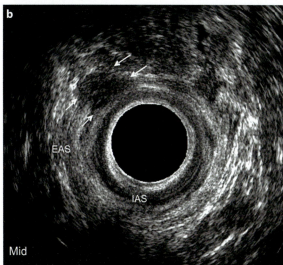

Fig. 6 a-c. Muscle injury due to left lateral episiotomy. **a** Low (*arrows*). **b** Mid: well-defined incomplete external anal sphincter (*EAS*) injury 11 o'clock (*arrows*). **c** Mid-sagittal: incomplete injury involving lateral muscle fibers of the EAS (*arrows*); intact internal anal sphincter (*IAS*). *PR* puborectalis muscle

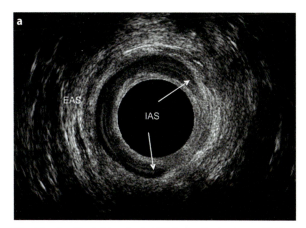

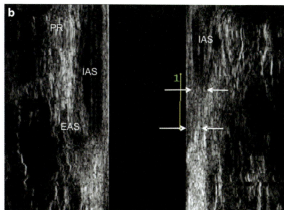

Fig. 7 a, b. Muscle injury due to left lateral sphincterotomy. **a** Mid: internal anal sphincter (*IAS*) defect 3 o'clock (*arrow*). **b** Coronal plane: IAS injured in its distal part (*arrows*). *PR* puborectalis muscle

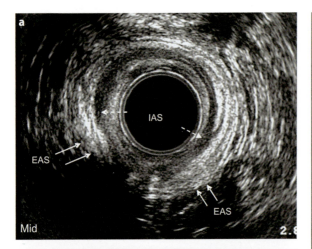

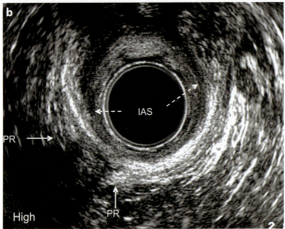

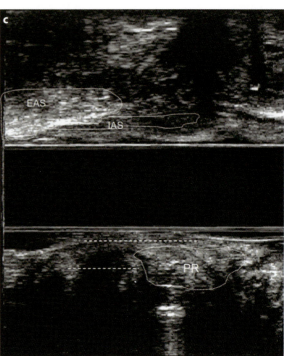

Fig. 8 a-c. Sphincter muscle defect following fistulotomy. **a** Mid: external anal sphincter (*EAS*) 5-8 o'clock (*solid arrows*) and internal anal sphincter (*IAS*) 5-9 o'clock (*interrupted-line arrows*); complete defects. **b** High: incomplete defect compromising the lateral part of the EAS 7-8 o'clock (*arrows*). Complete IAS defect 2-9 o'clock (*interrupted-line arrows*). **c** Sagittal and diagonal planes: complete damage to the posterior IAS (*upper interrupted line*). Posterior EAS-puborectalis (*PR*) muscle defect length (*lower interrupted line*); the remaining EAS-PR length

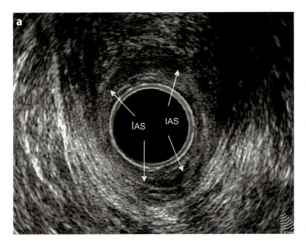

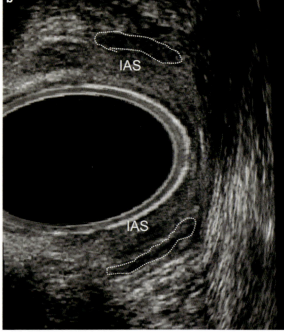

Fig. 9 a, b. Internal anal sphincter (*IAS*) fragmentation following manual anal dilatation. **a** Remaining muscle fibers (*arrows*), **b** (*circle*)

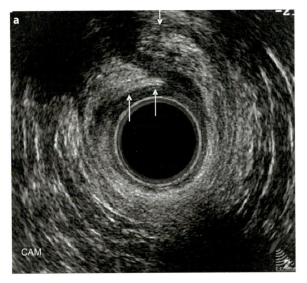 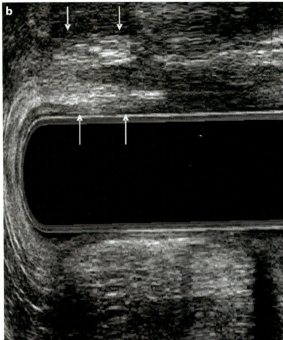

Fig. 10 a, b. Anterior sphincter repair. **a** Mid: internal anal sphincter (*IAS*) defect 12 o'clock (*arrow*). **b** Mid-sagittal: distal IAS injury (*arrows*)

References

1. Gold DM, Bartram CI, Halligan S et al (1999) Three-dimensional endoanal sonography in assessing anal canal injury. Br J Surg 86:365–370
2. Regadas SMM, Regadas FSP, Rodrigues LV et al (2005) Importância do ultra-som tridimensional na avaliação anorretal. Arq Gastroenterol 42:226–232
3. West RL, Dwarkasing S, Briel JW et al (2005) Can three-dimensional endoanal ultrasonography detect external and sphincter atrophy? A comparison with endoanal magnetic resonance imaging. Int J Colorectal Dis 20(4):328–333
4. Zetterstrom JP, Mellgren A, Madoff RD et al (1994) Perineal body measurement improves evaluation of anterior sphincter lesions during endoanal ultrasonography. Dis Colon Rectum 41:705–713
5. Bollard RC, Gardiner A, Lindow S et al (2002) Normal female anal sphincter: difficulties in interpretation explained. Dis Colon Rectum 45:171–175

6. Regadas FSP, Murad-Regadas SM, Lima DRM et al (2007) Anal canal anatomy showed by three-dimensional anorectal ultrasonography. Surg Endoscopy 21(12):2207–2211
7. Nielsen MB, Gammelgaard L, Pedersen JF (1994) Endosonographic assessment of the anal sphincter after surgical reconstruction. Dis Colon Rectum 37:434–438
8. Savoye-Collet C, Savoye G, Koning E et al (1999) Anal endosonography after sphincter repair: specific patterns related to clinical outcome. Abdom Imaging 24:569–573
9. Ignacio EA, Hill MC (2003) Ultrasound of the acute female pelvis. Ultrasound Q 19(2):86–98
10. Briel JW, Stoker J, Rociu E et al (1999) External anal sphincter atrophy on endoanal magnetic resonance imaging adversely affects continence after sphincteroplasty. Br J Surg 86:1322–1327

Commentary

Mario Pescatori

US identification of sphincter defects allows selection of patients whose fecal incontinence may be treated by means of a bulking-agents injection, a procedure mainly indicated in case of small internal sphincter disruption causing mild or moderate symptoms.

Multiparous women whose anal US shows an anterior lesion of the external sphincter may be clinically continent but are at risk of postoperative soiling in case they undergo fistulotomy, hemorrhoidectomy, rectocele repair, and low colorectal or ileo- or coloanal anastomosis. Anal US is therefore indicated in elderly and multiparous patients who are candidates for transanal and perineal operations with the aim of minimizing the risk of postoperative incontinence.

Internal sphincter defects have been reported following both the procedure for prolapse and hemorrhoids (PPH) and stapled transanal rectal resection (STARR) for obstructed defecation, possibly due to the large size of the stapling device. Such defects may occasionally require a bulking-agent injection or, more rarely, a sphincter reconstruction.

Patients who are operated for obstructed defecation via a transanal route may have US-detectable sphincter lesions prior to surgery due to muscle atrophy related to the chronic straining at stool, causing perineal descent and stretching of the pudendal nerves.

When planning a postanal repair for fecal incontinence in a patient with perineal descent and neurogenic incontinence, a preoperative anal US may reveal an unsuspected anterior lesion of the external sphincter. In this case, it may be worthwhile to associate an anterior sphincter reconstruction and an anterior levatorplasty to increase the chance of cure.

Finally, the reduced thickness of the internal sphincter, which may be evaluated by anal US, represents – together with the presence of perineal scars and decreased voluntary contraction – a negative predictor of outcome for patients undergoing pelvic floor rehabilitation for fecal incontinence.

CHAPTER 6

Transperineal Ultrasonography of Anatomic Defects in Fecal Incontinence

Harry Kleinübing Jr., Mauro S.L. Pinho

Abstracts

Highly accurate imaging of the anal sphincters is obtained by transperineal ultrasonography. This imaging technique is especially valuable in assessing women with anterior defects caused by obstetric injury.

Introduction

Transperineal ultrasonography, performed by positioning conventional transducers on the perineum, provides highly accurate images of anal sphincters. It is used to demonstrate anal sphincter defects and evaluate postoperative results of sphincter repair [1–5]. It is particularly useful in women to assess anterior defects resulting from obstetric injuries. Different anal sphincter section images, transverse or longitudinal, may be obtained by varying the position and angle of the transducer, as demonstrated in the following images (Figs. 1–5).

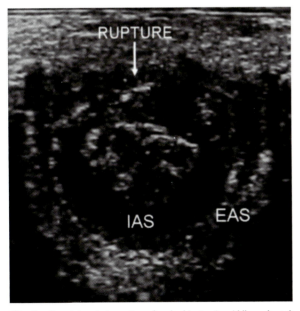

Fig. 1. Complete anterior rupture of anal sphincters in middle anal canal. *IAS* internal anal sphincter, *EAS* external anal sphincter

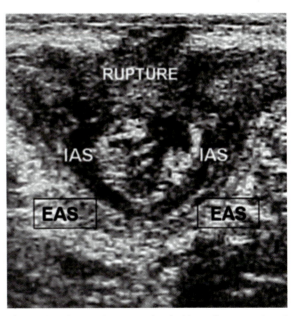

Fig. 2. Complete anterior rupture of anal sphincters in upper anal canal. *IAS* internal anal sphincter, *EAS* external anal sphincter

M. Pescatori, F.S.P. Regadas, S.M. Murad Regadas, A.P. Zbar (eds.), *Imaging Atlas of the Pelvic Floor and Anorectal Diseases*. ISBN 978-88-470-0808-3. © Springer-Verlag Italia 2008

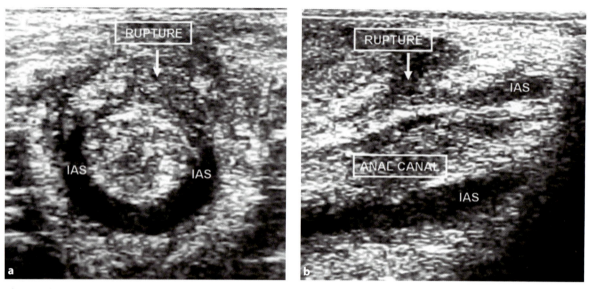

Fig. 3 a, b. Complete anterior rupture of anal sphincters in middle anal canal: **a** transverse section, **b** longitudinal section. *IAS* internal anal sphincter, *EAS* external anal sphincter

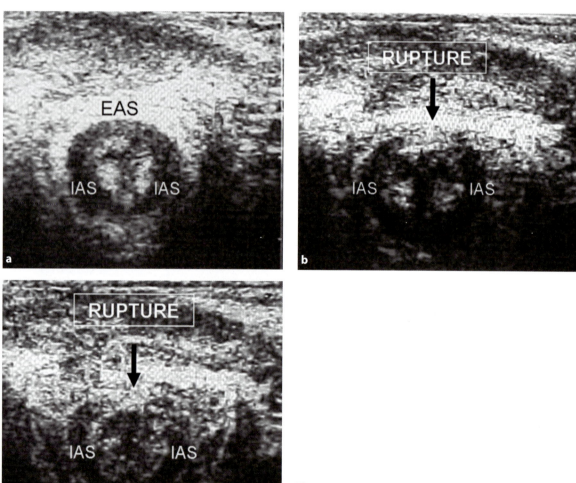

Fig. 4 a-c. Different levels of sectional images in the same patient: **a** normal lower anal canal, **b** internal sphincter rupture in middle anal canal, **c** increased internal sphincter rupture in upper anal canal. *IAS* internal anal sphincter, *EAS* external anal sphincter

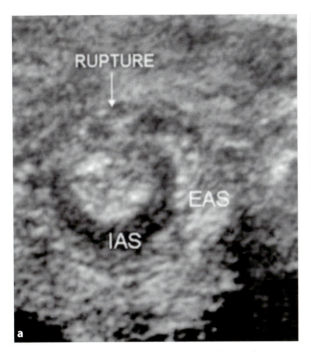 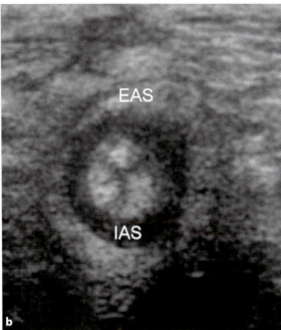

Fig. 5 a, b. **a** Complete anterior rupture of anal sphincters; **b** same patient after sphincter repair. *IAS* internal anal sphincter, *EAS* external anal sphincter

References

1. Peschers UM, Delancey JOL, Schaer GN, Schuessler B (1997) Exoanal ultrasound of the anal sphincter: normal anatomy and sphincter defects. B J Obstet Gynaecol 104:999–1003
2. Kleinübing H Jr, Jannini JF, Malafaia O (1997) Ultrasonografia transperineal: novo método de imagem da região anorretal. Presented at 1° Encontro Catarinense de Colo-Proctologia
3. Rubens DJ, Strang JG, Bogineni-Misra S, Wexler IE (1998) Transperineal sonography of the rectum: anato-my and pathology revealed by sonography compared with CT and MR imaging. AJR Am J Roentgenol 170:637–642
4. Kleinübing H Jr, Jannini JF, Malafaia O et al (2000) Transperineal ultrasonography: new method to image the anorectal region. Dis Colon Rectum 43:1572–1574
5. Roche B, Deléaval J, Fransioli A, Marti M-C (2001) Comparison of transanal and external perineal ultrasonography. Eur Radiol 11:1165–1170

CHAPTER 7

Magnetic Resonance Imaging of Anatomic Defects in Fecal Incontinence

Jaap Stoker, Andrew P. Zbar

Abstract

Endoanal probe technology provides high-resolution soft-tissue imaging for periluminal anal and rectal disease, most notably in complex perirectal sepsis and in patients presenting with fecal incontinence and sphincter damage. The trend is a movement away from direct sphincter repair toward sacral neuromodulation in external anal sphincter (EAS) injury. However, endoanal magnetic resonance imaging (EAMRI) has shown clear accuracy in the delineation of both EAS defects suitable for surgical treatment and in the definition of internal anal sphincter (IAS) damage potentially suitable for bioimplant deployment. Moreover, endoanal MR images have shown a correlation with histopathologically defined sphincter atrophy, which in turn has been predictive of relatively poor postsphincteroplasty outcomes. The role of EAMRI in the hierarchy of imaging modalities for use in an incontinence algorithm is somewhat unclear in the absence of comparative randomized clinical trials. However, it has a definitive place in defining sphincter atrophy in equivocal cases that are perhaps best treated nonoperatively or initially by temporary neuromodulatory stimulation.

Introduction

Accurate imaging of the anal sphincter is an essential part of assessment in patients presenting with fecal incontinence, prior to surgery for complex (or recurrent) perirectal sepsis where sphincter musculature is at risk and perhaps as a premonitory to complex reconstructive coloanal anastomosis [1]. Lately, there has been extensive evidence to show that endoanal magnetic resonance (EAMR) imaging is accurate in detecting external anal sphincter (EAS) defects potentially suitable for repair in patients presenting with fecal incontinence when compared with the traditional gold standards of endoanal ultrasonography (EAUS) [2–5] and surgery [6–10]. In environments without access to endoluminal MR technology, surface phased-array MRI may be an alternative, with relative accuracy in the detection of EAS defects [11–14], although there is reduced local spatial resolution using this technology.

Recently, there has been evidence to show that the longer-term functional outcome following sphincteroplasty for obstetric-related EAS defects (the principal cause of clinical fecal incontinence) is somewhat dependent upon the presence of attendant pudendal neuropathy [15–17] and that worse outcome is correlated with neuropathy-associated EAS atrophy [18]. EAMRI has been shown to accurately define EAS atrophy both in comparison with EAUS [19] and with operative findings [20], whereas there are technical limitations with EAUS in the definition of the external echogenic limits of the EAS musculature [21], grading of EAS atrophy [19], and with surgery in the objective definition of atrophy [22]. This chapter outlines the recommended role of EAMRI in assessing patients with fecal incontinence and discusses the basic MRI technique and its limitations and comparisons with other imaging modalities in determining potential operative candidates and in the objective delineation of EAS atrophy.

M. Pescatori, F.S.P. Regadas, S.M. Murad Regadas, A.P. Zbar (eds.), *Imaging Atlas of the Pelvic Floor and Anorectal Diseases*.
ISBN 978-88-470-0808-3. © Springer-Verlag Italia 2008

Endoanal Magnetic Resonance Imaging Technique

MRI has a high intrinsic contrast resolution and is therefore very well suited to visualize the muscular layers of the anal sphincter and adjacent structures. EAMRI has been independently described by two groups [23–26] using minimum field strengths of T1 and either a rectal coil or a dedicated anal cylindrical rigid coil. T2-weighted turbo spin echo (TSE) sequences are acquired in the axial and longitudinal planes, providing optimal soft-tissue contrast. These images are obtained parallel or orthogonal to the coil to reduce partial volume-averaging effects, with additional angulated axial sequences required because of the shift in direction of the anal canal when there is combined disease of the anus and rectum.

The highest spatial resolution at the anal sphincter is reached with an endoluminal coil, and several coil designs are used for that purpose. We utilize a dedicated endoanal coil with a 19-mm diameter. The coil holder is covered by a lubricated condom and inserted with the patient in the lateral decubitus position. The patient is subsequently turned to the supine position for image acquisition after correct coil positioning. Bowel relaxants (butyl scopolamine bromide, not approved for this application in the USA, or glucagon) can be given to reduce motion artifacts introduced by bowel contractions, with evidence to suggest that this endoluminal approach is acceptable for overall patient comfort even in the presence of painful anorectal disease when compared with manometry, EAUS, and defecation proctography [27]. A survey is performed to verify the coil position and plan the sequences. T2-weighted sequences, preferably TSE, are used with scan parameters optimized for anal sphincter visualization. [e.g., for 1.5-Tesla (T), repetition time (TR) 2,500 ms, echo time (TE) 70 ms, slice thickness 2–3 mm). In our experience, T1-weighted sequences without or with intravenous contrast medium do not seem to provide additional information. A combination of an axial and coronal T2-weighted TSE sequences will suffice in most cases examined for fecal incontinence. The examination may be combined with a dynamic MRI of the pelvic floor, as described by Fletcher and colleagues [28].

Normal Anal Sphincter Anatomy at MRI

The MR images in this chapter all comprise T2-weighted TSE sequences. On MRI, contrast is described in relation to the surrounding structures, as there are no absolute values for tissue contrast (as there are, for example, in computed tomography). For reference at T2-weighted sequences, fat or fluid are often used as relative signal intensities, which are in general very hyperintense (white), whereas very hypointense (black) structures such as fibrous tissue (e.g., tendon, aponeurosis) and cortical structures are used as further references.

The anal sphincter comprises several cylindrical layers, which are well appreciated on endoanal MRI (Fig. 1) [29], where there is some similarity to endosonography. The innermost layer is the relatively hyperintense subepithelium/submucosa (including the anal cushions), with a thin demonstrable hypointense muscularis mucosae layer (Fig. 2). Next to this is the cylindrical smooth muscle of the IAS, which is relatively hyperintense in comparison with the subepithelium. This muscle is the continuation of the circular muscular layer of the muscularis propria of the rectum. The following layer is the relatively hyperintense fat-containing layer that represents the surgical intersphincteric space. Through this space courses the relatively hypointense longitudinal layer, which is a continuation of the longitudinal layer of the muscularis propria [30]. The outermost layer is the relatively hypointense striated muscle of the EAS and the puborectalis muscle, which are separable (Fig. 1) [31]. The EAS forms the lower outer ring of

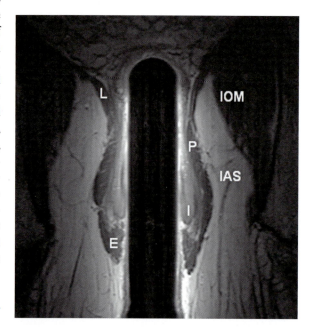

Fig. 1. Coronal T2-weighted endoanal magnetic resonance image showing the anal sphincter anatomy comprising the internal anal sphincter (*I*), external anal sphincter (*E*), puborectal muscle (*P*), and levator plate (*L*). The levator plate is attached to the internal obturator muscle (*IOM*). The anal sphincter is surrounded by the ischioanal space (*IAS*)

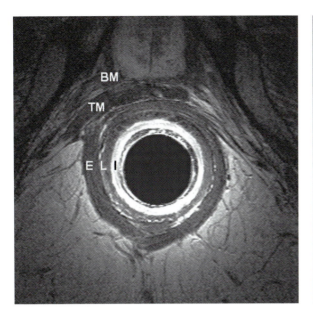

Fig. 2. Axial T2-weighted endoanal magnetic resonance image at the lower half of the anal sphincter showing the multilayered, concentric anatomy in a man. It comprises the internal anal sphincter (*I*), longitudinal layer (*L*) in the intersphincteric space, and the external anal sphincter (*E*). *TM* transverse perineal muscle, *BM* bulbospongiosus muscle

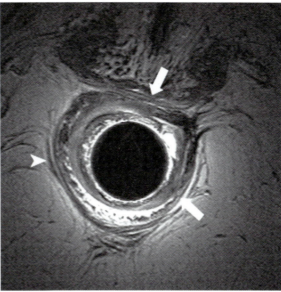

Fig. 3. Axial T2-weighted endoanal magnetic resonance image at the lower half of the anal sphincter in a woman with fecal incontinence demonstrates a defect and scar tissue (*low-signal-intensity area*) of the left anterolateral internal and external anal sphincters (*arrows*). The external anal sphincter is atrophied (*arrowhead*) (compare with Fig. 2)

the sphincter complex, whereas the sling-like puborectalis muscle forms the upper part of these images.

In a series of 100 normal volunteers, age- and gender-related differences were demonstrable on EAMRI [32], as women have a significantly shorter EAS than do men, both laterally (27.1 mm vs. 28.6 mm) and anteriorly (14.0 mm vs. 27.0 mm). This difference has anteriorly been shown with conventional [33] and three-dimensional (3D) EAUS as well [34]. Detectable age-related variations include a significant decrease in EAS thickness in men with advancing years. With age, there is a significant decrease in longitudinal muscle thickness and an increase in IAS thickness in both genders, as has previously been demonstrated with EAUS [35].

Endoanal Magnetic Resonance Imaging in Fecal Incontinence: Anal Sphincter Lesions

External Anal Sphincter Defects

EAS lesions are detected as alterations in the normal EAS anatomical integrity or as scarring, local atrophy, or a definitive defect. Scarring is identified by the replacement of relatively hypointense striated muscle by more hypointense fibrous tissue and disturbance of the multilayer morphology (Fig. 3).

Scar tissue can extend outside the expected border of the sphincter and on occasion can be very subtle. This may be the only finding, and it is most easily appreciated when scrutinizing the multilayered appearance of the EAS musculature, which becomes relatively obliterated. Local atrophy represents thinning or fatty degeneration of the EAS, whereas a defect is a discontinuity of the EAS ring often combined with an excess scar tissue. The term defect is somewhat relative in many cases, and in some of the available literature, it is more loosely used to indicate all four forms of local EAS damage. The full extent of this damage is best appreciated in a combined evaluation of the axial and longitudinal plane sequences. Secondary changes to the architecture of adjacent structures (longitudinal muscle, perianal fat) (Fig. 4) provide supportive evidence of a sphincter tear, where the contralateral side may be atrophic or normal when compared with the side of the tear.

Variations in normal anatomy of the anal sphincter may be misdiagnosed as sphincter defects, with constitutive differences in the EAS being observed. The lower edge of the EAS often does not form a complete ring and can easily be misdiagnosed as a defect at this level – an effect that has also been reported with endoanal sonography [36]. Such defects can present as bilateral crescents or as an anterior cap-like morphological appearance, forming a continuous ring at a slightly higher level. The posterior

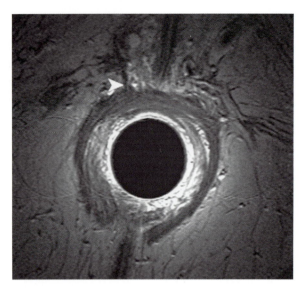

Fig. 4. Axial T2-weighted endoanal magnetic resonance image through lower edge of the anal sphincter in a woman with fecal incontinence shows subtle asymmetry of the right anterolateral external anal sphincter (compare to left anterolateral side), contiguous with some scar tissue in the perineal space (*arrowhead*)

part of the EAS may normally have prominent extensions to the anococcygeal ligament, suggesting a local defect in between these extensions. Symmetry, the absence of scar tissue and a normal layered morphology, all help in differentiating a normal variant from a defect.

Internal Anal Sphincter Defects

IAS defects are identified as either IAS discontinuity or as replacement of the normal smooth muscle by fibrous tissue with concomitant muscle thinning (Fig. 3). IAS defects are often found in combination with EAS defects, especially in women presenting with incontinence. Solitary IAS defects are more common in iatrogenic cases of incontinence, particularly following the newer forms of limited hemorrhoidectomy or after repeated surgeries for a complex perianal fistula [37].

Atrophy

External Anal Sphincter Atrophy

Recent publications on EAMRI imaging reemphasize the importance of EAS atrophy with its potential predictive clinical implications on sphincteroplasty outcome [10, 18, 22]. This entity had become somewhat neglected following the widespread introduction of endosonography and subsequent removal of electromyography from the workup in many institutions [38]. Until the introduction of EAMRI imaging, no endosonographic study addressed the issue of EAS atrophy. One of the technical problems with an endosonographic diagnosis of atrophy is that although the outer border of the EAS may be visible in control cases, it is no longer evident when there is substantial fat replacement of the muscle, as occurs in atrophy [39]. Accurate visualization of the EAS boundaries and its internal structure on EAMRI provides the unique opportunity to evaluate the presence of definitive sphincter lesions and define EAS atrophy in one examination.

Generalized EAS atrophy on EAMRI may present as overall thinning, fat-muscle replacement or both (Fig. 5). There are no objective criteria established for its diagnosis, although some guidelines can be provided based on an assessment of control data [20, 32, 40–42]. In severe EAS atrophy, hardly any muscle fibers are identified, although the fascial outer contours of the muscle can be intact. In limited EAS atrophy, some intertwining fat is seen among the muscle so that a considerable amount of muscle mass can still be identified. Moderate atrophy represents an intermediate situation between these two extremes, providing a potential for semiquantitative atrophy assessment. Here, mild atrophy represents <50% thinning/replacement, with severe atrophy representing >50% thinning or total muscle replacement with fat. Although a comparison with the puborectalis muscle or levator plate can also be made to objectify atrophy, this can be relatively inaccurate, as these muscles may atrophy concomitantly as part of an overall pudendal neuropathy. Accurate assessment of EAS atrophy on EAMRI can be made by quantitative measurements of the area of remaining EAS and of the percentage of fat content of the muscle [18, 22, 42, 43].

EAS atrophy on EAMRI is a finding that has been related to sphincter function in which maximal voluntary squeeze pressure correlates with EAS bulk but not with fat content [44]. In a series of 200 patients with moderate to severe fecal incontinence, EAS atrophy on EAMRI was depicted in 62% of patients, varying from mild to severe, with increasing levels of quantifiable atrophy correlating with impaired voluntary squeeze function [20]. In that study by our group, patients with severe atrophy had a lower maximal squeeze ($p = 0.003$) and squeeze increment pressure ($p < 0.001$) when compared with patients with mild atrophy.

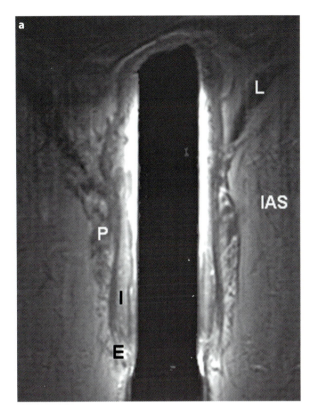 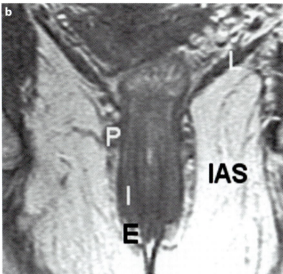

Fig. 5 a, b. **a** Coronal T2-weighted endoanal magnetic resonance image (MRI) showing extensive atrophy of the external anal sphincter (*E*) and puborectal muscle (*P*) (compare with Fig. 1) in a patient with fecal incontinence. The internal anal sphincter (*I*) and levator plate (*L*) are normal. *IAS* is-chioanal space. **b** Coronal T2-weighted MRI with external coil in the same patient as in **a** demonstrates identical findings: extensive atrophy of the external anal sphincter (*E*) and puborectal muscle (*P*) and normal internal sphincter (*I*) and levator plate (*L*). *IAS* ischioanal space

Internal Anal Sphincter Atrophy

IAS atrophy is defined as generalized thinning of the IAS, typically to a diameter of <2 mm on EAMRI. Atrophy of the IAS as a distinct entity with advancing age is recognized as an important degenerative process leading to passive incontinence [45]. Such IAS atrophy is also a specific principal finding in patients with scleroderma [46].

Endoanal Magnetic Resonance Imaging Accuracy in Determining Anal Sphincter Defects

Several studies have evaluated the accuracy of EAM-RI in detecting anal sphincter defects. Tears of both the IAS and EAS are readily visualized, with an accuracy of 95% for EAS lesions [6, 10, 18, 40]. Several types of sphincter lesions can be identified, including defects, scar tissue, and focal atrophy. The clinical relevance of this differentiation is at present unknown, and each finding can effectively be considered a defect that is either anatomical or functional [41]. The overall interobserver agreement for assessing sphincter integrity using EAMRI is strongest

if the sphincters are either both intact or both disrupted [5]. For individual sphincters, the interobserver agreement for defects is only fair for the EAS and moderate for the IAS and is somewhat dependent upon the radiologist's experience [14].

Endoanal Magnetic Resonance Imaging versus Endosonography

EAUS has a prominent place in the workup of patients with fecal incontinence [46]. Three comparative studies of EAUS and EAMRI in fecal incontinence have been published. In one study by our group reported by Rociu et al., EAUS and EAMRI imaging were compared with surgery in a retrospective single-center study of 22 patients presenting with sphincter defects [3]. In this series, comparison was made with surgical findings; EAMRI images were found to be the most accurate. EAS defects were detected with EAUS and EAMRI in 16 (73%) and 20 (91%) patients, respectively, with IAS defects detected in 15 (68%) and 17 (77%), respectively. A second prospective single-center study in 52 consecutive patients with fecal incontinence suggested that EAUS and endoanal MRI are comparable for EAS defects but that EAUS was superior for IAS defects [4]. In this study by Malouf and colleagues at St. Mark's Hospital, London, a comparison of imaging findings was made by consensus of a gastroenterologist and a surgeon familiar with EAUS. The differences between the results of both studies are at least partly related to differences in patient populations, study design, and the experience of the reading clinician with either technique.

More recently, a large comparative series was published by our group; Dobben et al. reported a multi-institutional study on 237 patients, including 214 women, presenting with fecal incontinence who were studied specifically for EAS defects using EAUS and EAMRI [6]. In that study, there was fair agreement between EAMRI and EAUS in 146 patients (61%; κ = 0.24) using the Bland-Altman differential method [47] and the McNemar correlation for comparison. Based on imaging findings and other considerations, 36 patients had an anterior anal sphincter repair (mean interval between imaging and surgery = 10 months), where at surgery, an EAS defect was found in 31 of the 36 patients (86%). There was no significant difference between EAUS and EAMRI in demonstrating sphincter defects (κ = 0.23: fair agreement), and the sensitivity and positive predictive value were 90% and 85%, respectively for EAUS and 81% and 89%, respectively, for EAMRI. Patients who had an EAS defect shown on EAUS tended to be significantly older than patients with an EAS defect depicted on both modalities. Each defect was assigned a score for its location on the anterior or anterolateral side of the EAS, with an allocation in 95% of cases by both modalities of a specific lesional site.

Magnetic Resonance Imaging Accuracy in Determining Anal Sphincter Atrophy

External Anal Sphincter Atrophy

Atrophy is characterized on EAMRI by generalized sphincter thinning and fat–muscle replacement (Fig. 5). EAMRI has demonstrated accuracy in this evaluation, which has been validated both surgically and histologically [18, 22]. In the study by Briel and colleagues assessing comparative sphincter histology, EAMRI demonstrated accuracy in evaluating EAS atrophy in 93% (14/15) cases [22]. The reproducibility of EAMRI for determining EAS atrophy

is somewhat dependent upon experience; the reported interobserver agreement is moderate and the intraobserver agreement is moderate to very good [42].

Endoanal Magnetic Resonance Imaging versus Endoanal Ultrasonography

EAUS has limitations in identifying EAS atrophy, as already indicated. In this setting, fatty infiltration cannot be adequately distinguished from normal muscle tissue, and the boundaries of the EAS are particularly difficult to accurately and repeatedly determine. In a comparative study by Briel et al. of 20 female patients, no cases of EAS atrophy were detected using EAUS, whereas EAS atrophy was demonstrated on EAMRI in eight cases of the patient cohort [18]. That study also showed that the finding of EAS atrophy on EAMRI was related to functional outcome following sphincteroplasty (*vide infra*). Two more recent studies, both including 18 patients, evaluated 3D EAUS in detecting EAS atrophy in comparison with EAMRI. In one study by West and colleagues [21], despite the multiplanar capability of 3D reconstruction from the axial images, the technique was unable to consistently demonstrate muscle atrophy and did not enhance the conventional endosonographic images. The other study by Cazemier et al., also with 18 patients, showed no significant difference between 3D EAUS and EAMRI in detecting EAS atrophy [19] with, however, poor agreement of atrophy grading between the two techniques. Comparisons in that study between 3D EAUS and EAMRI of sphincter thickness and length showed no statistically significant concordance between the two modalities, with no specific correlation between the measurements and the definition of EAS atrophy for either technique. Williams and colleagues, however, found that patients with a thin IAS (i.e., <2 mm) and/or a poorly defined EAS on EAUS were more likely to have EAS atrophy. They suggested that EAMRI should be considered in this group to determine whether the sphincter is grossly atrophic [43]. EAMRI can be considered the standard for detecting and grading EAS atrophy.

Internal Anal Sphincter Atrophy

The diagnosis of IAS atrophy is made on imaging when the internal sphincter measurement is generally <2 mm thick. No study of which we are aware has evaluated EAMRI accuracy in determining IAS atrophy. As the IAS is accurately demonstrated with both EAUS and EAMRI, this diagnosis can be established with either technique, and EAUS effectively remains the standard for IAS assessment.

Endoanal Magnetic Resonance Imaging and Treatment Outcome

External sphincter atrophy on EAMRI is a negative predictor of the outcome of sphincter repair [48, 49]. In the study by our group reported by Briel et al. [18], the presence of severe EAS atrophy as diagnosed on EAMRI in 8/20 cases prior to surgery correlated with a poor functional outcome following sphincteroplasty ($p = 0.004$). These findings were supported by a recent study of 30 patients presenting with fecal incontinence and an EAS defect treated by anterior anal repair [51], although patients with severe EAS atrophy were excluded from the analysis because of their overall short-term poor functional results. In that study by Dobben and colleagues, incontinence severity was objectively evaluated pre- and postoperatively using the Vaizey incontinence score [52], with all patients undergoing both EAMRI and EAUS before and after sphincter repair. Following surgery, the mean Vaizey score (scale 0–24) improved from 18 to 13 ($p < 0.001$), with the EAMRI showing that the baseline preoperative measurement of preserved EAS thickness correlated with a better functional outcome ($r = 0.42$; $p = 0.03$).

Importantly, however, the clinical outcome did not differ between patients with and without a persistent EAS defect ($p = 0.54$) or atrophy ($p = 0.26$) following surgery, where other studies showed a poor association between patient-reported function and endosonographic findings or manometric variables [53, 54]. Patients with a visible muscle overlap and <20% fat tissue replacement on EAMRI had, however, a significantly better outcome than patients with a non-visible, fat-replaced sphincter overlap. Those with a persistent EAS defect on EAUS had an overall worse functional outcome than those without a defect (17 scale points vs 10 scale points, respectively; $p = 0.003$). Given the deterioration in functional results with anterior sphincteroplasty over time [55] and the fact that 3D endoluminal US has shown that poor postoperative function may correlate with inadequate coronal length of anterior repair [56], there is as yet no data on the use of EAMRI to define the adequacy of anterior sphincteroplasty or as an indicator for selective operative use of levatorplasty in these patients. EAMRI can, however, serve as a preoperative technique to identify suitable candidates for sphincteroplasty by identifying and grading external sphincter atrophy.

Alternatives to Endoanal Magnetic Resonance Imaging Technology

Endovaginal Magnetic Resonance Imaging

Endovaginal MRI (EVMRI) has been used to evaluate the anal sphincter without distension by an endoanal coil. The increased distance between the anal sphincter and the coil has, however, proven to be a substantial disadvantage, although it has not been specifically evaluated in the immediate postsphincteroplasty patient [25, 57]. No studies have so far evaluated or validated EVMRI in detecting EAS defects, and the technique is generally not used in clinical practice for this purpose.

External Phased-Array Coils

Initial studies on the role of external phased-array-coil MRI in the workup of fecal incontinence have been reported. The potential advantages of this approach are simpler examination, with an overall wider availability and experience using this technology without the need for the introduction of – or the cost of – an endoluminal coil. Earlier studies have shown that the pelvic-floor anatomy can be adequately demonstrated using an external coil [10–13]. In two specific studies, comparison was made between external phased-array MRI and EAMRI in patients presenting with fecal incontinence and selected with both EAS defects and muscle atrophy [14, 42]. The MRI techniques did not significantly differ in depicting EAS and IAS defects [14], with a concordance in 25/30 patients (83%) for depicting EAS defects and in 28/30 patients (93%) for IAS defects. The interobserver agreement for EAS defects was moderate to good for EAMRI but only poor to fair for external phased-array MRI, in which considerable experience is required to ascertain sphincter structures and the sphincteric resolution is more limited. Intraobserver agreement ranged from fair to very good for both imaging techniques, reflecting specific familiarity of some radiologists with either modality.

The findings for EAS atrophy were comparable where the techniques did not significantly differ in their ability to depict EAS atrophy, showing generally good agreement, with a κ factor = 0.72 (Fig. 5) [42]. For atrophy, interobserver agreement was moderate using EAMRI (κ = 0.53–0.56) and moderate to good using external phased-array MRI (κ = 0.55–0.8). Intraobserver agreement was moderate to very good with EAMRI (κ = 0.57–0.86) and fair to very good with external phased-array MRI (κ = 0.31–0.86).

Overall, it would seem that given the limited availability of endoanal coils, external phased-array MRI could be a valid alternative for clinical use in demonstrating EAS defects and atrophy, provided that – given its moderate learning curve – there is sufficient experience available [14, 42, 56].

Conclusion: The Role of EAMRI in Fecal Incontinence

In the workup of patients with fecal incontinence, EAUS can be used as a primary imaging technique, given the comparable results when compared with EAMRI in detecting sphincter defects, the widespread availability of EAUS, and the lower costs. There is no doubt, however – based on some seminal trials concerning the diagnostic capability in detecting both EAS and IAS defects in comparison with US and with surgery – that EAMRI technology is accurate; it certainly has a role as a second-line technique when disruption of the EAS has been diagnosed. Then, its role in defining and diagnosing EAS atrophy can both direct sphincter repair and provide some prognostic information. External MRI might prove to be a suitable alternative. The prevalence (and definition) of EAS atrophy in a given patient population presenting with fecal incontinence to a specialist center will partially define the role of this new technology and may justify an economic stance toward its use in some centers of first-line EAMRI examination. There are no data, however, supporting the early (or routine) introduction of EAMRI into the algorithm as a cost-beneficial exercise based on its predictive value for those undergoing either sphincteroplasty or sacral neuromodulation. EAMRI definition of atrophy may need to be measured against an agreed-upon qualitative or quantitative histological standard of the diagnosis in operated cases – a standard of sphincter examination for which there is no consensus. Equally, it is accepted that there is no data yet suggestive of the benefit of EAMRI in directing additional operative procedures in selected incontinent patients (most notably anterior levatorplasty) or in the specific evaluation of postsphincteroplasty patients regardless of their reported functional outcome.

References

1. Zbar AP, Armitage NC (2006) Complex perirectal sepsis: clinical classification and imaging. Tech Coloproctol 10:83–93
2. Stoker J, Hussain SM, Lameris JS (1996) Endoanal magnetic resonance imaging versus endoanal sonography. Radiol Med (Torino) 6:738–741
3. Rociu E, Stoker J, Eijkemans MJ et al (1999) Fecal incontinence: endoanal US versus endoanal MR imaging. Radiology 212:453–458
4. Malouf AJ, Williams AB, Halligan S et al (2000) Prospective assessment of accuracy of endoanal MR imaging and endosonography in patients with fecal incontinence. AJR Am J Roentgenol 175:741–745
5. Malouf AJ, Halligan S, Williams AB et al (2001) Prospective assessment of interobserver agreement for endoanal MRI in fecal incontinence. Abdom Imaging 26:76–78
6. Dobben AC, Terra MP, Slors JFM et al (2007) External anal sphincter defects in patients with fecal incontinence. Comparison of endoanal MR imaging and endoanal US. Radiology 242:463–471
7. Deen KI, Kumar D, Williams JG et al (1993) Anal sphincter defects: correlation between endoanal ultrasound and surgery. Ann Surg 218:201–205

8. deSouza NM, Hall AS, Puni R et al (1996) High resolution magnetic resonance imaging on the anal sphincter using a dedicated endoanal coil: comparison of magnetic resonance imaging with surgical findings. Dis Colon Rectum 39:926–934
9. Myenberger C, Bertschinger P, Zala GF, Buchmann P (1996) Anal sphincter defects in fecal incontinence: correlation between endosonography and surgery. Endoscopy 28:217–224
10. deSouza NM, Puni FR, Zbar A et al (1996) MR imaging of the anal sphincter in multiparous women using an endoanal coil: correlation with in vitro anatomy and appearances in fecal incontinence. AJR Am J Roentgenol 167:1465–1471
11. Beets-Tan RG, Beets GL, van der Hoop AG et al (1999) High-resolution magnetic resonance imaging of the anorectal region without an endocoil. Abdom Imaging 24:576–581
12. Morren GL, Beets-Tan RG, van Engelshoven JM (2001) Anatomy of the anal canal and perianal structures as defined by phased-array magnetic resonance imaging. Br J Surg 88:1506–1512
13. Beets-Tan RG, Morren GL, Beets GL et al (2001) Measurement of anal sphincter muscles: endoanal US, endoanal MR imaging, or phased-array MR

imaging? A study with healthy volunteers. Radiology 220:81–89

14. Terra MP, Beets-Tan RGH, van der Hulst VPM et al (2005) Anal sphincter defects in patients with fecal incontinence: endoanal versus external phased array MR imaging. Radiology 236:888–995

15. Jacobs PP, Scheuer MM, Kuijpers JH, Vingerhoets MH (1990) Obstetric fecal incontinence: role of pelvic floor denervation and results of delayed sphincter repair. Dis Colon Rectum 33:494–497

16. Gilliland R, Altomare DF, Moreira H Jr., Oliveira L, Gilliland JE, Wexner SD (1998) Pudendal neuropathy is predictive of failure following overlapping anterior sphincteroplasty. Dis Colon Rectum 41:1516–1522

17. Shu-Hung Chen A, Luchtefeld MA, Senagore AJ, MacKeigan JM, Hoyt C (1998) Pudendal nerve latency – does it predict outcome of anal sphincter repair? Dis Colon Rectum 41:1005–1009

18. Briel JW, Stoker J, Rociu E, Lameris JS, Hop WJC, Schouten WR. External anal sphincter atrophy on endoanal magnetic resonance imaging adversely affects continence after sphincteroplasty (1999) Br J Surg 86:1322–1327

19. Cazemier M, Terra MP, Stoker J et al (2006) Atrophy and defects detection of the external anal sphincter: comparison between three-dimensional anal endosonography and endoanal magnetic resonance imaging. Dis Colon Rectum 49:20–27

20. Terra MP, Deutekom M, Beets-Tan RG et al (2006) Relationship between external anal sphincter atrophy at endoanal magnetic resonance imaging and clinical, functional, and anatomic characteristics in patients with fecal incontinence. Dis Colon Rectum 49:668–678

21. West RL, Dwarkasing S, Briel JW et al (2005)Can three-dimensional endoanal ultrasonography detect external anal sphincter atrophy? A comparison with endoanal magnetic resonance imaging. Int J Colorectal Dis 20:328–333

22. Briel JW, Zimmerman DD, Stoker J et al (2000) Relationship between sphincter morphology on endoanal MRI and histopathological aspects of the external anal sphincter. Int J Colorectal Dis 15:87–90

23. deSouza NM, Puni R, Gilderdale DJ, Bydder GM (1995) Magnetic resonance imaging of the anal sphincter using an internal coil. Mag Reson Q 11:45–56

24. Stoker J, Hussain SM, van Kempen D et al (1996) Endoanal coil in MR imaging of anal fistulas. AJR Am J Roentgenol 166:360–362

25. Zbar AP, deSouza NM (2001) The anal sphincter. In: deSouza NM (ed). Endocavitary MRI of the pelvis. Harwood Academic, London, pp 91–109

26. Stoker J, Rociu E, Zwamborn AW et al (1999) Endoluminal MR imaging of the rectum and anus: technique, applications, and pitfalls. RadioGraphics 19:383–398

27. Deutekom M, Terra MP, Dijkgraaf MG et al (2006) Patients' perception of tests in the assessment of faecal incontinence. Br J Radiol 79:94–100

28. Fletcher JG, Busse RF, Riederer SJ et al (2003) Magnetic resonance imaging of anatomic and dynamic defects of the pelvic floor in defecatory disorders. Am J Gastroenterol 98:399–411

29. Stoker J (2003) The anatomy of the pelvic floor and sphincters. In: Bartram CI, DeLancey JO, Halligan S et al (eds) Imaging pelvic floor disorders. Springer, Berlin

30. Lunniss PJ, Phillips RKS (1992) Anatomy and function of the anal longitudinal muscle. Br J Surg 79:882–884

31. Fucini C, Elbetti C, Messerini L (1999) Anatomical plane of separation between the external anal sphincter and puborectalis muscle: clinical implications. Dis Colon Rectum 42:374–379

32. Rociu E, Stoker J, Eijkemans MJC, Laméris JS (2000) Normal anal sphincter anatomy and age- and sex-related variations at high-spatial-resolution endoanal MR imaging. Radiology 217:395–401

33. Sultan AH, Kamm M A, Hudson CN et al (1994) Endosonography of the anal sphincters: normal anatomy and comparison with manometry. Clin Radiol 49:368–374

34. Williams AB, Bartram CI, Halligan S et al (2001) Multiplanar anal endosonography: normal anal canal anatomy. Colorectal Dis 3:169–174

35. Burnett SJ, Bartram CI (1991) Endosonographic variations in the normal internal anal sphincter. Int J Colorect Dis 6:2–4

36. Bollard RC, Gardiner A, Lindow S et al (2002) Normal female anal sphincter: difficulties in interpretation explained. Dis Colon Rectum 45:171–175

37. Zbar AP, Beer-Gabel M, Chiappa AC, Aslam M (2001) Fecal incontinence after minor anorectal surgery. Dis Colon Rectum 44:1610–1623

38. Tjandra JJ, Milsom JW, Schroeder T, Fazio VW (1993) Endoluminal ultrasound is preferable to electromyography in mapping anal sphincteric defects. Dis Colon Rectum 36:689–692

39. Enck P, Heyer T, Gantke B et al (1997) How reproducible are measures of the anal sphincter muscle diameter by endoanal ultrasound? Am J Gastroenterol 92:293–296

40. Rociu E, Stoker J, Zwamborn AW, Laméris JS (1999) Endoanal MR imaging of the anal sphincter in fecal incontinence. RadioGraphics 19:S171–S177

41. Terra MP, Stoker J (2006) The current role of imaging techniques in fecal incontinence. Eur Radiol 16:1727–1736

42. Terra MP, Beets-Tan RG, van der Hulst VPM et al (2006) MR imaging in evaluating atrophy of the external anal sphincter in patients with fecal incontinence. AJR Am J Roentgenol 187:991–999

43. Williams AB, Bartram CI, Modhwadia D et al (2001)Endocoil magnetic resonance imaging quantification of external anal sphincter atrophy. Br J Surg 88:853–859

44. Williams AB, Malouf AJ, Bartram CI et al (2001) Assessment of external anal sphincter morphology in id-

iopathic fecal incontinence with endocoil magnetic resonance imaging. Dig Dis Sci 46:1466–1471

45. Vaizey CJ, Kamm MA, Bartram CI (1997) Primary degeneration of the internal anal sphincter as a cause of passive faecal incontinence. Lancet 349(9052):612–615

46. Daniel F, De Parades V, Cellier C (2005) Abnormal appearance of the internal anal sphincter at ultrasound: a specific feature of progressive systemic sclerosis? Gastroenterol Clin Biol 29:597–5999

47. Rao SS (2004) Diagnosis and management of fecal incontinence. American College of Gastroenterology Practice Parameters Committee. Am J Gastroenterol 99:1585–1604

48. Altman DG (1999) Practical statistics for medical research. CRC, Boca Raton

49. Baig MK, Wexner SD (2000). Factors predictive of outcome after surgery for faecal incontinence. Br J Surg 87:1316–1320

50. Starck M, Bohe M, Valentin L (2006) The extent of endosonographic anal sphincter defects after primary repair of obstetric sphincter tears increases over time and is related to anal incontinence. Ultrasound Obstet Gynecol 27:188–197

51. Dobben AC, Terra MP, Deutekom M et al (2007) The role of endoluminal imaging in clinical outcome of overlapping anterior anal sphincter repair in patients with fecal incontinence. AJR Am J Roentgenol 189:W70–W77

52. Vaizey CJ, Carapeti E, Cahill JA, Kamm MA (1999) Prospective comparison of faecal incontinence grading systems. Gut 44:77–80

53. Saranovic D, Barisic G, Krivokapic Z et al (2007). Endoanal ultrasound evaluation of anorectal diseases and disorders: technique, indications, results and limitations. Eur J Radiol 61:480–489

54. Hill K, Fanning S, Fennerty MB, Faigel DO (2006) Endoanal ultrasound compared to anorectal manometry for the evaluation of fecal incontinence: a study of the effect these tests have on clinical outcome. Dig Dis Sci 51:235–240

55. Evans C, Davis K, Kumar D (2006) Overlapping anal sphincter repair and anterior levatorplasty: effect of patient's age and duration of follow-up. Int J Colorectal Dis 21:795–801

56. Gold DM, Bartram CI, Halligan S et al (1999) Three-dimensional endoanal sonography in assessing anal canal injury. Br J Surg 86:365–370

57. Tan IL, Stoker J, Zwamborn AW et al (1998) Female pelvic floor: endovaginal MR imaging of normal anatomy. Radiology 206:777–783

58. Hoeffel C, Arrive L, Mourra N et al (2006) Anatomic and pathologic findings at external phased-array pelvic MR imaging after surgery for anorectal disease. RadioGraphics 26:1391–1407

Commentary

Geraldo Magela G. Cruz

Figure 1 demonstrates a very interesting angle of view with endoanal magnetic resonance imaging (EAMRI) of the entire musculature of the anal region as well as the perianal spaces. In EAMRI T2-weighted turbo spin-echo sequence, fat and fluid are in general hyperintense and represented in *white*. Structures such as muscle and tendons and aponeurosis are very hypointense and are represented in *black*. This sequence shows the normal anal sphincter anatomy in a very conspicuous manner, demonstrating the several cylindrical layers that comprise both anal sphincters. The appearance of the region's anatomical musculature is very clear, with special reference to the internal (IAS) (*I*) and external (EAS) (*E*) anal sphincters, the puborectal muscle (*P*), the levator plate (*L*), and the internal obturator muscle (*IOM*) to which it is attached. Continuity of the IAS with the muscularis propria of the rectum is very well demonstrated. The difference in intensity with the submucosa is clearly marked along both structures – IAS and muscularis mucosae. Also, the hyperintense fat-containing intersphincteric space is well delimitated between both and represents the surgical intersphincteric space. The anal sphincters are surrounded externally by the ischioanal space (hyperintense area). By these views, one can determine that EAMRI is a valuable method to show any alteration of the musculature of this region, which means a possible lesion of one or both anal sphincters.

Figure 2, clearly shows the IAS (*I*) and the EAS (*E*) on EAMRI. The outer layer in relation to the IAS (*I*) is the relatively hyperintense fat-containing layer – the surgical intersphincteric space. The most inner layer is the hyperintense submucosa tissue, including the anal cushions, with a very thin hypodense layer of muscle (muscularis mucosae). The IAS is relatively hyperintense in comparison with the submucosa. The outer hypodense layer is the striated EAS muscle (*E*), which is well defined.

Figure 3 clearly shows an EAS defect on axial EAMRI. Fibrous tissue presents as an area of low signal intensity. This identifies the presence of scar tissue in the low-signal-intensity area of the left anterolateral IAS and the EAS (*arrows*) as local atrophy or a definitive defect. The EAS is atrophied (*arrowhead*). The hypointense scar is clearly identified by the replacement of relatively hypointense striated muscle of the EAS by a more conspicuous hypointense fibrous tissue. Although this defect is obvious in this axial sequence, it can be much better identified by the coronal MRI shown in Figure 5.

Figure 5a clearly shows extensive atrophy of the EAS (*E*) and the puborectal muscle (*P*). In this image, EAS atrophy is characterized by generalized sphincter thinning and fat-muscle replacement. In Figure 5b, the atrophy can be nicely appreciated on the MR images obtained by an external coil.

CHAPTER 8

Two- and Three-dimensional Ultrasonography in Abscess and Anal Fistula

Sthela M. Murad Regadas, F. Sérgio P. Regadas

Abstract

Three-dimensional anorectal ultrasound presents an important role in the evaluation of cryptoglandular disease of the anal canal. It clearly shows the location, extent of the abscess cavity, and relation to the sphincter muscles and rectal wall, making classification possible, which is particularly important for the complex abscess. It is also particularly useful for evaluating anorectal fistulas, as it identifies primary and secondary tracts, internal opening, and adjacent cavities. This information facilitates surgical planning, consequently preventing recurrence and fecal incontinence.

Introduction

Three-dimensional anorectal ultrasound is an important imaging technique in evaluating and classifying anorectal abscesses and fistula.

Anorectal Abscess

Anorectal ultrasound clearly shows location and extent of the anorectal abscess cavity and its relation to sphincter muscles and the rectal wall, making classification possible. Abscesses appear as nonhomogenous hypoechoic areas due to inflammatory processes and are associated with more hypoechogenic areas corresponding to liquid in the cavity, whereas hyperechogenicity suggests residual air.

Ultrasound scanning is particularly indicated in early inflammatory processes or during the absorption stage, when proctological examination alone cannot determine whether therapy should be conservative or surgical (Fig. 1). Ultrasonography is likewise useful to determine the location and extent of large abscesses in relation to sphincter muscles and in the choice of treatment approach (Fig. 2a, b). As the three-dimensional scanning mode shows the extent of the injury in relation to the length and circumference of the anal canal, it is particularly indicated for complex abscesses located above the levator muscle (Fig. 2c). In such cases, ultrasound findings for the rectum and perirectal fat should be taken into account as well.

The complete view of the anal canal and rectum provided by three-dimensional scanning is helpful when evaluating extensive inflammatory and infectious processes, as it shows the boundaries of the cavity with the tract draining into the anal canal but without the external communication, i.e., without all the components of the fistula complex (Fig. 3). It is also well tolerated, because the scanning procedure is quick and images may be analyzed a posteriori. Ischiorectal abscesses in deep lateral locations require greater focal distance to view the lateral boundaries. The examination may be inconclusive in patients with Fournier's syndrome due to the presence of fibrosis and excessive muscle decay.

Anorectal Fistula

Anorectal ultrasound makes it possible to identify the entire fistula complex (primary and secondary tract, internal openings, and adjacent cavities), facilitating surgical planning and conse-

M. Pescatori, F.S.P. Regadas, S.M. Murad Regadas, A.P. Zbar (eds.), *Imaging Atlas of the Pelvic Floor and Anorectal Diseases*. ISBN 978-88-470-0808-3. © Springer-Verlag Italia 2008

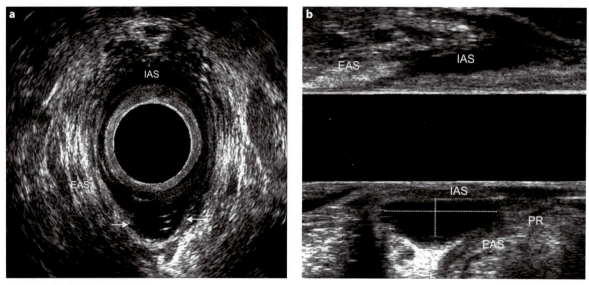

Fig. 1 a, b. Male patient. Posterior intersphincteric abscess (*arrows*). **a** Axial plane: mid anal canal (MAC). **b** Midsagittal plane: cavity size is 1.6 cm × 0.5 cm (*lines*), involving the lower anal canal and MAC. *IAS* internal anal sphincter, *EAS* external anal sphincter, *PR* puborectalis muscle

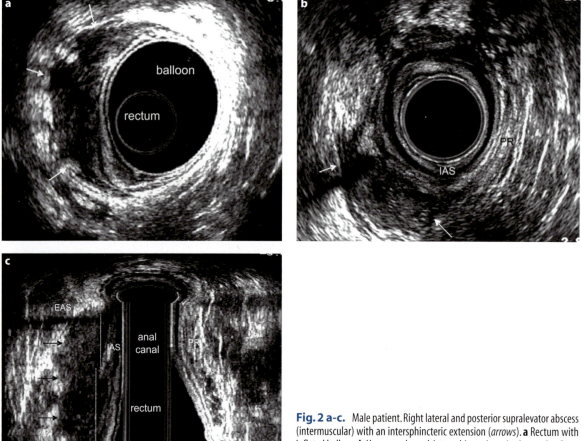

Fig. 2 a-c. Male patient. Right lateral and posterior supralevator abscess (intermuscular) with an intersphincteric extension (*arrows*). **a** Rectum with inflated balloon. **b** Upper anal canal: intersphincteric cavity (*arrows*). **c** Coronal plane: abscess cavity involving the lower rectum as far as the median anal canal (*arrows, lines*). *IAS* internal anal sphincter, *EAS* external anal sphincter, *PR* puborectalis muscle

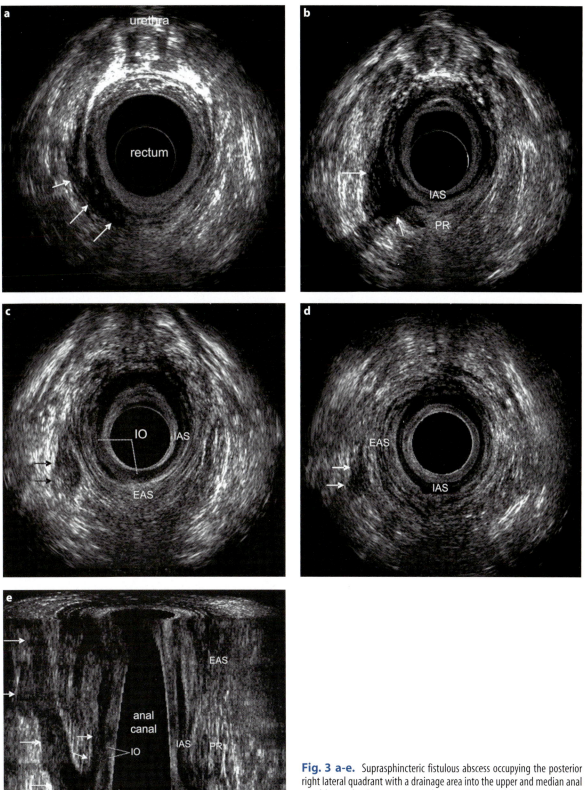

Fig. 3 a-e. Suprasphincteric fistulous abscess occupying the posterior right lateral quadrant with a drainage area into the upper and median anal canal (*arrows*). **a** Lower rectum: submucosa is involved. **b** Upper anal canal: intersphincteric cavity (*arrows*). **c** Mid anal canal (MAC): break in the internal anal sphincter (*IAS*) between 6 and 7 o'clock (*lines*), corresponding to the site of the internal opening (*IO*), which is located 3.0 cm from the anal margin. **d** MAC: tract is located outside the striated muscles (*arrows*). **e** Coronal with diagonal plane. *EAS* external anal sphincter, *PR* puborectalis muscle

quently preventing recurrence and fecal incontinence. In fact, it has been shown that recurrence is often due to failure to identify secondary tracts (20–30%) and internal openings (32–53%) [1, 2]. The more complex fistulas may be difficult to visualize when scanning is limited to the axial plane. However, the three-dimensional scanning mode allows accurate viewing and classification of the entire extent of the fistulous tract and its relation to the sphincter muscles, the exact position of the internal opening in relation to the anal margin, and any secondary tracts and/or cavities (Fig. 4). When associated with the diagonal plane, the fistulous tract may be examined at different depths. In addition, this type of transducer employs frequencies up to 16 MHz and a focal distance up to 6.2 cm and makes it possible to review the acquired images in real time.

If the external opening is patent, hydrogen peroxide (H_2O_2) should be applied through a fine polyethylene catheter to confirm findings and identify any previously ignored secondary tracts, specially in the presence of associated fibrosis. The scan is performed in two steps by administering 0.1–3.0 ml of 10.0% H_2O_2 at normal pressure (first step) and heightened pressure (second step). Fistulous tracts typically appear as hypoechoic areas, but echogenicity increases as a result of bubble formation due to the contact between H_2O_2 and tissue [3] (Fig. 5). The contrast should be carefully titered to prevent bubble formation inside the anal canal and rectum that might impair sound propagation and adequate visualization or induce acoustic shadowing deep beyond the enhanced image, thereby losing all the information acquired. Santoro and Fortling [4] used H_2O_2 and volume-rendered three-dimensional imaging adjusted to low brightness and high contrast, thus making it easier to follow fistulous tracts into semitransparent dark cavities.

The internal fistulous opening appears on the image as a rupture in the internal anal sphincter (IAS) (in the absence of previous sphincterotomy) and subepithelium tissue. When the use of H_2O_2 is precluded, a hypoechoic patch is visualized continuous with the fistulous tract (Fig. 4). When, however, H_2O_2 is applied, a hyperechoic area is clearly observed in the subepithelium crossing the IAS toward the endoprobe (Fig. 5b, d, e).

Based on the classification proposed by Parks [5], anorectal fistulas appear with the following ultrasound features:
1. *Intersphincteric*. The fistulous tract is located in the intersphincteric space, with the distal part between the external anal sphincter (EAS) and the subepithelial surface (Fig. 5). Secondary tracts, tract extent, and adjacent cavities may be identified, and tracts may be defined as straight, curved, or horseshoe shaped (Fig. 6).
2. *Transsphincteric*. The tract crosses the EAS and IAS (Fig. 7). According to the point at which the tract crosses the EAS, fistulas may be classified as high, medium, or low.
3. *Extrasphincteric*. The tract is located in the ischiorectal fossa (lateral to the sphincter muscles), whereas the internal opening is in the rectum, corresponding to an area of lost uniformity in the rectal layers. It is best seen with the transducer in rectal mode, distending the rectal wall (Fig. 8).
4. *Suprasphincteric*. The internal fistulous opening may be seen associated with the intersphincteric tract extending toward the rectum and crossing over the puborectalis muscle distally, lateral to the sphincter muscles, through the ischiorectal fossa. The most distal part of the rectum should also be evaluated to rule out involvement of rectal wall layers (Fig. 9).

The percentage of sphincter muscle to be sectioned during surgery must be previously determined. To calculate this percentage, the total length of the compromised sphincter is measured, as is the distance from the distal part of each muscle to the point where it is crossed by the fistulous tract. These measurements are used in surgical planning and help prevent fecal incontinence (Fig. 10).

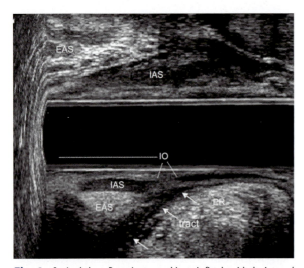

Fig. 4. Sagittal plane. Posterior transsphincteric fistula with the internal opening (*IO*) located 2.8 cm from the anal margin (*lines*) (without hydrogen peroxide). *EAS*, external anal sphincter; *IAS*, internal anal sphincter; *PR*, puborectalis muscle

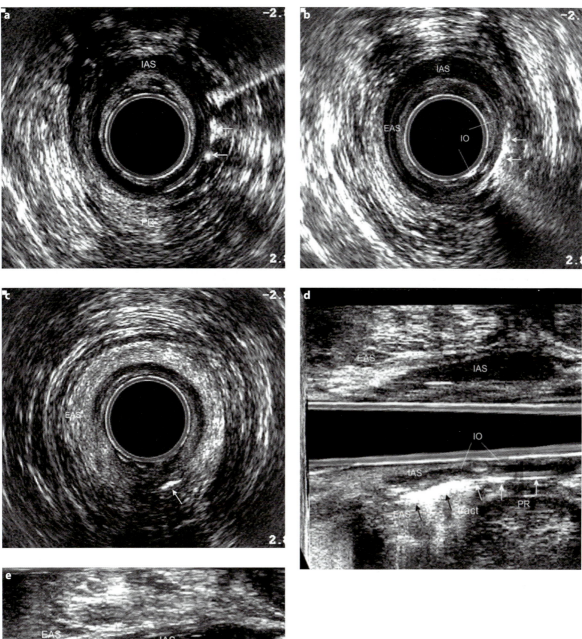

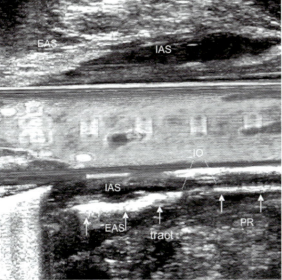

Fig. 5 a-e. Male patient with hydrogen peroxide injection. Posterior and left lateral intersphincteric (*arrows*) fistula located between 3 and 5 o'clock, with a secondary tract proximal to the internal opening (*IO*). **a** Upper anal canal: secondary tract proximal to the IO (*arrows*). **b** Mid anal canal: fistulous tract (*arrows*) and IO between 3 and 5 o'clock. **c** Lower anal canal: fistulous tract (*arrows*). **d** Intersphincteric tract with a secondary extension proximal (*arrows*) to the IO, located 2.5 cm from the anal margin. **e** Volume rendered mode. *EAS* external anal sphincter, *IAS* internal anal sphincter, *PR* puborectalis muscle

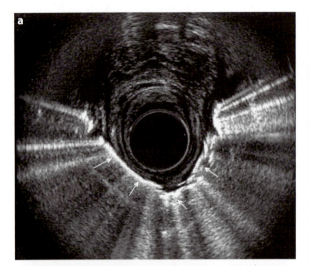

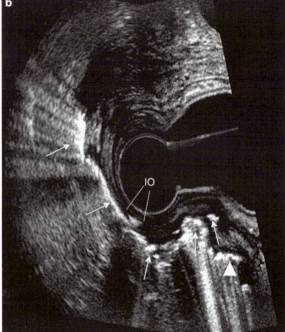

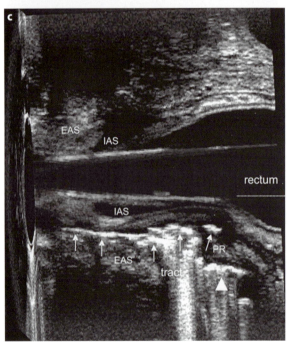

Fig. 6 a-c. Female patient with hydrogen peroxide injection. Horseshoe intersphincteric fistula located at 7 o'clock, with two secondary tracts beyond (proximal to) the internal opening (*IO*) (*arrows*). **a** Upper anal canal: horseshoe tract (*arrows*). **b** Sagittal with diagonal planes: primary horseshoe intersphincteric tract (*white arrows*) with proximal secondary inter- and transsphincteric tract (*white arrowhead*); IO at 7 o'clock. **c** Sagittal with diagonal planes: intersphincteric tract with a proximal secondary intersphincteric tract (*white arrows*) associated with a high secondary transsphincteric tract (*white arrowheads*). *EAS* external anal sphincter, *IAS* internal anal sphincter, *PR* puborectalis muscle

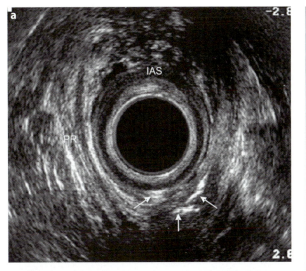

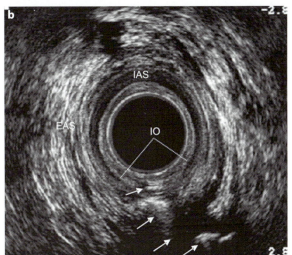

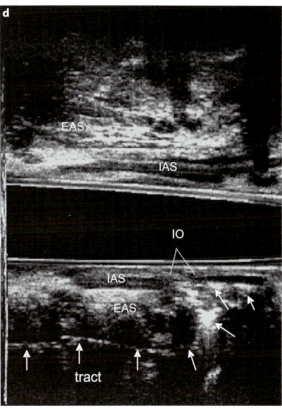

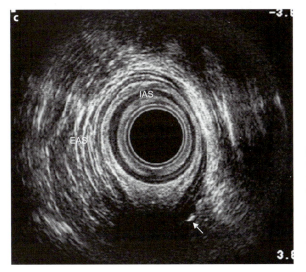

Fig. 7 a-d. Male patient with hydrogen peroxide injection. Posterior transsphincteric fistula between 5 and 7 o'clock, with a secondary tract beyond (proximal to) the internal opening (IO). **a** Upper anal canal: secondary tract beyond (proximal to) the IO (*arrows*). **b** Mid anal canal: tract (*arrows*) and IO are located between 5 and 7 o'clock. **c** Lower anal canal: transsphincteric tract (*arrows*). **d** Transsphincteric tract with a secondary intersphincteric tract (*arrows*) beyond (proximal to) the IO, which is located 3.1 cm from the anal margin. *EAS* external anal sphincter, *IAS* internal anal sphincter, *PR* puborectalis muscle

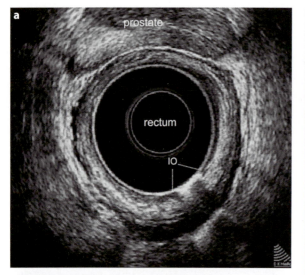

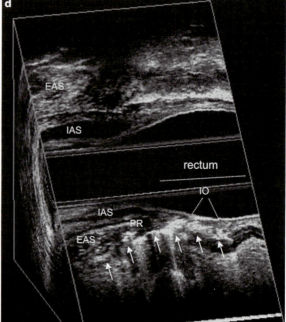

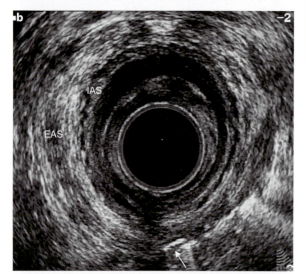

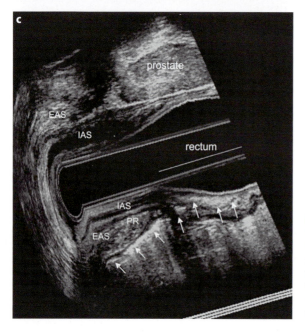

Fig. 8 a-d. Male patient with hydrogen peroxide injection. Posterior and left lateral extrasphincteric fistula. **a** Lower rectum: internal opening (*IO*) is located at 5 o'clock. **b** Mid anal canal: tract extends through the ischioanal space (*white arrow*). **c, d** Coronal with diagonal planes: tract is located in the ischioanal space, extending from the perianal skin to the rectum lumen, without anal canal involvement (*white arrows*); IO is located in the lower rectum. *EAS* external anal sphincter, *IAS* internal anal sphincter, *PR* pub-orectalis muscle

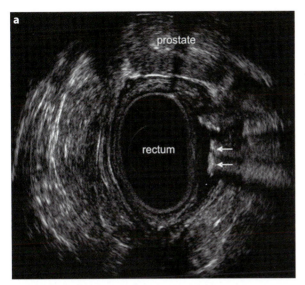

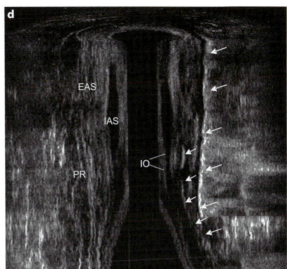

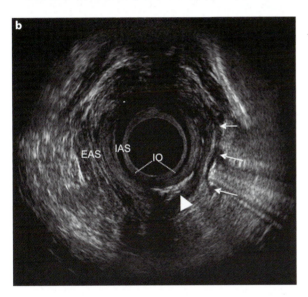

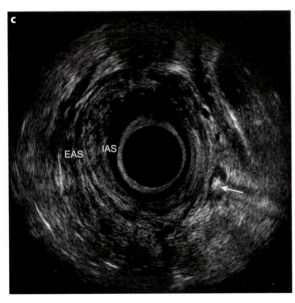

Fig. 9 a-d. Male patient with hydrogen peroxide injection. Posterior and left lateral suprasphincteric fistula. **a** Lower rectum: tract is located above the puborectalis muscle (suprasphincteric fistula) (*arrows*). **b** Mid anal canal: tract extends through the ischioanal fossa (*arrows*) and through the intersphincteric space (*arrowhead*); internal opening (*IO*) is located between 6 and 7 o'clock. **c** Lower anal canal: fistulous tract is visualized in the ischioanal space (*arrow*). **d** Coronal with diagonal planes: tract (*arrows*) and IO are simultaneously visualized. *EAS* external anal sphincter, *IAS* internal anal sphincter, *PR* puborectalis muscle

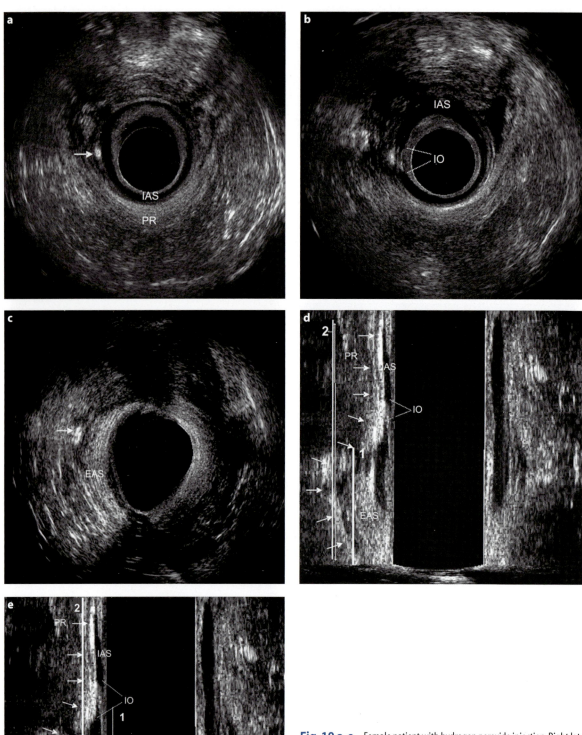

Fig. 10 a-e. Female patient with hydrogen peroxide injection. Right lateral transsphincteric fistula located at 3 o'clock, with a secondary tract beyond (proximal to) the internal opening (*IO*) (*arrows*). **a** Upper anal canal (UAC): intersphincteric secondary tract (*arrow*) beyond (proximal to) the IO. **b** UAC and mid anal canal: fistulous tract and IO are visualized at 3 o'clock (*lines*). **c** Lower anal canal: transsphincteric fistulous tract (*arrow*). **d** Length between the point where the muscle is crossed by the fistulous tract (*arrows*) and the distal border of the external anal sphincter (*EAS*) (anal margin) (*1*). Striated muscle length [EAS – puborectalis (*PR*) muscle] (*2*). **e** Length between the IO and the distal border of the internal anal sphincter (*IAS*) (*1*). Smooth muscle length (*IAS*) (*2*)

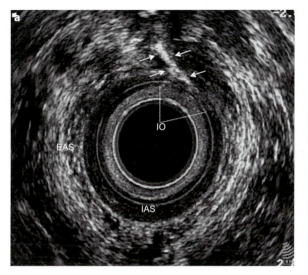

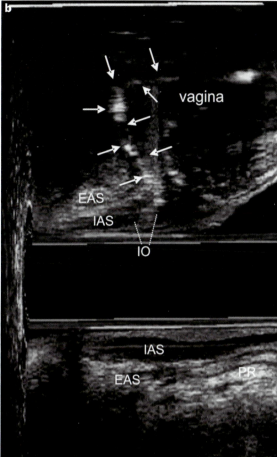

Fig. 11 a, b. Anovaginal fistula, hydrogen peroxide injection. Tract extends through the internal anal sphincter (*IAS*) and external anal sphincter (*EAS*) (*arrows*), with an opening into the vagina. *IO* internal opening

Anorectal-Vaginal Fistula

Ultrasound can show the fistulous tract and its relation to the anal canal or rectum and helps evaluate the anatomic integrity of the sphincter muscles for improved surgical planning and preventing recurrence and fecal incontinence [6, 7].

Identifying the opening in the vagina and the injection of H_2O_2 help visualization of the tract, especially at the point where it crosses the perineal body and in cases of associated fibrosis (Fig. 11). The transducer may subsequently be introduced into the vagina to confirm or expand findings.

References

1. Seow-Choen, Phillips RKS (1991) Insights gained from the management of problematic anal fistulae at St. Mark's Hospital, 1984–1988. Br J Surg 78:539–541
2. Sangwan YP, Ronsen L, Riether RD et al (1994) Is simple fistula in ano simple? Dis Colon Rectum 37:885–889
3. Lunniss PJ, Barker PG, Sultan AH et al (1994) Magnetic resonance imaging of fistula in ano. Dis Colon Rectum 37:708–718
4. Santoro GA, Fortling B (2007) The advantages of volume rendering in three-dimensional endosonography of the anorectum. Dis Colon Rectum 50(3):359–368
5. Parks AG, Gordon PH, Hardcastle JD (1976) A classification of fistula-in-ano. Br J Surg 63:1-12
6. Sudol-Szopinska I, Jakubowski W, Szczepkowski M (2002) Contrast-enhanced endosonography for the diagnosis of anal and ano-vaginal fistulas. J Clin Ultrasound 30(3):145–150
7. Stocker J, Rociu E, Schouten WR, Lameris JS (2002) Anovaginal and rectovaginal fistulas: endoluminal sonography versus endoluminal MR imaging. AJR AM J Roentgenol 178(3):737–741

CHAPTER 9

Computed Tomography and Magnetic Resonance Imaging in Abscess and Anal Fistula

Adrian E. Ortega, Hector Lugo-Colon, Alberto Diaz-Carranza, Howard S. Kaufman

Abstract

Cryptoglandular infection represents one of the oldest known surgically treated conditions and to this day continues to bewilder even the most experienced colorectal surgeons. Computed tomography (CT) and magnetic resonance imaging (MRI) are both valuable modalities with which to evaluate acute anorectal infections; however, they both have advantages and disadvantages in this setting. For example, CT scanning is readily available 24 hours a day in most major hospitals, and whereas it is perhaps most valuable when excluding ongoing concomitant infections, it has a very limited role in evaluating anal fistula. MRI is more effective than CT in evaluating soft-tissue structures, and the different MRI techniques now available, such as body-coil MRI, phased-array MRI, high-resolution MR fistulography, and subtraction fistulography, increases MRI utility for evaluating recurrent and complex anal fistulas. In fact, the current state of the art suggests that MRI is the gold standard for imaging such condition in most centers throughout the world.

Introduction

Cryptoglandular disease has a natural history consisting of acute and chronic phases. The acute stage is represented by perirectal abscess in its five anatomic presentations. The chronic phase manifests as fistula in ano in its five anatomic trajectories (Fig. 1). Historically, physicians have relied primarily on physical diagnosis to predict the anatomic location of the disease process. Surgeons have been content with this approach because the same empiric approach holds that the majority of cryptoglandular diseases results in simple infralevator infections. Moreover, the chronic phase of the disease develops in only 25–50% of individuals with an antecedent anorectal infection. This mindset needs to be increasingly questioned in light of the increased information obtainable from adjunctive imaging. Table 1 lists the frequency of anorectal infections according to anatomic location/trajectory [1].

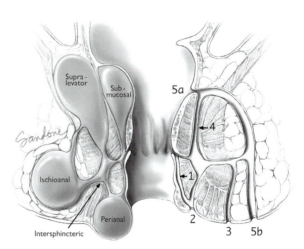

Fig. 1. Obstruction of a cryptoglandular process can result in five types of infections: perianal, ischioanal (ischiorectal), intersphincteric, supralevator, and submucosal. An intersphincteric abscess may lie completely isolated between the internal and external sphincters or extend above and below the sphincter complex. Similarly, a submucosal abscess may present either beneath the rectal mucosa or as a perianal abscess. Progression to a chronic phase may result in one of five types of anal fistula: *1* superficial, *2* intersphincteric, *3* transsphincteric, *4* supralevator, and extrasphincteric *5a* with or *5b* without an infralevator transsphincteric component. Abdomino-pelvic infections may reach extrapelvic sites by either extra- or intersphincteric routes

M. Pescatori, F.S.P. Regadas, S.M. Murad Regadas, A.P. Zbar (eds.), *Imaging Atlas of the Pelvic Floor and Anorectal Diseases*. ISBN 978-88-470-0808-3. © Springer-Verlag Italia 2008

Table 1. Incidence of various types of anorectal infections. From [1]

Type of Abscess	n = 1,023	Percent
Perianal	437	34.6
Ischiorectal	233	22.8
Intersphincter	219	21.4
Supralevator	75	7.3
Submucosal	59	5.8

One third of anorectal infections are simple and located at the anal margin, i.e., perianal abscesses. The unilateral ischioanal (ischiorectal) abscess may be dealt with in a straightforward manner. However, unilateral or bilateral ischioanal abscesses may result from an obstructed posterior midline cryptoglandular complex producing a posterior infection in at least one of four spaces: (1) the superficial postanal space, (2) the deep postanal space, (3) the supralevator space above the insertions of the pubococcygeus and iliococcygeus muscles onto the lateral sides of the coccyx, and (4) from an abdominopelvic etiology coursing through the presacral (retrorectal) space (Fig. 2) [2].

Four types of anorectal infections may extend above the surgical canal, i.e., above the sphincter mechanism. The top of the anal sphincter complex

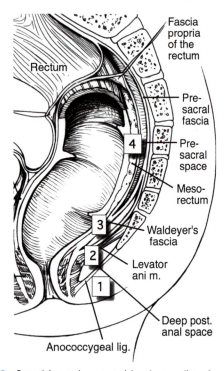

Fig. 2. Potential posterior spaces giving rise to unilateral or bilateral ischioanal infections: *1* superficial postanal space, *2* deep postanal space, *3* supralevator space, *4* presacral space. Modified from [2], with permission from Elsevier

posterolaterally is represented by the distal/cephalad edge of the puborectalis (PR) muscle. Clinically, they are detectable as a bulge or extramucosal pseudotumor above the puborectalis muscle on digital rectal examination. Infections coursing above the levator complex will produce a mass effect in the rectum. They may arise from a (1) submucosal, (2) intersphincteric, or (3) extrasphincteric route of infection. The fourth manifestation of a supralevator abscess occurs when an abdominopelvic infection breaks through retrorectal (presacral) planes reaching one or both ischioanal spaces. Infections above the levator diaphragm may extend though the medial border of the ischial spine bordered by the fascia of the obturator internus muscle through the potential foramen known as Alcock's canal. This region is also the space where intrapelvic pudendal nerves, arteries, and veins become extrapelvic on their way to supply the external sphincter, puborectalis muscle, and other perineal structures.

Acute anorectal infection presents surgeons with anatomic challenges surpassed only by the potential variations present in the management of chronic anal fistula. Sir Allan Parks provided surgeons with the most comprehensive landmark description and classification of anal fistula [3]. Practicing surgeons may find variations not described by Parks. The distribution of anal fistula according to the Parks classification is presented in Table 2 [4].

The Parks classification of anal fistula was truly remarkable because it demonstrated a significant prevalence of complex fistula. However, the compelling question that remains is: "Why does the average, well-trained, conscientious, surgeon not see the type of pathology seen by a master of proctologic surgery"? Specialized centers see a concentration of advanced disease, creating a significant selection bias. This argument lies beside the aphorism that "surgeons only see what they know, and all else goes unrecognized". Whereas Goodsall's rule remains a cornerstone in the clinical evaluation of anal fistula, it proves disappointingly inadequate in predicting the course of anal fistula. The preponderance of the evidence suggests that Goodsall's rule is highly predictive when surgeons en-

Table 2. Park's classification of anal fistula

Type	Percent
Superficial	16
Intersphincteric	56
Transsphincteric	21
Supralevator	4
Extrasphincteric	3
	100%

counter posterior hemispheric external openings. The majority of these trajectories will communicate with a curvilinear primary opening in the posterior midline (>90%). External openings found in the anterior hemisphere of the anal margin follow a direct radial course in only 50% of cases. The overall accuracy of Goodsall's rule is slightly better in men than women [5] and is far from being the gold standard in the twenty-first century. Proper identification of the fistulous tract remains a challenge. Injection techniques are also limited to an 80% accuracy rate. However, digital palpation for the primary crypt at the intersphincteric groove may be as accurate as 95% in experienced hands [6]. What remains completely unknown is the prevalence of accessory cephalad fistulous trajectories and/or collections extending away from the primary tract between internal and external opening. For example, an apparently simple, low intersphincteric fistula may have a cephalad intersphincteric component not recognized by the surgeon. The clinical significance of such a finding is also unknown. A more poignant example occurs when a unilateral transsphincteric tract is expertly treated only to have the patient return with contralateral disease. Current surgical practice often requires a more advanced diagnostic armamentarium.

Clinical Evaluation

History and physical examination are important tools in evaluating perirectal infection. Conceptually, it is useful to divide perirectal infections into simple and complex categories. Perianal and unilateral ischioanal infections are simple abscesses. Horseshoe abscesses should be considered complex because they occupy a minimum of three anatomic spaces: right and left ischioanal, and at least one posterior postanal, supralevator, or presacral space. Infections tracking through and/or above the sphincters as well as those originating in the abdomen or pelvis are, by definition, complex.

Patients with perianal infections tend to report acute, rapid-onset, and intense sustained pain at the anal margin. Their pain is usually unrelated to bowel movements. Swelling, erythema, and tenderness are characteristic and easily recognizable on physical examination. Infections in the ischioanal fossa can be much more subtle. Patients present after several days of vague pain that only in its latest stages reaches severe acuteness. Skin changes may be totally absent in the early stages. Bidigital examination is required to detect these infections. The examiner needs to palpate the anal canal and the ischioanal fossa simultaneously with his or her index finger on the inside and thumb on the outside. Fullness in the ischioanal fossa con-

firms the diagnosis. In its late states, ischioanal infections may be associated with a large mass effect, swelling, erythema, edema, tenderness, skin breakdown, and/or drainage of frank pus.

Pain on defection suggests a submucosal or intersphincteric process extending above the sphincter complex. Fullness in the rectum is a critical finding suggesting a supralevator abscess, which may course via a submucosal, intersphincteric, or extrasphincteric route. An extrasphincteric supralevator abscess is usually associated with fullness projecting into the rectum and in one or both ischioanal fossae. The diagnosis of an abdominopelvic origin should be considered when patients report antecedent abdominal, pelvic, or back pain, which may be associated with tenesmus. Purulence within the rectum suggests a supralevator abscess achieving partial drainage into the rectum. Imaging can be useful in the presence of horseshoe abscesses. An infected posterior midline gland may decompress into one of four posterior spaces: (1) superficial postanal space anterior to the anococcygeal ligament, (2) the deep postanal space above the anococcygeal ligament, (3) the supralevator space bordered by insertions of the pubococcygeus and ileococcygeus muscles on to the lateral aspects of the coccyx, and (4) the presacral space above the confluence of the presacral fascia and the fascia propria of the rectum. Suppurative processes in either the superficial or deep postanal spaces can extend directly to both ischioanal fossae. Processes above the levators can pass through either the right or left Alcock canal to reach the ischioanal fossae. Adjunctive imaging of horseshoe abscesses can guide the surgeon to the correct posterior space. For example, a horseshoe abscess originating in the superficial postanal space should not require division of the superficial component of the external sphincter and/or the anococcygeal ligament.

Adjunctive imaging with either computed tomography (CT) or magnetic resonance imaging (MRI) should be considered when a supralevator or abdominopelvic abscess is suspected. Fullness in the rectum or purulent discharge within the rectum are also indications for additional diagnostic imaging. CT and MRI should also be considered in patients with histories of Crohn's disease, rectal cancer undergoing radiation, diverticulitis, tuboovarian abscess, and/or patients with abdominal, pelvic, or back pain (Table 3). Occasionally, patients previously undergoing incision and drainage of a perirectal abscess re-present for medical attention due to persistence of symptoms. In this setting, imaging is useful in excluding an undrained collection and/or distinguishing it from the subtherapeutic treatment of an infection commonly seen in diabetic patients. Immuno-

Table 3. Indications for adjunctive imaging in anorectal infection

- Suspicion of supralevator extension
  - Rectal fullness
  - Soft, extraluminal pseudotumor
  - Transrectal purulent drainage
  - Tenesmus
- Suspicion of abdominopelvic source
  - Lower abdominal/pelvic/back pain
- Horseshoe abscess with rectal pain, tenderness, or fullness
- Unilateral ischioanal abscess with rectal fullness, pain, or tenderness
- Recurrent abscess
- Comorbid conditions
  - Crohn's disease
  - Anal or rectal malignancy with concurrent radiation
  - Turbo ovarian abscess
  - Diverticulitis
  - Rectovaginal fistula with or without previous radiation
  - Persistent symptoms following incision and drainage of an abscess
  - Neutropenia
  - Urinary Retention

compromised patients often require prolonged treatment of the associated cellulitis in addition to incision and drainage. Finally, anorectal infections in neutropenic patients can be difficult to evaluate clinically. They tend to present with minimal physical signs and commonly have minimal purulence. CT and MRI can be useful in this setting to locate the presence and extent of cryptoglandular infection. The finding of fat stranding and/or gas in the tissues confirms the diagnosis and should direct treatment.

CT versus MRI in Acute Anorectal Infections and their Sequelae

Both CT scanning and MRI are useful in evaluating acute anorectal infections. CT scanning has three principal advantages over MRI: (1) it is relatively ubiquitous in most major hospitals, (2) surgeons are more accustomed to the axial views of the pelvis than viewing this region in axial, coronal, and sagittal views, and (3) CT is more likely to be available on a 24-h basis in most centers. MRI is far better suited than CT scan to distinguish soft-tissue structures, so anatomic detail is greater with MRI. A variety of signals are used in MRI, including T1- and T2-weighted images and fat-saturation techniques. MRI interpretation has an associated learning curve, which is optimally mastered with good communication between radiologists and surgeons. Both modalities are useful in evaluating acute cryptoglandular infection.

CT scans have a very limited role in evaluating anal fistula. It is most useful to exclude ongoing concomitant infections. Fistulography is of limited value

and is mentioned only for historical reasons. Its main limitation and utility is the interest of the examiner. The absence of a three-dimensional perspective also limits its role. Finally, fistulous tracts are often fibrotic. Injection techniques may fail to elucidate the entire tract because of insufficient pressure head on contrast infusion. Two-dimensional ultrasonography is similarly limited by its lack of spatial orientation. Three-dimensional ultrasonography has significant advantages but is also associated with a significant learning curve. The current state of the art suggests that MRI is the gold standard for imaging anal fistula in the majority of centers throughout the world. In an outcome-based reference standard study, Buchanan et al. compared physical diagnosis, ultrasound, and MRI in 104 patients. The overall accuracy of these modalities was 61%, 81%, and 90%, respectively [7].

A variety of techniques may be employed in MRI. Body-coil MRI is the most standard and readily available. Phased-array MRI may provide more detailed and accurate information compared with body-coil MRI. High-resolution MR fistulography or subtraction fistulography is another technique under evaluation in some centers. The superiority of any one MRI technique remains to be seen. Little information is available on the cost-effectiveness of liberal application of MRI technology to primary anal fistula. However, there seems little doubt about the utility of MRI in evaluating recurrent and complex fistulas. In the largest study of consecutive patients with recurrent anal fistula, Buchanan et al. examined 71 patients with MRI. The findings were revealed to the surgeons perioperatively. The surgeon was free to act on the imaging findings at his or her discretion. The authors found a postoperative relapse rate of 16% for patients treated by surgeons who always re-explored if MRI findings suggested missed disease. The recurrence rate was 57% for surgeons who always ignored imaging, believing their clinical assessment to be superior. The authors concluded that preoperative MRI in patients with complex recurrent disease could reduce recidivism by approximately 75% [8].

Impressions on the State of the Art

CT and MRI have significant utility in evaluating complex anorectal infections. Careful history and physical examination generally provide sound indications for adjunctive imaging in this setting. Horseshoe abscesses represent potentially complex anatomic infections. Their evaluation and treatment should not be relegated to the most junior member of the surgical service. The chronic phase of cryptoglandular infection represents one of the oldest known surgically treated conditions, which continues to perplex and confound even expert surgeons. MRI should be considered in the presence of inflammatory bowel disease and recurrent anal fistula. The utility of three-dimensional ultrasonography in expert hands vis-à-vis MRI is an important subject that requires careful study. However, given the wider availability of MRI compared with three-dimensional ultrasonography, MRI should be considered the gold standard study in evaluating complex/recurrent disease in most centers throughout the world (Figs. 1–13).

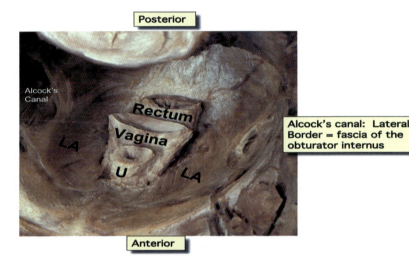

Fig. 3. Anorectal infections may reach the supralevator and/or retrorectal spaces via Alcock's canal. This extrapelvic foramen occurs at the lateral border of the obturator internus muscle and fascia. Similarly, extrapelvic infections in the ischioanal spaces may break through to supralevator and retro (presacral) sites via these bilateral virtual orifices. The pudendal nerves, arteries, and veins course through Alcock's canal on their way to supply the external sphincter, puborectalis muscle, and other perineal structures. *LA* levator ani, *U* urethra

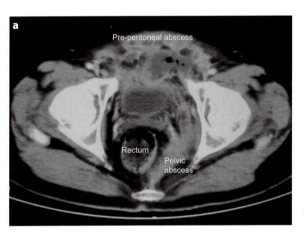

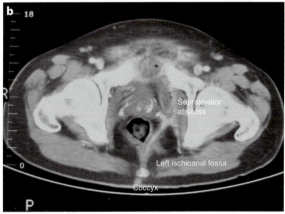

Fig. 4 a, b. Computed tomography of an infected urachal cyst coursing from the abdominal wall behind the rectum (**a**) to the left ischioanal fossa (**b**)

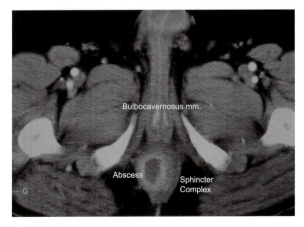

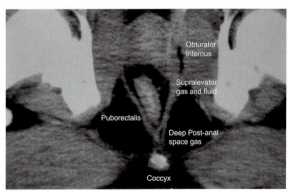

Fig. 6. Computed tomography of a supralevator abscess originating in the deep postanal space extending on the left medial to the obturator internus muscle

Fig. 5. Computed tomography of intersphincteric infralevator abscess

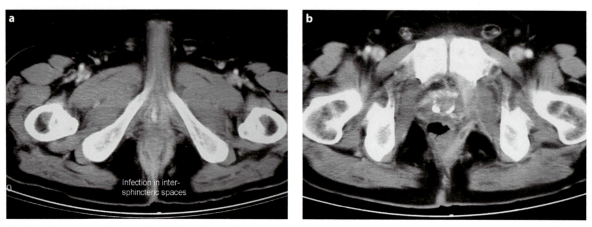

Fig. 7 a, b. Computed tomography of a bilateral intersphincteric abscess (**a**) extending into supralevator space (**b**)

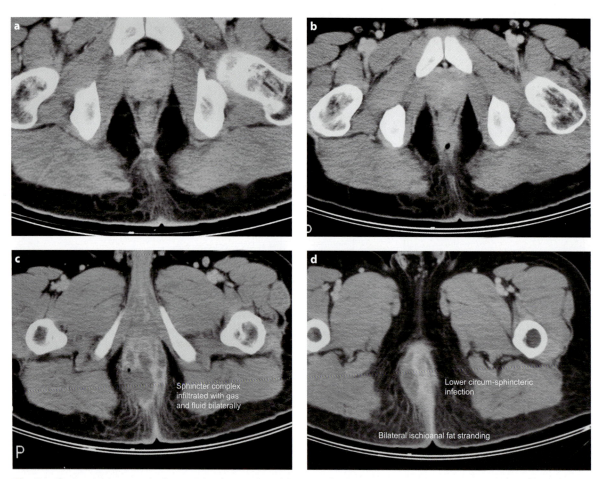

Fig. 8 a-d. Computed tomography demonstrating the normal tip of the coccyx showing the insertion of the pubococcygeus (**a**). Gas is present in the next lower cut within the superficial postanal space (**b**). There is extensive gas and fluid infiltration in the upper (**c**) and lower (**d**) sphincter complex as well as bilateral ischioanal fat stranding

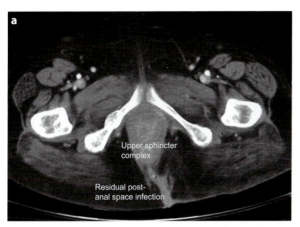
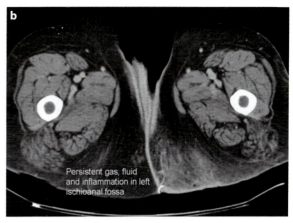

Fig. 9 a, b. Computed tomography in a subtherapeutically drained horseshoe abscess. The initial surgery drained only the bilateral ischioanal fossae. Persistent post-anal-space infection is present (**a**). There is also residual infection and gas in the left ischioanal fossa (**b**). This diabetic patient required re-exploration with drainage of the postanal and left ischioanal regions

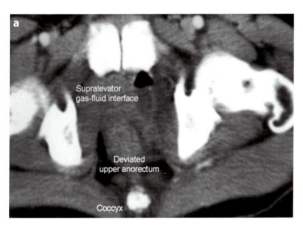
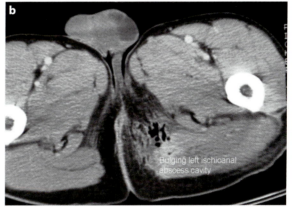

Fig. 10 a, b. Combined left supralevator (**a**) and ischioanal abscesses (**b**) in a Crohn's patient with a concomitant extrasphincteric fistula. The combination of both collections is highly suggestive of an extrasphincteric course. The examiner will palpate fullness within both the rectum and the affected ischioanal fossa

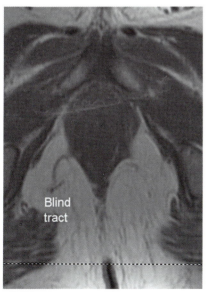

Fig. 11. Axial magnetic resonance image of a transsphincteric blind-ended fistula tract on the *right* in a patient with a history of recurrent fistulas

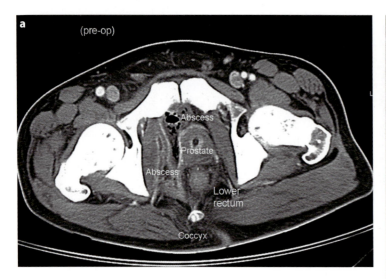

Fig. 12 a, b. Computed tomography in a patient with a supralevator abscess in the setting of an established combined high extrasphincteric and low transsphincteric fistula (**a**). The supral-evator abscess was drained with a catheter, whereas the lower transsphincteric fistula was treat-ed with a cutting seton. Postoperative magnetic resonance imaging with catheter in place (**b**)

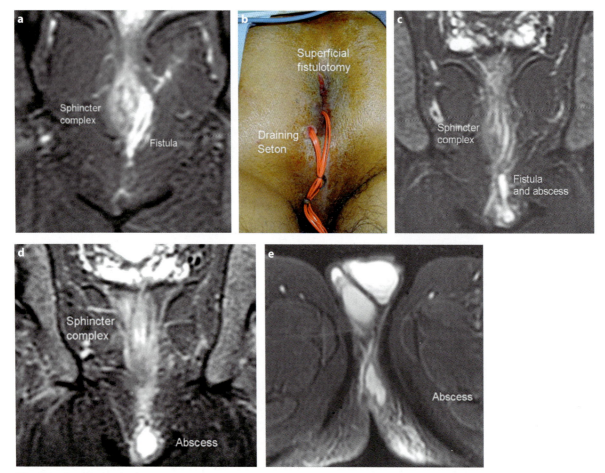

Fig. 13 a-h. (*Continued →*)

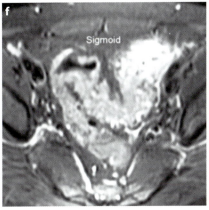 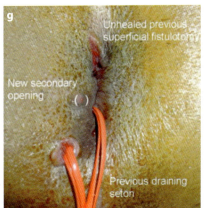 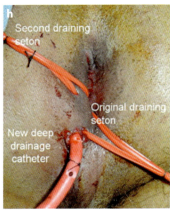

Fig. 13 a-h. Coronal magnetic resonance imaging (MRI) demonstrating a fistula in a patient with Crohn's disease (**a**). The patient is treated with a draining seton as well as a posterior midline superficial fistulotomy (**b**). The same patient presents with recurrent pain 2 months later: coronal MRI views demonstrating a persistent deeper fistula (**c**) and abscess cavity (**d**). Axial MRI views of the abscess cavity (**e**) and abdomen (**f**) demonstrating severe edema, luminal narrowing, and inflammation of the sigmoid colon. Re-examination of this patient reveals an unhealed posterior midline fistulotomy wound, a new secondary opening, and the original seton in place (**g**). He is treated with a second draining seton as well as a drainage catheter placed into the deeper abscess cavity (**h**)

References

1. Ramanujam PS, Prasad ML, Abcarian H et al (1984) Perianal abscesses and fistulas: a study of 1023 patients. Dis Colon Rectum 27:593–597
2. Kaiser AM, Ortega AE (2003) Anorectal anatomy. Surg Clin N Am 82(6):1125–1138
3. Parks AG, Gordon PH, Hardcastle JD (1976) A classification of fistula-in-ano. Br J Surg 63:1–12
4. Bartram C, Buchanan G (2003) Imaging in anal fistula. Radiol Clin N Am 31:443–457
5. Cirocco WC, Reilly JC (1992) Challenging the predictive accuracy of Goodall's rule for anal fistulas. Dis Colon Rectum 35:537–542
6. Gonzalez-Ruiz C, Kaiser AM, Vukasin P et al (2006) Intraoperative physical diagnosis in the management of anal fistula. Am Surg 72(1):11–15
7. Buchanan GN, Bartram CI, Williams AB et al (2004) Clinical examination, endosonography, and MR imaging in preoperative assessment of fistula in ano: comparison with outcome-based reference standard. Radiology 233(3):674–681
8. Buchanan G, Halligan S, Williams A et al (2002) Effect of MRI on clinical outcome of recurrent fistula-in-ano. Lancet 360:1661–1662

Commentary

Lusmar Veras Rodrigues

The authors describe the basic and conceptual aspects of anorectal fistulas and draw attention to the essential role of clinical history and physical examination in diagnosing the different presentations of the disease. It is clearly demonstrated that the disease evolves from an initial acute stage (abscess) to a chronic condition (fistula) and that acute-stage symptoms can provide information on the topography and, consequently, complexity of the inflammatory process. The authors also stress that Goodsall's rule has exceptions, especially when the external opening is located anteriorly, and that the rule is best applied to male patients. The fistulas are described in relation to the sphincter complex based on the Parks classification. Inflammatory processes are shown to be simple if occupying a single perianal quadrant, whereas suprasphincteric, pelvic, or abdominal processes or fistulas with multiple tracts involving two or more perianal quadrants are defined as complex.

The authors explain that routine CT scanning and MRI is indicated in complex rather than in simple inflammatory processes, as well as in cases of recurrent fistulas or abscesses, in immunodepressed patients and in patients with ill-defined symptoms. Finally, three-dimensional ultrasonography is shown to be a useful and accurate tool in the diagnosis of this disorder though requiring a long learning curve. The authors conclude by stressing that MRI is considered the gold standard at state-of-the-art clinics around the world for cases of recurrence and complex inflammatory processes.

Indeed, everyday clinical experience shows cryptogenic processes (abscesses and fistulas) to be simple in more than 80% of cases, whereas complex cases may require multiple surgical approaches and may be associated with high recurrence rates. We have worked with three-dimensional ultrasonography for 3 years and use it routinely as a preoperative procedure in patients of this type, attaining more than 90% accuracy in both the acute and chronic stages, though we do not use MRI with intrarectal coil, an examination comparable with three-dimensional ultrasonography. On the other hand, we indicate CT in acute cases when the patient's condition does not allow for proper ultrasound scanning or in pelvic and abdominal processes out of reach of the ultrasound scanner. With the aid of these complementary tools, in addition to clinical data and careful physical examination, complex cases have been referred to surgery less empirically and with more satisfactory results.

CHAPTER 10

Staging and Follow-up of Anal Canal Neoplasms with 2- and 3-D Ultrasonography

Sthela M. Murad Regadas, F. Sérgio P. Regadas

Abstract

Here we discuss the importance of the three-dimensional ultrasonography in evaluating malignant tumor of the anal canal as it allows quantifying the extent of tumor invasion into the sphincter muscles, adjacent tissues, and rectum, identifying lymph nodes as well. This modality is very useful in evaluating chemoradiotherapy response and selecting safe biopsy sites in case of suspicion of early recurrence.

Introduction

Malignant neoplasia of the anal region represents 1–2% of all cases of large-bowel cancer, corresponding to 0.6/100,000 inhabitants. The disease most commonly affects patients in their 50s and 60s. Tumors tend to be located in the anal canal in women (5:1) and on the anal margin in men (4:1) [1, 2]. Diagnosis requires detailed clinical examination, evaluation of the risk factors, proctological examination, and the histopathology finding. By digital rectal examination, the site, length, and circumference of tumor involvement may be determined, and attachment to adjacent structures may be appreciated subjectively. On the other hand, pretreatment anorectal ultrasound scanning, an important method for evaluating malignant tumors of the anal canal, allows quantification of the extent of tumor invasion into the sphincter muscles, adjacent tissues, and rectum and identification of compromised lymph nodes. This makes the examination the mainstay for evaluating response to chemo/radiotherapy [3, 4].

Ultrasonographic staging of neoplasms was first proposed by the *Union Internationale Contre le Cancer* (UICC) in 1987 and is based on criteria of tumor size and degree of invasion [5]:

uT1 – Tumor restricted to the mucous membrane
uT2 – Tumor compromising the internal anal sphincter (IAS)
uT3 – Tumor compromising the external anal sphincter (EAS)
uT4 – Tumor invading adjacent structures
N0 – Lymph nodes unaffected
N1 – Lymph nodes affected

Based on the satisfactory responses obtained in 94.5% of cases, it is now generally held that uT1- and uT2-type tumors smaller than 4.0 cm should be treated with radiotherapy alone. For uT2-type lesions larger than 4.0 cm and for uT3- and uT4-type lesions, treatment should include both radio- and chemotherapy [4, 5]. Other authors favor the TNM classification (modified in 1985), according to which tumors are staged based on the degree of invasion alone [6]:

uT1 – Tumor restricted to the submucosal layer
uT2a – Tumor compromising the IAS
uT2b – Tumor compromising the EAS
uT3 – Perianal tissue affected
uT4 – Adjacent structures affected
N0 – Lymph nodes unaffected
N1 – Lymph nodes affected

Imaging Characteristics

Echographically, tumor stages are characterized as follows:

uT1: A hypoechoic area in the subepithelial (mucosal-submucosal) tissue due to thickening, with the IAS preserved (Fig. 1)

M. Pescatori, F.S.P. Regadas, S.M. Murad Regadas, A.P. Zbar (eds.), *Imaging Atlas of the Pelvic Floor and Anorectal Diseases*. ISBN 978-88-470-0808-3. © Springer-Verlag Italia 2008

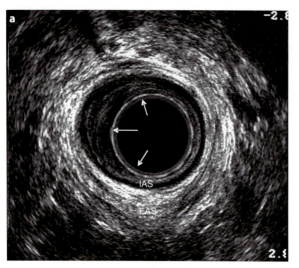 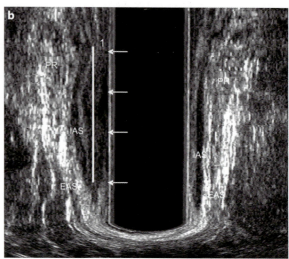

Fig. 1 a, b. Male patient. uT1 tumor occupying half the anal canal, located at the right lateral quadrant. The subepithelial (mucosa-submucosa) is thicker. The hypoechoic layer [internal anal sphincter (*IAS*)] is intact. **a** Axial plane: mid anal canal (*arrows*). **b** Coronal plane: lesion length is 4.2 cm, involving the upper and mid anal canal (*arrows*). *EAS* external anal sphincter

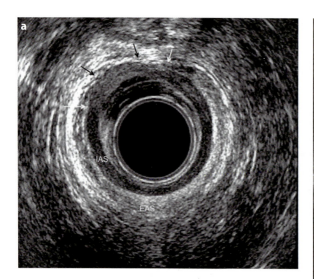 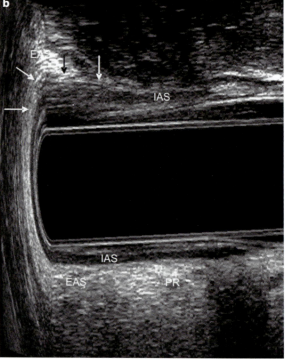

Fig. 2 a, b. Female patient. uT2b tumor located at the right lateral quadrant. Hypoechoic area covering the entire width of the internal anal sphincter (*IAS*) and partially the external anal sphincter (*EAS*). **a** Axial plane: mid anal canal (*arrows*). **b** Sagittal plane: lesion length is 1.7 cm (*1*) involving the middle anal canal (*arrows*). *PR* puborectalis muscle

uT2a: Invasion of the IAS evidenced by hypoechoic area representing disruption or thickening of the musculature

uT2b: Hypoechoic area covering the entire width of the IAS and affecting the EAS and puborectalis (PR) muscle (Figs. 2, and 3a-d)

uT3: Hypoechoic area covering the entire width of the sphincter muscles and affecting the perianal fat (Figs. 4 and 5)

uT4: Adjacent structures affected (Fig. 6a-e)

If the lower rectum has been affected, the examination should include scanning in the rectal mode

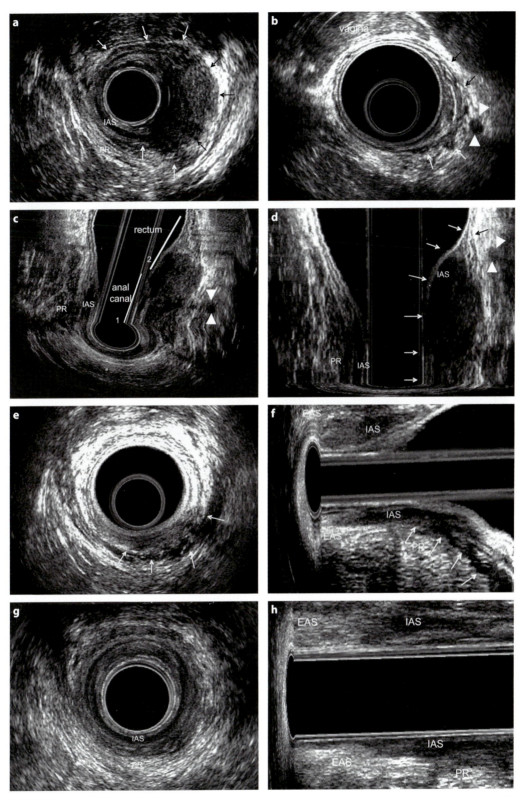

Fig. 3 a-h. Female patient. Upper anal canal. **a** Axial plane: preradiotherapy uT2bN1 tumor located at the left anterolateral quadrant invading the internal anal sphincter (*IAS*) and puborectalis (*PR*) muscle (*arrows*); vaginal wall is intact. **b** Axial plane: lesion extends to lower rectum (*arrows*); lymph node appears with echogenicity similar to the primary tumor, suggesting metastasis (*arrowheads*). **c, d** Coronal plane: lesion length is 5.2 cm (*1*) involving the upper anal canal and lower rectum (*2*) (*arrows*). There are two malignant lymph nodes in the perianal (**c**) and perirectal (**d**) fat (*arrowheads*). **e** Axial plane, **f** sagittal plane: 50 days after radiotherapy, showing slightly hypoechogenic area involving the *IAS* and *PR*, suggesting inflammation – fibrosis (*arrows*). **g** Axial plane, **h** sagittal plane: 80 days after radiotherapy, showing regression of the inflammatory process

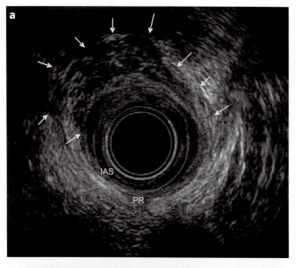

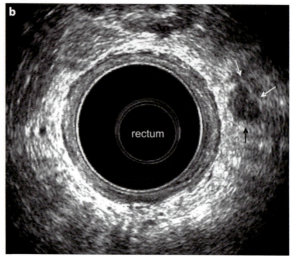

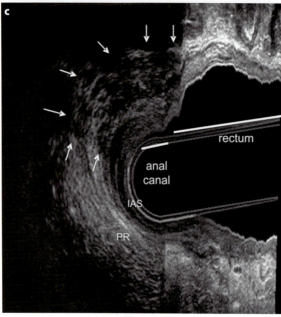

Fig. 4 a-c. Female patient. uT3N1 tumor located at the right anterolateral quadrant. Hypoechoic area covering the entire width of the sphincter muscles and affecting the perianal fat. Vaginal wall is intact. **a** Axial plane: upper anal canal; internal anal sphincter (*IAS*), puborectalis (*PR*) muscle, and perianal fat is invaded (*arrows*). **b** Axial plane: lymph node appears with an echogenicity similar to the primary tumor, suggesting metastasis located in the perirectal fat of the lower rectum (*arrows*). **c** Sagittal plane: tumor involves the upper anal canal, extending to the lower rectum (*arrows*)

with a balloon for an evaluation of the rectal-wall layers. The lymph nodes are located in the perianal or perirectal fat proximally or distally to the lesion. Thus, the more proximal the transducer is to the lesion, the greater the chances for a complete tumor evaluation. To distinguish between inflammation and metastasis, the following aspects need to be observed: 1) rounded lymph nodes with irregular borders and tumor-like (hypoechoic) echogenicity suggest the presence of metastasis (it should also be kept in mind that the larger the lymph node, the more likely it is to harbor a metastasis); 2) oval lymph nodes with regular borders and a central hyperechoic area (corresponding to the hilum) are suggestive of inflammation.

Postradio-/chemotherapy ultrasound scanning may be performed after 6-8 weeks and then periodically, depending on the case, until response to therapy has been established. During this period, the patient may also need to be submitted to proctological examinations. Radiotherapy-induced edema, inflammation, and fibrosis resolve completely after approximately 4 months [6]. Less invasive tumors may appear to have regressed completely upon first follow-up examination if the anatomical structures are clearly distinguishable at the former tumor location. However, reduced-size lesions, ill-defined and slightly hypoechoic areas may be observed as a result of the radio/chemotherapy effects (edema, inflammation, fibrosis) or even presence of residual tumor.

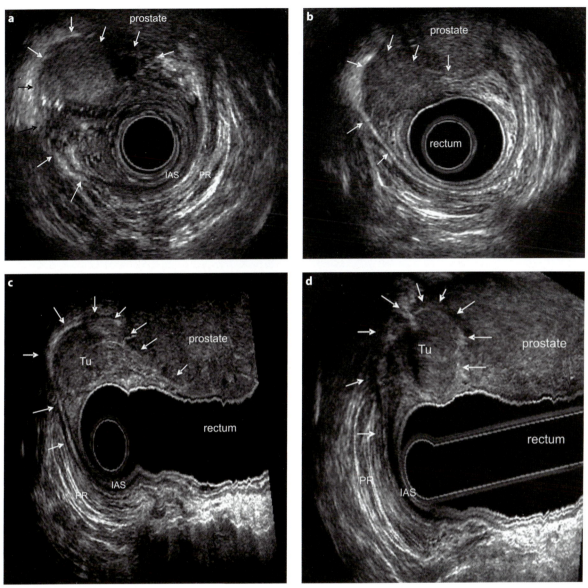

Fig. 5 a-d. Male patient: uT3 tumor located at the right anterolateral quadrant, invading the internal anal sphincter (*IAS*), puborectalis (*PR*) muscle, and perirectal fat but without involving the hypertrophic prostate (*arrows*). **a** Axial plane: upper anal canal; a cleavage plane is seen between prostate and the lesion (*hyperechoic line*). **b** Axial plane: hypertrophic prostate (*arrows*). **c, d** Sagittal with diagonal planes: tumor involves the upper anal canal and lower rectum (*arrows*). *Tu* tumor

However, the continuous size reduction of such images seen during subsequent exams, defining the anatomic structures and visualizing all rectal layers, represents complete tumor regression (Fig. 3).

The presence of residual tumor (incomplete response) is evidenced by the persistence of well-defined hypoechoic image or by its enlargement on the subsequent exams and/or in the absence of cleavage planes with affected adjacent structures (Fig. 6). When a residual tumor is suspected due to the persistence of a hypoechoic image from the first follow-up examination, an excisional biopsy should be per-

formed for definitive diagnosis. In this case, ultrasound scanning is helpful in selecting an appropriate biopsy site and preventing muscle injury (Fig. 6). Between the fourth and fifth months, patients experience complete regression of radiotherapy effects (edema and fibrosis). At this point, any change in the image may suggest recurrence. Periodic ultrasound scanning during follow-up can provide early diagnosis of subclinical neoplasms not observed on earlier examinations (Fig. 7).

When response to radio/chemotherapy is complete, follow-up examinations are performed every 6 months,

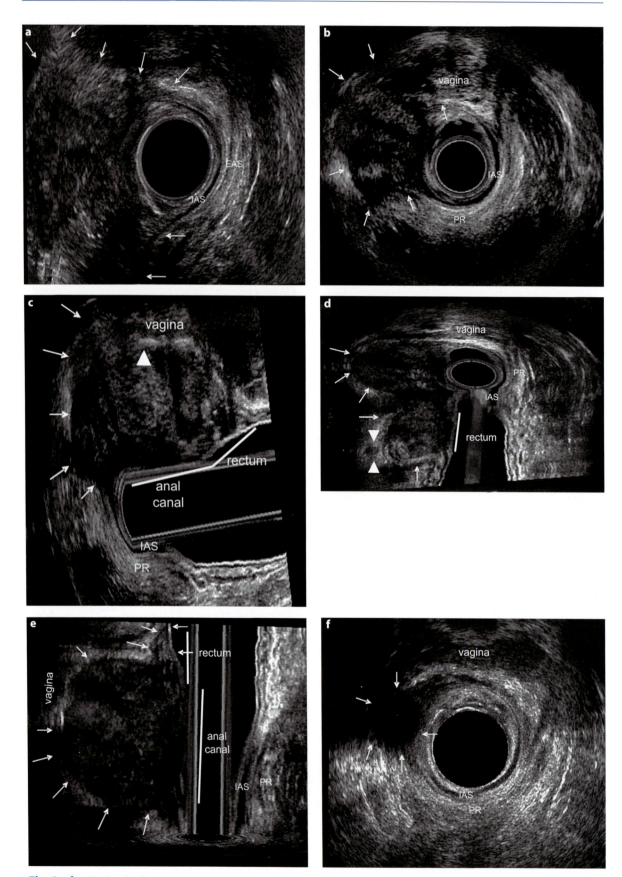

Fig. 6 a-h. (*Continued* →)

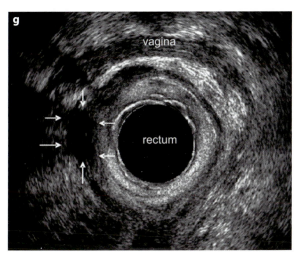
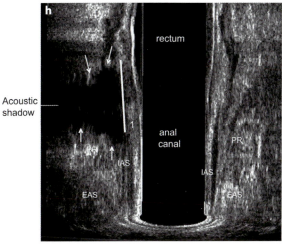

Fig. 6 a-h. Female patient. **a** Axial plane: mid anal canal; uT4N1 preradiotherapy located at the right anterolateral quadrant, invading the internal anal sphincter (*IAS*), external anal sphincter (*EAS*), and perianal fat (*arrows*). **b** Axial plane: upper anal canal; tumor invading the IAS, puborectalis (*PR*) muscle, perianal fat, and vagina wall (*arrows*). **c** Sagittal with diagonal planes: lesion extends to lower rectum, invading the outer hyperechoic layer (perirectal fat) (*arrows*) and vagina wall (*arrowhead*). **d** Coronal with diagonal planes: lymph node is located in the perirectal fat adjacent to the rectal lesion. It appears with the same tumor echogenicity (metastasis) (*arrowhead*). **e** Coronal with diagonal planes: lesion length is 5.4 cm, involving middle/upper anal canal and lower rectum (*arrows*). **f, g** Axial; and **h** coronal planes: 50 days after radiotherapy, showing hypogenic, well-defined area involving the IAS, PR, and rectal wall at the right lateral quadrant, suggesting residual tumor (*arrows*). Lesion length is 1.5 cm (*1*). Posterior acoustic shadow produced by inflammatory process. Excisional biopsy revealed residual tumor

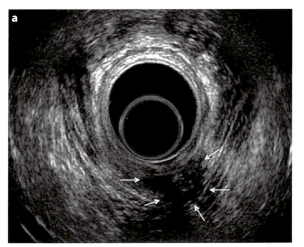
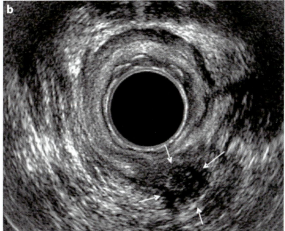

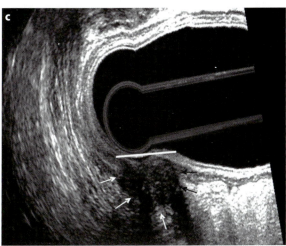

Fig. 7 a-c. Recurrence. Hypoechoic lesion located at the left posterolateral quadrant involving the internal anal sphincter (*IAS*), puborectalis (*PR*) muscles and extending to lower rectal wall. **a, b** Axial plane (*arrows*). **c** Sagittal plane: lesion length is 1.4 cm

or even more frequently, during the first 2 years, then annually until the fifth year. The most appropriate scanning modality is three-dimensional anorectal ultrasound because of the possibility of evaluation in multiple planes, accurate measurement of circumferential and longitudinal tumor extension, and real-time review in ambiguous cases. In a study comparing the two- and three-dimensional scanning modalities,

Christensen et al. [7] demonstrated the superiority of the latter in lesion staging due to the possibility of evaluation in multiple planes and in real time. Ultrasound scanning makes it possible to follow the evolution of neoplasms of the anal canal, choose a suitable treatment approach, establish response to treatment, confirm complete response, or select safe biopsy sites in case of suspicion of early recurrence.

References

1. Stearns MW Jr, Urmacher C, Sternberg SS et al (1980) Cancer of the anal canal. Curr Probl Cancer 4:1–44
2. Greenlee RT, Murray T, Bolden S, Wingo PA (2000) Cancer statistics. CA Cancer J Clin 50:7–33
3. Goldman S, Glimelius B, Norming U et al (1988) Transanorectal ultrasonography in anal carcinoma: a prospective study of 12 patients. Acta Radiol 29:337–341
4. Giovanini M, Bordou VJ, Bar Clay R et al (2001) Anal carcinoma: prognostic value of endorectal ultrasound. Results of a prospective multicenter study. Endoscopy 33(3)231–236
5. International Union Against Cancer (1997) Digestive system tumours. In: Sobin LH, Wittekind C (eds) TNM classification of malignant tumours. 5th edn. Wiley-Liss, New York, pp 51–59
6. Tarantino D, Bernstein MA (2002) Endoanal ultrasound in the staging and management of squamosus cell carcinoma of the anal canal: potential implications of a new ultrasound staging system. Dis Colon Rectum 45(1):16–22
7. Christensen AF, Nielsen MB, Engelholm SA et al (2004) Three-dimensional anal endosonography may improve staging os anal cancer compared with two-dimensional endosonography. Dis Colon Rectum 47:341–345

Commentary

Herand Abcarian

This chapter deals with classification of cancers of the anal canal and the value of two-dimensional and especially three-dimensional endoanal ultrasonography in staging and the follow-up of regression, complete response, or recurrence of the disease. Assessing the primary tumor or its evolution with radiation or chemoradiation therapy, by digital rectal examination, and by endoscopy is very subjective. Also, it is difficult to tell anal-wall infiltration, edema, or scarring secondary to treatment from tumor persistence or recurrence. In cases of recurrence deep in the wall of the anal canal, e.g., external sphincter, it would take weeks or months before any mucosal lesion arises suspicion that warrants biopsy. If persistence or recurrence is suspected, a needle biopsy is desirable, but if the lesion is not sampled accurately, a negative biopsy may mislead the treating physician and delay definitive therapy. With endoanal ultrasonography, evolution of the disease under treatment can be assessed in real time. If there is any doubt or suspicion, a needle biopsy can be obtained, with accuracy, from a deeper needle lesion, thus avoiding false negative biopsy or injuring the adjacent tissues.

CHAPTER 11

Staging and Follow-up of Anal Canal Neoplasm with Magnetic Resonance

Pedro C. Basilio, Alice Brandão, Rosilma Gorete Lima Barreto

Abstract

Anal cancer is a rare condition with several etiologic agents, including human papilloma virus (HPV) and other infectious agents. Oncogenes and carcinogens are also involved in anal cancer genesis. Among contributory factors are homosexuality with anal-receptive intercourse, immunosuppression, Crohn's disease, and chronic anorectal disease. Staging systems, treatment regimens, and particularly indications for magnetic resonance imaging, are outlined in this chapter along with depictions of primary anal cancer and lymphatic spread and images documenting clinical response to chemoradiation.

Introduction

Anal canal cancer is an uncommon neoplastic disease that accounts for only a small percentage (4%) of all cancers of the lower alimentary tract [1]. In the USA, 5,070 new cases are expected for the year 2008, corresponding to 680 deaths [2]. The incidence of anal cancer is rising, with statistical data suggesting that anal-receptive intercourse as part of routine sexual practice leads to a higher percentage of human papilloma virus (HPV) infection, accounting for an increased risk for squamous anal carcinoma in this patient population [2]. The histogenesis of anal cancer implicates the HPV virus as well as other infectious agents, including herpes simplex virus (HSV-2), HIV, chlamydia, and *Neisseria gonorrhoeae* [3]. Oncogenes and carcinogens are also involved, with commonly cited factors including homosexuality and anal-receptive intercourse, immunosuppression, Crohn's disease [4], and chronic anorectal disease as the most prevalent associations. Cigarette smoking interacting with HPV is currently under investigation for anal cancer genesis.

Epidermoid (squamous cell) carcinoma is the most common histological variant, representing about 80% of anal cancer cases seen. Somewhat less common is the cloacogenic (or basaloid/transitional cell) carcinoma, with rare variants including anal adenocarcinoma (originating from anal glands or from chronic fistula in ano), anal melanoma, and primary anal lymphoma [5–7]. Squamous anal cancer is a curable disease when diagnosed early and adequately treated. The best prognosis is achieved in anal cutaneous lesions located at the anal margin < 2 cm in maximal diameter [8], with no lymph node involvement. Lately, neoadjuvant chemoradiation is the treatment of choice according to the best evidence-based regimens modeled on the Nigro Wayne State protocol, which offers the highest chances of disease remission [9].

Anatomy

Anus is a word derived from the Greek meaning "end" and refers to the last 4–6 cm of the digestive tract [9]. Anal cancer topography is divided into the anal canal and the anal margin. Anal canal limits are surgically defined between the anorectal ring (transitional epithelium) and the anal verge (squamous epithelium). On the other hand, anatomists define the anal canal as the region extending from the anal verge to the dentate or pectinate line. The anal margin initiates at the anal opening and comprises the skin in

M. Pescatori, F.S.P. Regadas, S.M. Murad Regadas, A.P. Zbar (eds.), *Imaging Atlas of the Pelvic Floor and Anorectal Diseases*. ISBN 978-88-470-0808-3. © Springer-Verlag Italia 2008

the perianal area. Tumors in these two locations have different prognoses and occasionally alternate treatment regimens.

Recently, endoanal magnetic resonance imaging (MRI) probes have been able to enhance image details of the anal canal to better study sphincter radiologic anatomy, especially the internal sphincter (Figs. 1–3) [10–12].

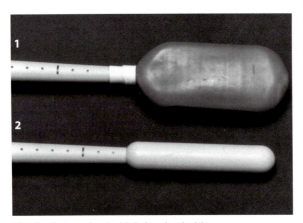

Fig. 1. Endorectal probe (*1*). Endoanal probe (*2*)

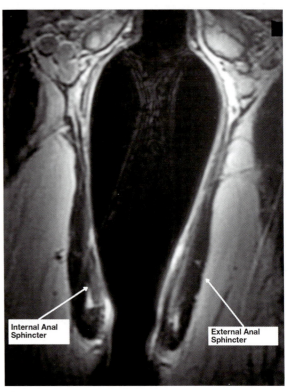

Fig. 2. Coronal plane. Normal sphincter muscle appearance

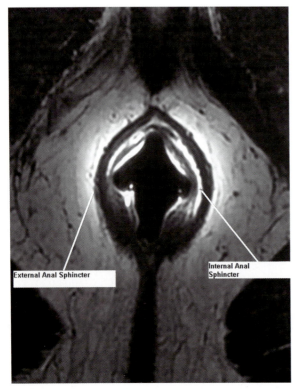

Fig. 3. Transverse plane: normal sphincter muscle appearance (*arrows*)

Staging System

To classify anal canal and anal margin lesions, the World Health Organization uses the following definitions: "Anal canal neoplasms are defined as lesions arising from the anorectal ring proximally (including the anal transitional zone) to the dentate line distally. Anal margin neoplasms are defined as those lesions arising distal to the dentate line to the junction of perianal skin with the hair-bearing skin of the buttock". Unfortunately, the dentate line is not usually seen in MRI, so this provides little discriminatory detail for prognostic purposes.

The clinical staging system for such tumors is somewhat controversial. However, in 1978, the Union Internationale Contre le Cancer (UICC) developed a staging system incorporating the anal canal and anal margin tumors as well as a clinical pathological staging system after surgery [13]. In 1987, the American Joint Committee on Cancer (AJCC) adopted the same staging system, although tumors of the anal canal and anal margin were considered separate despite stages I (Tables 1 and 2) and II being identical for the two malignancies [14].

Table 1. Carcinoma of the anal canal staging. Data from [3]

AJCC/UICC stage	Primary tumor	Regional lymph nodes	Distant metastasis
Stage 0	Tis	N0	M0
Stage I	T1	N0	M0
Stage II	T2	N0	M0
	T3	N0	M0
Stage IIIA	T4	N0	M0
	T1-3	N1	M0
Stage IIIB	T4	N1	M0
	Any T	N2-3	M0
Stage IV	Any T	Any N	M1

AJCC American Joint Committee on Cancer, *UICC* Union Internationale Contre le Cancer

Table 2. Carcinoma of anal margin staging. Data from [3]

AJCC/UICC stage	Primary tumor	Regional lymph nodes	Distant metastasis
Stage 0	Tis	N0	M0
Stage I	T1	N0	M0
Stage II	T2	N0	M0
	T3	N0	M0
Stage III	T4	N0	M0
	Any T	N1	M0
Stage IV	Any T	Any N	M1

AJCC American Joint Committee on Cancer, *UICC* Union Internationale Contre le Cancer

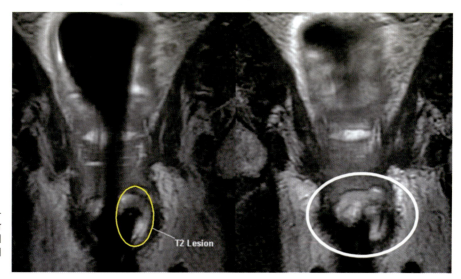

Fig. 4. Coronal T2-weighted image. Hyperintense T2-stage tumor of the anterior left-lower anal canal extending into external anal sphincter (*circle*)

Tumor Classification: Size

According to the AJCC/UICC staging system, a T1 lesion is considered as a lesion < 2 cm in greatest dimension, a T2 tumor being between 2–5 cm in size (Figs. 4 and 5), and a T3 cancer > 5 cm in maximal dimension. A T4 cancer is different for both cancers; T4 tumors of the anal canal invade the vagina and/or urethra or bladder. Involvement of the sphincter musculature in isolation does not characterize a T4 malignancy. Conversely, in anal margin lesions, T4 cancers invade deep extradermal structures, most notably the skeletal muscle or bone (Fig. 6). Overall tumor dimensions have a significant impact on prognosis and survival. Patients with tumors classified as T1 and T2 have >80% 5-year cancer-specific survival, whereas those with T3 and T4 lesions have <20% cancer-specific survival at 5 years [15].

Lymph Node Involvement

Lymph node involvement is a significant negative prognostic variable in anal carcinoma outcome. About 30% of patients operated upon have metastatically involved lymph nodes. Lymph node spread can occur in three principal directions. From the inferior anal canal, lymphatic drainage can lead to the inguinal nodes. From the upper anal canal, lymphatic flow goes to the superior hemorrhoidal and mesorectal nodes. The third direction for lymphatic drainage

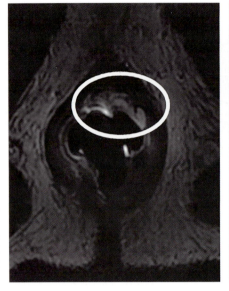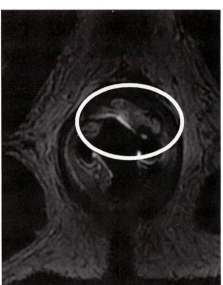

Fig. 5. Anal cancer with external anal sphincter infiltration. Axial T2-weighted image. Hyperintense left side inferior anal canal nodule with sphincter involvement (*circle*)

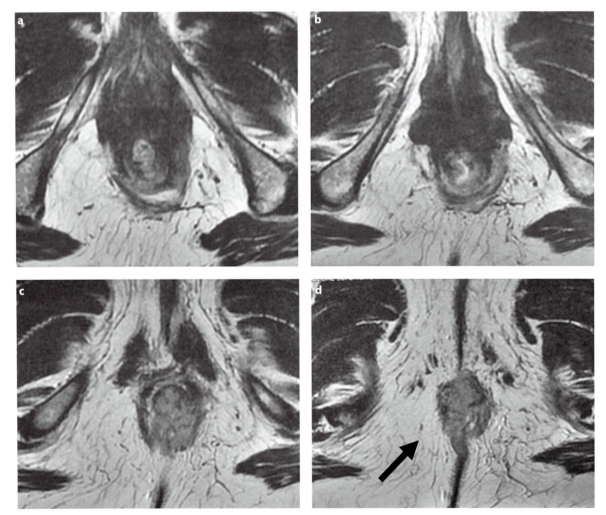

Fig. 6 a-d. Anal margin tumor infiltrating dermal structure. Transaxial T2-weighted image from the **a-d** lower anal canal to the anal margin. **d** Posterior hyperintense infiltrating tumor extending into right side dermal layer (*arrow*)

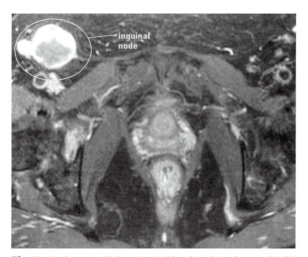

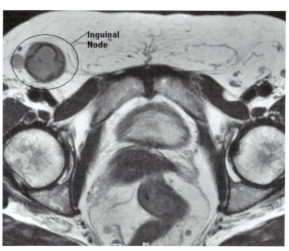

Fig. 7. Anal cancer with large inguinal lymph node involvement (*circle*). Transaxial T1-weighted postcontrast image through the inguinal level clearly showing enlarged heterogenous right lymph node

Fig. 8. Anal cancer with inguinal lymph node involvement (N1) (*circle*). Transaxial T2-weighted image showing heterogenous and enlarged lymph nodes

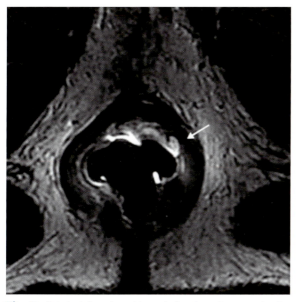

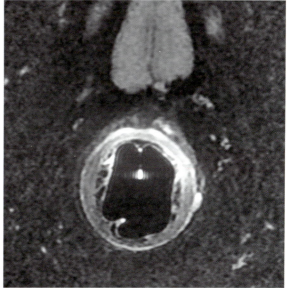

Fig. 9. Anterior left anal canal tumor before chemotherapy and radiotherapy (*arrow*). Axial T2-weighted endoanal probe image. Note the left anterior hyperintense lesion. Note external anal sphincter extension

Fig. 10. Anal canal cancer after chemotherapy and radiotherapy. Axial T2-weighted image with fat saturation. The lesion is not identifiable. The anterior left wall is thinner and hyperintense, suggesting changes due to radiation therapy

is toward the internal iliac nodal group through the hypogastric lymph vessels and laterally to obturator nodes [16].

In accordance with the AJCC/UICC staging systems for anal canal cancers, N1 stage is associated with perirectal nodal involvement, N2 stage corresponds to unilateral internal iliac and/or inguinal lymph nodes (Figs. 7 and 8), and N3 stage is defined as combined positive perirectal and inguinal nodal disease and/or bilateral internal iliac and/or bilateral inguinal lymph node involvement. For cancers of the anal margin, the same system is utilized, although a difference lies in the N1 classification in that there is ipsilateral inguinal node involvement only.

There are several factors that influence the rate of lymph node metastasis. Tumors up to 4 cm in size have an overall lymphatic metastasis rate of 20% at presentation. Tumors measuring between 4 and 6 cm and larger than 6 cm have a probability of lymph node metastasis of 30% and 50%, respectively. Moreover, tumor location also determines prognosis and the likelihood of nodal disease at presentation where tumors of the upper third of the anal canal have a probability of 30% of having lymphatic metastasis and tumors of middle third of the anal canal have approximately a 25% incidence of nodal positivity. Tumors located in the lower third of the anal canal rarely, if ever, spread to the lymphatic system [17].

Conclusion

In conclusion, MRI is probably best indicated to evaluate local regional spread of tumors located in the low rectum and anal canal and to identify recurrence following chemoradiation as well as sphincter infiltration. An advantage in this group is the ability of enhanced MRI to differentiate between cancer recurrence and radiation response [18]. MRI appears to be a very promising modality for assessing treatment responsiveness in anal tumors (Figs. 9 and 10), and perineal recurrence can also be diagnosed using this technique [19].

References

1. Ministério da Saúde. Instituto Nacional de Câncer. Registro de Câncer (2008) Câncer do ânus. www.inca.gov.br. Cited 23 Feb 2008
2. National Cancer Institute, US Institutes of Health (2008) Anal Cancer www.cancer.gov. Cited 23 Feb 2008
3. Savoca EP, Wong WD (1995) Anal carcinoma: anatomy, staging, and prognostic variables In: Cohen AM, Winawer SJ, Friedman MA, Gunderson LL (eds). Cancer of the colon rectum and anus. McGraw-Hill, pp 1013–1020
4. Ball CS, Wujanto R, Haboubi NY et al (1988) Carcinoma in anal Crohn's disease: discussion paper. J Roy Soc Med 81:217–219
5. Getz SB Jr, Ough YD, Patterson RB et al (1981) Mucinous adenocarcinoma developing in chronic anal fistula: report of two cases and review of the literature. Dis Colon Rectum 24:562–566
6. Jensen SL, Shoukouh-Amiri MH, Hagen K et al (1988) Adenocarcinoma of the anal ducts: a series of 21 cases. Dis Colon Rectum 31:268–272
7. Minsky BD, Hoffman JP, Kelsen DP (2001) Cancer of the anal region. In: DeVita VT Jr, Hellman S, Rosenberg SA (eds). Cancer: Principles & Practice of Oncology, 6th edn. Lippincott, Williams & Wilkins, Philadelphia, pp 1319–1342
8. Heitland W (1997) Anal and perianal tumors. Ther Umsch 54:202–204
9. Martenson JA, Lipsitz SR, Lefkopoulou M et al. (1995) Results of combined modality therapy for patients with anal cancer (E7283). An Eastern Cooperative Oncology Group study. Cancer 76(10):1731–1736
10. Zbar AP, deSouza NM, Strickland N et al (1998) Comparison of endoanal magnetic resonance imaging and computerized tomography in the preoperative staging of rectal cancer: pilot study. Techn Coloproctol 2:61–66
11. Gualdi GF, Casciani E, Guadalaxara A et al (2000) Local staging of rectal cancer with transrectal ultrasound and endorectal magnetic resonance imaging: comparison with histologic findings. Dis Colon Rectum 43:338–345
12. Indinnimeo M, Cicchini C, Stazi A et al (2000) Magnetic resonance imaging using endoanal coil in anal canal tumors after radiochemotherapy or local excision. Int Surg 85:143–146
13. Spiessl B, Beahrs OH, Hermanek P et al (1992) UICC TNM Atlas. Illustrated guide to the TNM/pTNM classification of malignant tumors. Springer-Verlag, Berlin pp 87–95
14. Anal canal (2002) In: American Joint Committee on Cancer: AJCC cancer staging manual, 6th edn. Springer, New York, pp 125–130
15. Goldman S, Auer G, Erhardt K et al (1987) Prognostic significance of clinical stage, histologic grade, and nuclear DNA content is squamous-cell carcinoma of the anus. Dis Colon Rectum 30:444–448
16. Shank B, Warren EE, Marshall SF (2000) Neoplasms of the anus. In: Holland JF, Frei E (eds) Cancer medicine, 5th edn. Decker, Hamilton, pp 1521–1529
17. Veidenheimer MC (1995) Epidermoid carcinoma of the anus – primary surgical therapy. In: Cohen AM, Winawer SJ, Friedman MA, Gunderson LL (eds) Cancer of the colon rectum and anus. McGraw-Hill, New York, pp 1023–1024
18. Roach SC, Hulse PA, Moulding FJ et al (2005) Magnetic resonance imaging of anal cancer. Clin Radiol 60:1111–1119
19. Scherrer A, Reboul F, Martin D et al (1990) CT of malignant anal canal tumors. RadioGraphics 10:443–445

SECTION III

Rectal and Perirectal Diseases

CHAPTER 12

Two- and Three-dimensional Ultrasonography in Benign and Malignant Rectal Neoplasms

Sthela M. Murad Regadas, F. Sérgio P. Regadas

Abstract

Ultrasound (US) scanning plays an important role in locoregional tumor staging and has been shown to be efficient in detecting parietal invasion and metastasized perirectal lymph nodes. This chapter discusses the role of anorectal US in evaluating the extent of tumor invasion in the rectal wall, sphincter muscles, and perirectal lymph nodes; the extent of tumor invasion following radiotherapy; and detecting early local recurrence in the rectal wall or perirectal lymph nodes. The three-dimensional scanning mode enables the examiner to stage lesions in multiple planes, measure tumor length, and determine the distance between the distal tumor border and the sphincter muscles for comparison with measurements taken after radiotherapy. This is an important aspect to consider when planning surgical resection with or without sphincter saving. In addition, the three-dimensional scanning mode is safer, as it makes it possible to review the images posteriorly, in real time, as required by some lesions.

Introduction

The digital rectal examination is essential for diagnosing rectal neoplasm and provides information on site, number of involved quadrants, and tumor mobility/fixation. However, the method is subjective and restricted to evaluating rectal-wall invasion. Staging rectal tumors is essential to determine the best treatment approach to prevent recurrence and preserve sphincter function. Ultrasound (US) scanning plays an important role in locoregional staging and has been shown to be efficient in detecting parietal invasion and metastasized perirectal lymph nodes in 69–96% and 64–83% of cases, respectively [1–4]. The efficiency of the US evaluation is examiner dependent, and variation may reflect a learning curve. Established indications include:

1. Determine the extent of tumor invasion in the rectal wall, sphincter muscles, and perirectal lymph nodes
2. Evaluate extent of tumor invasion following radiotherapy
3. Detect early local recurrence in the rectal wall or perirectal lymph nodes
4. Detect extrarectal neoplasms and determine their relation to rectal-wall layers
5. Make biopsy of suspect lymph nodes or sites with images suggestive of postradiotherapy residual tumors or early recurrence with ambiguous proctological findings.

The multiplane three-dimensional scanning mode enables the examiner to stage lesions in multiple planes, measure tumors longitudinally, and determine the distance between the distal tumor border and the proximal border of the sphincter muscles for comparison with measures taken after radiotherapy. Quadrants differ both in relation to tumor occupation and sphincter-muscle configuration (muscle bundles are arranged asymmetrically). This is the most important aspect to consider when planning surgical resection with or without sphincter saving. In addition, the three-dimensional scanning mode is safer, as it makes it possible to review the images posteriorly, in real time, as required by some lesions.

M. Pescatori, F.S.P. Regadas, S.M. Murad Regadas, A.P. Zbar (eds.), *Imaging Atlas of the Pelvic Floor and Anorectal Diseases*.
ISBN 978-88-470-0808-3. © Springer-Verlag Italia 2008

Ultrasonographic Staging

In 1985, Hildebrandt and Feifel [5] proposed using US scanning for staging rectal tumors based on the TNM classification:

uT0 – Noninvasive lesion affecting the mucous membrane and the muscularis mucosa
uT1 – Submucosal invasion
uT2 – Invasion of the circular and longitudinal muscle layers
uT3 – Invasion of perirectal fat
uT4 – Invasion of adjacent organs
N0 – Uncompromised lymph nodes
N1 – Compromised lymph nodes.

Muscularis mucosa and muscle layers are represented by hypoechoic (dark) images. Thickened layers suggest tumor invasion or involvement. Submucosal layer and perirectal fat are represented by hyperechoic (light) images. Tumor invasion appears as a disruption or irregularity.

1. Benign neoplasia: characterized by a thickened muscularis mucosa layer and an intact submucosal layer (Figs. 1 and 2)
2. Severe dysplasia, adenocarcinoma in situ: hypoechoic areas surrounded by homogenous image, characteristic of adenoma (Fig. 3)
3. uT1-type lesion: disruption (irregularity) is observed in the second hyperechoic (submucosal) layer (Figs. 4 and 5)

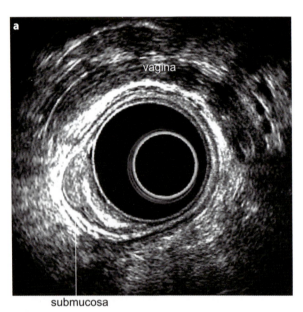

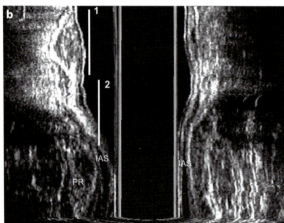

Fig. 1 a, b. uT0: Lesion expands the inner hypoechoic layer and is surrounded by the uniform middle hyperechoic layer representing the submucosa. **a** Axial plane: villous adenoma in the right posterior lateral rectal wall; **b** coronal plane: lesion length is 1.9 cm (*1*), located 1.7 cm from the internal anal sphincter (*IAS*) and puborectalis (*PR*) muscle (*2*)

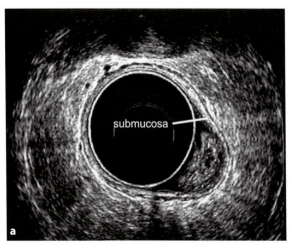

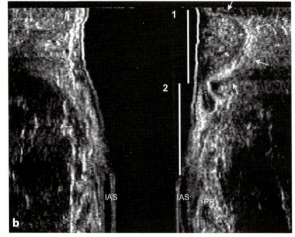

Fig. 2 a, b. uT0: Small polyp in the left posterior lateral rectal wall. Submucosa is intact. **a** Axial plane; **b** coronal plane: lesion length is 1.7 cm (*1*), located 2.0 cm from the internal anal sphincter (*IAS*) and puborectalis (*PR*) muscle (*2*)

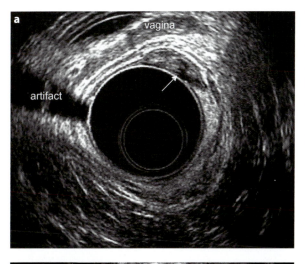

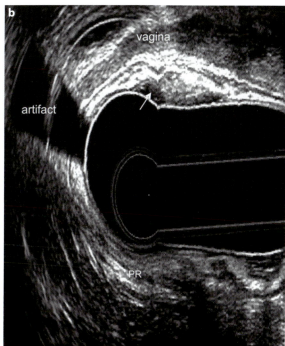

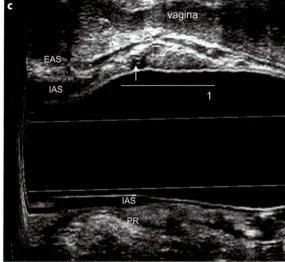

Fig. 3 a-c. uT0: Female patient with severe dysplasia in the anterior rectal wall. Thickened muscularis mucosa layer with hypoechoic area (*arrows*). The submucosa layer is intact. **a** Axial plane: feces in the rectal lumen (*artifacts*); **b, c** sagittal with coronal planes: lesion length is 2.0 cm (*1*), located at the level of the puborectal (*PR*) muscle. *EAS* external anal sphincter, *IAS* internal anal sphincter

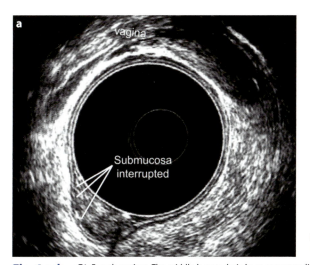

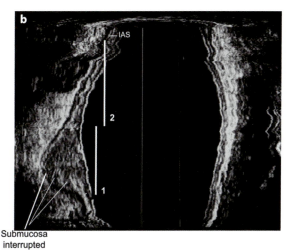

Fig. 4 a, b. uT1: Female patient. The middle hyperechoic layer corresponding to submucosa is interrupted at several points. The hypoechoic layer representing the muscularis propria is intact. **a** Axial plane; **b** coronal plane: lesion length is 2.1 cm (*1*), located in the right lateral posterior rectal wall 2.4 cm from the internal anal sphincter (*IAS*) and puborectalis muscle (*2*)

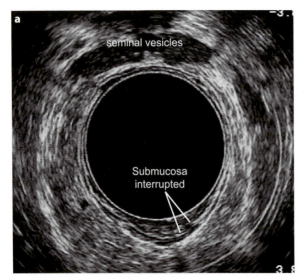

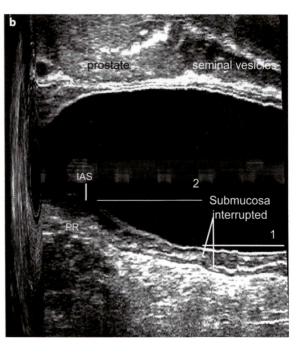

Fig. 5 a, b. uT1: Female patient with a small tumor in the posterior quadrant of the rectal wall. **a** Axial plane: tumor is located at the level of the seminal vesicles; **b** sagittal plane: lesion length is 2.0 cm (*1*), located 2.2 cm from the internal anal sphincter (*IAS*) and the puborectalis (*PR*) muscle (*2*)

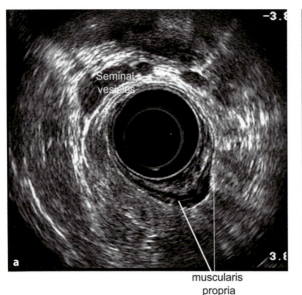

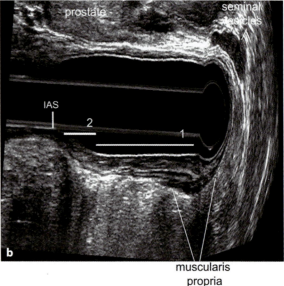

Fig. 6 a, b. uT2: Tumor located at the level of the seminal vesicles and prostate. The hyperechoic layer corresponding to submucosa is completely broken and the hypoechoic layer representing the muscularis propria is thickened. The outer hyperechoic layer (perirectal fat) is intact. **a** Axial plane; **b** sagittal plane: lesion length is 3.4 cm (*1*), located 0.4 cm from the internal anal sphincter (*IAS*) and puborectalis (*PR*) muscle (*2*)

4. uT2-type lesion: complete disruption of the submucosal layer associated with thickening of the musculature and intact perirectal fat (Figs. 6–8)
5. uT3-type lesion: irregularities (spicules) in the last hyperechoic layer (corresponding to perirectal fat) (Fig. 9)
6. uT4-type lesion: characterized by invasion of adjacent structures (Figs. 10 and 11)

7. Perirectal lymph nodes: observed in the perirectal fat proximally or distally to the lesion and measuring >1.0 mm. Size, echogenicity, and shape help distinguish between inflammatory and metastatic forms. When observed in the perirectal fat in the form of rounded and hypoechoic (or tumor-like) areas with irregular borders, lymph node metastasis should be suspected (Fig. 9).

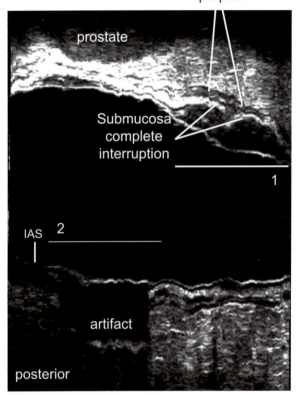

Fig. 7. uT2: Sagittal plane: lesion length is 2.3 cm (1), located 2.4 cm from the posterior internal anal sphincter (IAS) and puborectalis muscle (2)

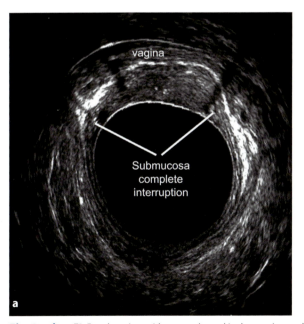

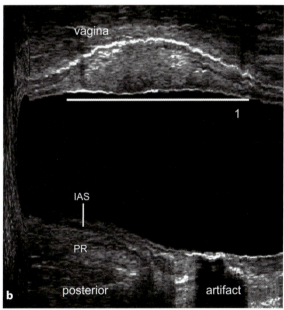

Fig. 8 a, b. uT2: Female patient with a tumor located in the anterior quadrant of the lower rectum and anorectal junction at the level of the puborectalis (PR) muscle and internal anal sphincter (IAS) posteriorly. The second hypoechoic layer (muscular propria) is thickened and the outer hyperechoic layer (perirectal fat) is intact. a Axial plane; b sagittal plane: lesion length is 4.7 cm (1), located in the anterior lower rectum and anorectal junction without involving the anterior IAS due to the anal canal anatomic configuration (see Chap. 2)

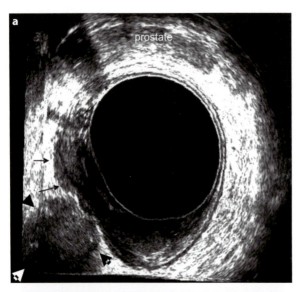

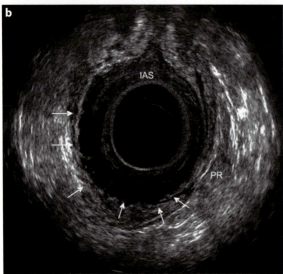

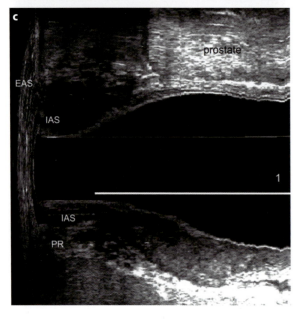

Fig. 9 a-c. uT3: Male patient with a tumor occupying 70% of the rectal wall (right lateral posterior quadrant). The hyperechoic layer corresponding to the perirectal fat shows irregularity (*arrows*). **a** Three-dimensional section: malignant lymph nodes at the level of the prostate (*arrowheads*); **b** axial plane: tumor invading the internal anal sphincter (*IAS*) and puborectalis (*PR*) muscle in the upper and middle anal canal (*arrows*); **c** sagittal plane: lesion length is 4.7 cm (*1*), involving the lower rectum and the anal canal and invading the IAS and PR muscle (*arrows*). *EAS* external anal sphincter

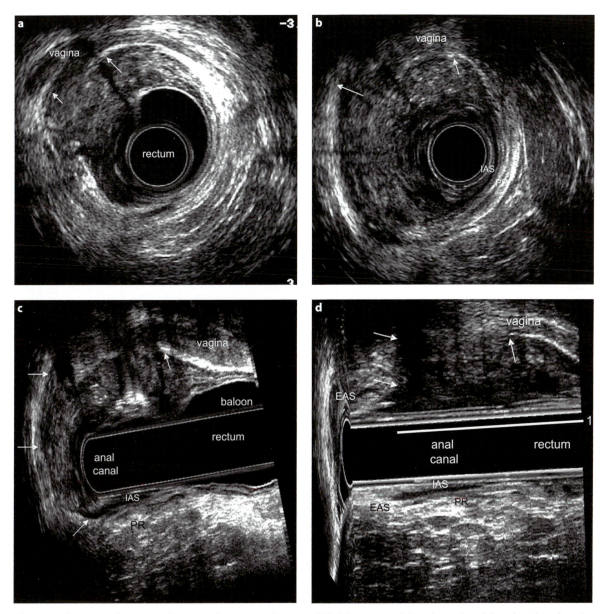

Fig. 10 a-d. uT4: Female patient with large rectal cancer occupying nearly 80% of the lower rectal circumference (especially at the right and anterior quadrants), invading the vaginal wall. **a** Upper anal canal: tumor infiltrating the internal anal sphincter (*IAS*), puborectalis (*PR*) muscle, perianal fat, and vagina (*arrows*); **b** vaginal-wall invasion (*arrows*) **c, d** sagittal with coronal planes: lesion length is 5.2 cm (*1*) extending to the middle anal canal with vaginal invasion. *EAS* external anal sphincter

In contrast, oval structures with regular borders and a hyperechoic area in the center (corresponding to the hilum) suggest inflammatory lesions (Fig. 12). In general, however, the larger the lymph nodes, the more likely they are to contain metastases [6, 7]. They are easily distinguished from blood vessels because the latter assume a longitudinal or branch-like form when the transducer is moved in the two-dimensional mode or in multiplane view.

Limitations of Ultrasonographic Staging of Neoplasms

The patient and the transducer must be adequately prepared in order to produce useful images with a minimum of artifacts and the best possible definition of rectal layers and/or perirectal tissues. Other factors may interfere with the accuracy of US staging of neoplasms:

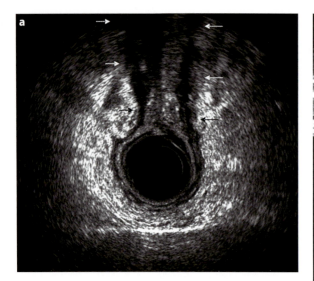

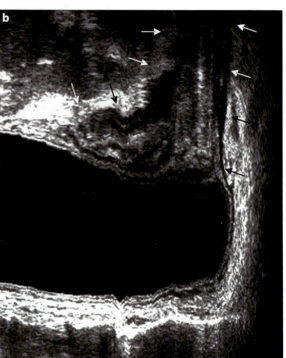

Fig. 11 a, b. uT4: Extensive anterior rectal tumor surpassing the rectal wall. Inability to visualize the outer boundary (*arrows*) even when increasing the focal distance to 6.2 cm; located proximal to the seminal vesicles. **a** Axial plane; **b** sagittal plane: it can be impossible to position the endoprobe proximal to locally advanced tumor due to lumen narrowing. Rectal balloon cannot be completely distended

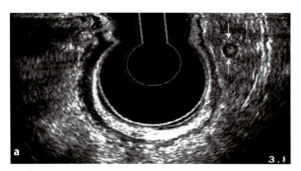

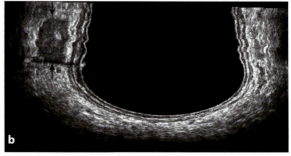

Fig. 12 a, b. Inflammatory lymph nodes: oval structures with central hyperechoic area (hilum). **a** One-year follow up of a rectal cancer (female patient): small, inflammatory lymph node (central hyperechoic area); **b** rectal cancer follow-up (male patient) demonstrating an enlarged lymph node associated with a pelvic abscess

- Large lesions can produce attenuated areas such as posterior acoustic shadows (shadows behind tumors), making staging difficult.
- If lesions are very small and the balloon is excessively distended around the transducer, lesions may be compressed and overstaged.
- If the air that is often retained on the surface of ulcerous lesions becomes interposed between the lesion and the transducer and the balloon is distended, a posterior acoustic shadow (shadow behind tumor) may be produced (Fig. 13). Air, calcium, and bone produce highly attenuated images and differ from soft tissues with regard to acoustic impedance. Thus, when sound waves go through these structures, they are attenuated and intense-

ly reflected so that no echo is produced below the structures, making the echographic evaluation impossible. The air may also produce a reverberation due to the reflection of the echo received by the transducer, leading to a series of densely juxtaposed reflexes that coalesce behind the lesion, making it impossible to view it completely. One such reverberation is the so-called "comet tail".

Severely inflamed lesions make it hard to distinguish between inflammatory parietal thickening and tumor invasion. In addition, the inflammatory reaction can produce attenuated areas (shadows) behind the lesion, making staging inaccurate. Peritumoral inflammation from the lesion often leads to US overstaging, as it makes the invasion seem larger than it

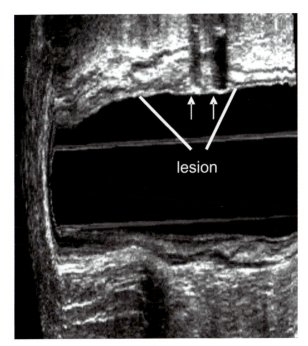

Fig. 13. Sagittal with diagonal planes: Female patient with small, ulcerous lesion. Posterior acoustic shadow produced by air retained on the surface of ulcerous lesions (*arrows*) reducing the accuracy for tumor staging

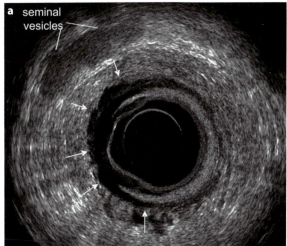

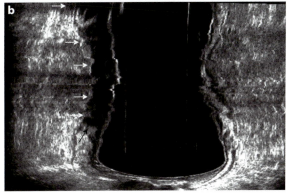

Fig. 14 a, b. uT3: Rectal tumor accompanied by lumen narrowing invading the hyperechoic layer representing the perirectal fat (*arrows*). **a** Axial plane: it is not possible to distend completely the balloon; **b** coronal plane: it can be impossible to insert the transducer through tumor lumen to evaluate it proximally; tumor is too long

is [8, 9]. Understaging is generally observed in cases of minimally invasive lesions and causes retention of tumor tissue, early recurrence, and shortened survival. Tumor biopsies can produce inflammatory reactions such as edema and fibrosis and even intratumoral hemorrhage, resulting in hypoechoic patches compromising interpretation. The examination should therefore be performed at least 15 days after the biopsy.

Regardless of stage, stenosing tumors represent a challenge to endorectal US scanning (Fig. 14). Even when it is possible to bypass them, the balloon cannot be completely distended, and the images acquired tend to be ambiguous.

The lesion site in relation to the anal canal may influence interpretation, especially when located in the upper third of the rectum/rectosigmoid junction and the anorectal junction. It is more difficult to center and maintain the transducer perpendicular when the lesions are located more proximally, and folds are often formed in the rectal wall. Lesions should be completely evaluated beginning at the most proximal point. Staging lesions located at the anorectal junction can be difficult because the balloon cannot be fully distended around the transducer, creating an acoustic interface without compressing the lesion excessively and, when not sufficiently distended, mucosal folds are formed. The problem is ultimately due to the excessive width of the rectal lumen.

Limitations of Ultrasonographic Staging of Lymph Nodes

1. Evaluating perirectal tissue may be inadequate due to artifacts (shadows and reverberation), insufficient preparation of the rectum, or the endoprobe.
2. Lateral pelvic lymph nodes cannot be evaluated because they exceed the focal distance of the transducer.

Staging after Radio/Chemotherapy

Changes in the rectal wall produced by radiation make it very difficult, if not impossible, to distinguish individual layers and therefore to restage lesions. However, in studies using US scanning to evaluate lesion regression in response to radiotherapy, disappearance of lymph nodes or overall

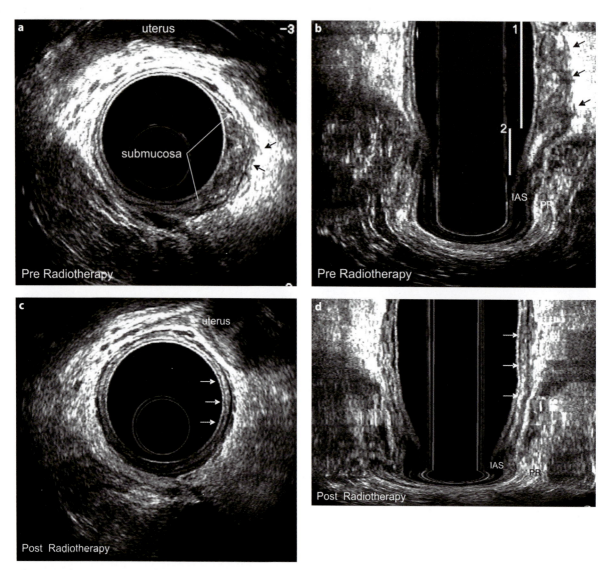

Fig. 15 a-d. uT3: Rectal cancer, female patient. Located on the left rectal wall. **a** Axial plane: preradiotherapy; complete disruption of the submucosal layer associated with thickening of the musculature and irregularities at the hyperechoic layer corresponding to perirectal fat (*arrows*); **b** coronal plane: lesion length is 3.2 cm (*1*), located 1.5 cm from the left lateral part of the internal anal sphincter (*IAS*) and puborectalis (*PR*) muscle (*2*) (*arrows*); **c** axial plane: postradiotherapy; **d** coronal plane: postradiotherapy; rectal-wall layers and/or sphincter muscles are clearly distinguishable (*arrows*). Pathological findings: complete tumor regression (pT0N0)

response varied from 75% to 92% [10–12] in relation to other imaging techniques and anatomical/pathological findings. By evaluating patients with malignant rectal neoplasms using high-resolution, automatic, three-dimensional US scanning before and after radiotherapy and comparing the results with anatomical/pathological findings, criteria may be established for postradiotherapy US analysis of lesions:

1. Complete regression of lesions: rectal-wall layers and/or sphincter muscles are clearly distinguishable where the tumor has previously been located (Fig. 15).

2. Residual lesions: certain patterns are observed depending on the extent of tumor regression and the association with the inflammatory process.

Heterogeneous image with hyperechoic areas due to residual tumor associated with hypoechoic areas due to the inflammatory process. Anatomical disorder is observed associated with parietal thickening at the tumor borders, and rectal-wall layers cannot be distinguished (Fig. 16).

Similar to image before radiotherapy, but more hypoechoic due to inflammation. Rectal wall layers are distinguishable at former tumor location, and restaging is possible in the absence of inflammation-induced

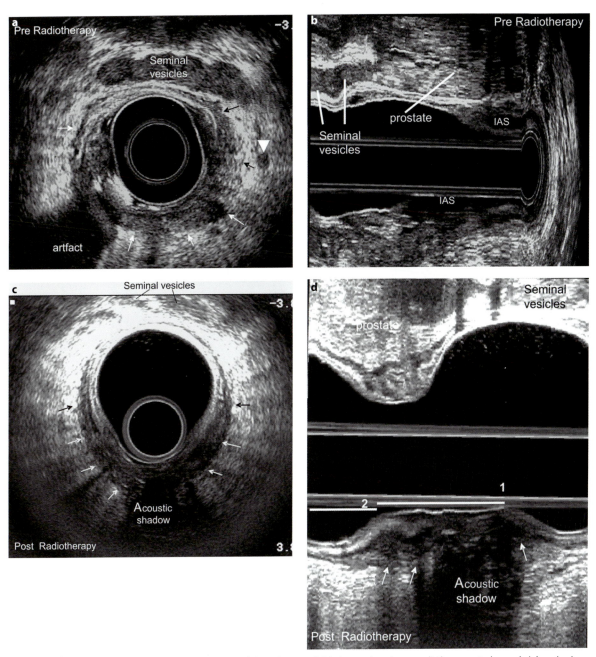

Fig. 16 a-d. uT3: Rectal cancer occupying the posterior rectal circumference. **a** Axial plane: male patient preradiotherapy; outer hyperechoic layer (perirectal fat) shows irregularity (*arrows*); big tumor produces artifacts (posterior acoustic shadows) behind lesion; lymph node appears with echogenicity similar to the primary tumor, suggesting strongly metastatic disease (*arrowhead*); **b** sagittal plane; lesion length >6.0 cm (*1*) and extends from lower rectum to anal canal, invading the internal anal sphincter (*IAS*) and puborectalis (*PR*) muscle (*arrows*); **c** axial plane: postradiotherapy; residual lesion with partial tumor regression; anatomical disorder; hyperechoic areas due to residual tumor (*arrows*) associated with hypoechoic areas due to inflammation producing posterior acoustic shadows; **d** sagittal plane: lesion length is 2.9 cm (*1*), located 1.7 cm from the IAS and PR muscle posterolaterally (*2*) (*arrows*). Pathological findings: residual tumor

anatomical disorder. The circumference and length of the lesion may be decreased, and the distance between the distal border of the tumor and the proximal border of the sphincter muscles may have increased. Even if tumor invasion is not circumferential, it is recommended measuring the distance from its distal border to the sphincter muscles in all quadrants, as the sphincter muscles are asymmetrically distributed (Fig. 17).

Inconclusive image characterized by parietal thickening with indistinguishable rectal wall layers at former tumor location. The existence of residual tumors cannot be ruled out (Fig. 18).

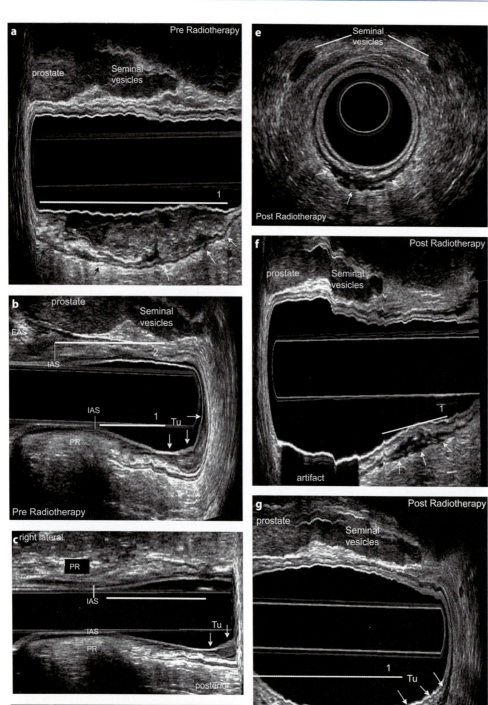

Fig. 17 a-g. uT3: Rectal cancer; male patient. Located on the posterior rectal wall. **a** Sagittal plane: preradiotherapy (*arrows*); lesion length is 5.7 cm (*1*); **b** sagittal plane: tumor is located 2.0 cm from the posterior internal anal sphincter (*IAS*) and puborectalis (*PR*) muscle (*1*) (*arrows*) and 3.1 cm from the anterior IAS (*2*); **c** sagittal with coronal planes: tumor is located 2.7 cm from the right lateral part of the IAS and PR muscle; **d** sagittal with coronal planes: tumor is located 2.6 cm from the left lateral part of the IAS and PR muscle (*1*); **e** axial plane: postradiotherapy; residual lesion, large tumor regression (*arrows*); **f** sagittal plane: postradiotherapy; lesion length is 1.5 cm (*1*); **g** sagittal plane: postradiotherapy; distance between the distal border of the tumor to the sphincter muscles is increased (4.3 cm posteriorly) (*1*). Pathological findings: residual tumor. *Tu* tumor, *EAS* external anal sphincter

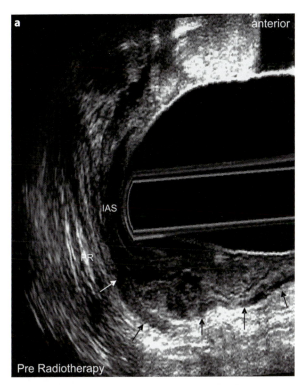

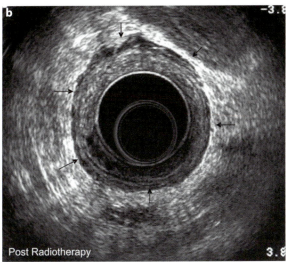

Fig. 18 a, b. uT3: Female patient. Rectal tumor invading the internal anal sphincter (*IAS*) and puborectalis (*PR*) muscle in upper anal canal. **a** Sagittal plane: preradiotherapy upper anal canal (*arrows*); **b** axial plane: postradiotherapy; circumferential parietal thickening (*arrows*). The existence of residual tumors cannot be ruled out. Pathological findings: residual tumor

Identification of Early Recurrence

Early recurrence is characterized by tumor-like hypoechoic images, with the widest portion outside the rectal wall (Fig. 19). The initial examination becomes an important reference during follow-up, since fibrosis and especially local sepsis and postsurgical anatomical distortions can influence interpretation. Tumor recurrence may be detected even when the lesion is enveloped by fibrous tissue.

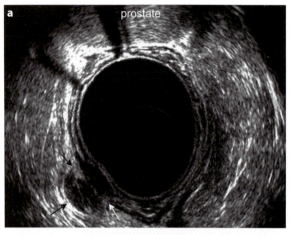

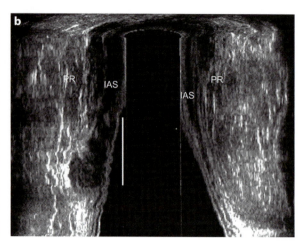

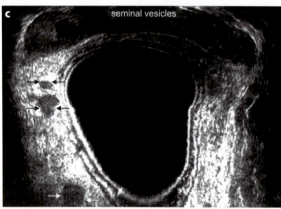

Fig. 19 a–c. Recurrence: Hypoechoic lesion with the widest portion outside the rectal wall (right lateral posterior). **a** Axial plane (*arrows*); **b** coronal plane: lesion length is 1.6 cm (*1*) located at the level of the internal anal sphincter (*IAS*) and puborectalis (*PR*) muscle (right lateral posterior) (*arrows*); **c** coronal plane: showing three malignant lymph nodes (*arrows*)

References

1. Hildrebandt U, Feifel G (1985) Preoperative staging of rectal cancer by intrarectal ultrasound. Dis Colon Rectum 28:42–46
2. Garcia-Aguilar J, Pollack J, Lee SH et al (2002) Accuracy of endorectal ultrasonography in preoperative staging of rectal tumors. Dis Colon rectum 45:10–15
3. Beynon J, Mortensen NJMcC, Foy DMA et al (1989) Preoperative assessment of mesorectal lymph node involvement in rectal cancer. Br J Surg 76:276–279
4. Dattala A, Albertin A, Parisi A et al (2000) Sensitivity and specificity of transrectal ultrasonography in the preoperative staging and postoperative follow up in rectal neoplasms. experience with 100 clinical cases. Chir Ttal 52:67–72
5. Hildrebant U, Fiefel G (1985) Preoperative staging of rectal cancer by intrarectal ultrasound. Dis Colon Rectum 28:42–46
6. Katsura Y, Yamada K, Ishizawa T et al (1992) Endorectal ultrasonography for the assessment of wall invasion and lymph node metastasis in rectal cancer. Dis Colon Rectum 35:362–368
7. Milsom JW, Graffner, H (1990) Intrarectal ultrasonography in rectal cancer staging and evaluating pelvic disease. Clinical uses of intrarectal ultrasound. Ann Surg 212:602–606
8. YamashitaY, Machi J, Shirouzu K et al (1988) Evaluation of endorectal ultrasound for the assessment of wall invasion of rectal cancer: report of a case. Dis Colon Rectum 31:617–623
9. Hulsmans FJ, Tio TL, Fockens P et al (1994) Assessment of tumor infiltration depth in rectal cancer with transrectal sonography: caution is necessary. Radiology 190:715–720
10. Gavioli M, Bagni A, Piccagli I et al (2000) Usefulness of endorectal ultrasound after preoperative radiotherapy in rectal cancer Comparison between sonographic and histopathologic changes. Dis Colon Rectum 43:1075–1083
11. Juska P, Pavalkis D, Pranys D (2004) Preoperative radiation with chemotherapy for rectal cancer: its impact on downstaging of disease and the role of endorectal ultrasound. Medicina (Kaunas) 40(1):46–53
12. Liersch T, Langer C, Jakob C et al (2003) Preoperative diagnostic procedures in locally advanced rectal carcinoma (> or = N+). What does endoluminal ultrasound achieve at staging and restaging (after neoadjuvant radiochemotherapy) in contrast to computed tomography? Chirurg 74(3):224–234

Commentary

Herand Abcarian

Ultrasonographic assessment of benign and malignant lesions of the rectum is discussed in detail in Chapter 12. The authors describe accurate disease staging and point out the important factors limiting examination accuracy. These include very large lesions casting posterior acoustic shadow, very small lesions that may be compressed by the probe, air retained over ulcerated tumors, stenosing lesions interfering with probe insertion, and high lesions causing difficulty in centering the transducer. Also, inflammation can be misinterpreted for invasion and hypoechoic images, and hematoma secondary to needle biopsy can interfere with staging. The authors suggest at least 15 days between biopsy and ultrasonography. As to factors limiting lymph node evaluation, insufficient cleansing of the rectum may limit evaluating perirectal fat, and lateral pelvic lymph nodes exceed the focal distance of the transducer.

After treatment with radiation or chemotherapy, US will demonstrate lesion regression. In cases of complete response, all layers previously affected will be seen as distinct normal layers. Redundant or recurrent lesions will appear as hypoechoic areas and indistinguishable layers. The suspected area can be pinpointed for accurate biopsy.

The value of three-dimensional US in axial planes is that it demonstrates the actual lesion size and distance from the anal verge or rectal wall as well as adjacent organ involvement, which will help guide the surgeon in planning the appropriate extirpative operation for the patient.

CHAPTER 13

Magnetic Resonance Imaging in Benign and Malignant Rectal Neoplasms

Pedro C. Basilio, Alice Brandão, Rosilma Gorete Lima Barreto

Abstract

Magnetic resonance imaging (MRI) is an accurate method for preoperative rectal cancer staging. The similarity with anatomy provides surgeons a clear view of local regional rectal cancer spread. Information detected through MRI is important to carefully plan adequate surgical management for each particular rectal cancer case. Data on cancer local status before neoadjuvant chemoradiation can be compared with posttreatment status to evaluate the magnitude of downstaging. Lymph node status should also be studied and taken into consideration whenever surgical treatment for rectal cancer is indicated, even before the number and lymph node volume regression occurs as a result of preoperative treatment regimens. Images acquired after neoadjuvant treatment are equally important to define surgical strategy. Imaging techniques and incidences as well as their surgical implications are contemplated in this chapter.

Introduction

According to the National Cancer Institute (NCI) Brazil, approximately 945,000 new cases of colorectal cancer are diagnosed every year worldwide, corresponding to the fourth most common type of cancer and the second most common type in developed countries [1]. In the USA, 41,420 new rectal cancer cases were expected for 2007 [2]. Adenocarcinoma accounts for 90–95% of malignant rectal neoplasias and therefore is the main focus of this chapter [3]. Rectal cancers usually arise in adenomatous polyps undergoing malignant transformation.

As patients are initially asymptomatic, developing permanent screening programs for early colorectal cancer detection is necessary. Whenever symptoms are present, the most common is low intestinal bleeding associated with change in bowel habits. Rectal cancer prognosis is clearly related to locoregional staging (depth of rectal wall invaded and type and number of lymph node involvement). MRI plays an important role in choosing the surgical approach, as it shows the distance between the mesorectum involved and the rectal fascia before the neoadjuvant radiotherapy as well as lymph node image status [4]. Surgeons should be extremely careful to dissect the mesorectal fascia over the site, with an exiguous tumor-free margin demonstrated by MRI. In such findings, the lateral part of the rectum, adjacent structures, and obturator fossa dissection should be considered. MRI is also particularly useful to evaluate tumor staging after neoadjuvant therapy. In addition, pelvic MRI is a helpful tool in rectal cancer follow-up and is indicated in patients with clinical symptoms of recurrence, such as rectal or perineal pain associated with high carcinoembryonic antigen (CEA) levels. The preoperative staging procedures include digital rectal examination, computed tomography (CT) scan or MRI of the abdomen and pelvis, endoscopic evaluation with biopsy, and endorectal ultrasound (EUS).

Staging System

MRI in rectal neoplasm is often helpful to clarify the nature and architecture of these tumors. It shows pre-

M. Pescatori, F.S.P. Regadas, S.M. Murad Regadas, A.P. Zbar (eds.), *Imaging Atlas of the Pelvic Floor and Anorectal Diseases.*
ISBN 978-88-470-0808-3. © Springer-Verlag Italia 2008

cisely the rectal wall layers infiltrated, as well as perirectal fat, lymph node, and adjacent organ involvement. MRI is an excellent method to accurately stage rectal cancer.

The current staging system was based on Dukes classification established in 1930 in the UK, and modified by Astler and Cooler in 1954, and finally correlating to the unified American Joint Committee on Cancer and Union Internationale Contre le Cancer (AJCC/UICC) TNM staging system [5] (Table 1). The purpose of these modifications was to determine the best treatment approach to obtain the best results.

MRI in the axial plane results in an image that closely reproduces what can be seen in transversal pathology specimens, detailing rectum and perirectal fat (Fig. 1). This image is obtained through a sagittal plane (Fig. 2). Rectal cancer image protocol usu-

ally comprises images in axial and coronal planes and in different technical sequences (Fig. 3). A circumferential lesion with clear sphincter involvement is well demonstrated (Fig. 4). To better visualize anatomic structures involved and degree of involvement, an endorectal probe should be utilized to magnify and clarify the anatomy as well as measure the distance to the anal verge (Figs. 5 and 6).

Studies have been developed evaluating the accuracy of MRI to identify the limit of the outermost parts of the tumor to the adjacent mesorectal fascia (as the potential circumferential resection margin in total mesorectal excision). Such images show 100% sensitivity and 88% specificity, confirming the important role of MRI in rectal cancer staging (Figs. 7–9). MRI is currently the only imaging technique with accuracy in predicting whether or not it is likely that a tumor-free margin can be achieved [6, 7].

Table 1. Rectal cancer staging

AJCC/UICC stage	Primary tumor	Regional lymph nodes	Distant metastasis	Dukes	Astler Coller
Stage 0	TIS	N0	M0		
Stage I	T1	N0	M0	A	
	T2	N0	M0	A	B1
Stage II	T3	N0	M0	B	B2
	T4	N0	M0	B	B3
Stage III	Any T	N1	M0	C	C1
	Any T	N2	M0	C	C2
	Any T	N3	M0	C	C3
Stage IV	Any T	Any N	M1	C	D

AJCC American Joint Committee on Cancer, *UICC* Union Internationale Contre le Cancer

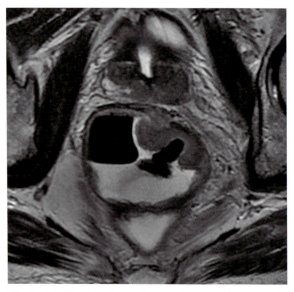

Fig. 1. Axial T2-weighted image. Rectum and mesorectal fat. Isointense lesion in left upper quadrant of the rectum. Note some liquid in the rectal lumen

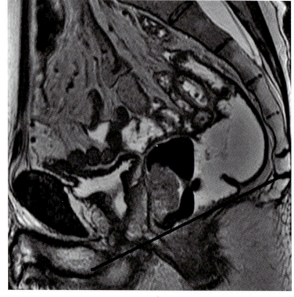

Fig. 2. Sagittal plane. Pelvis. T2-weighted image postprostatectomy

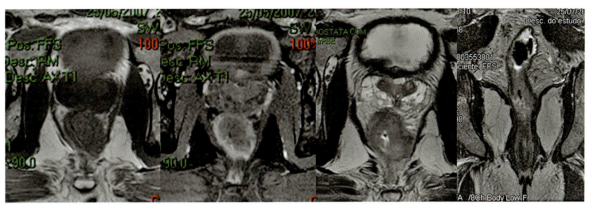

Fig. 3. Axial plane. Pelvis. T1-weighted image with fat suppression after contrast; T2-weighted and in coronal plane

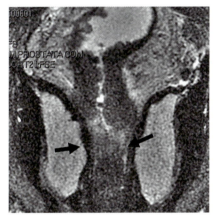

Fig. 4. Coronal T2-weighted image. Large circumferential mid- and lower-rectal tumor involving the internal anal sphincter (*arrows*)

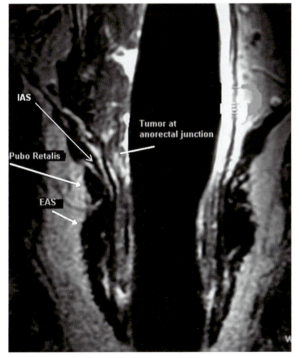

Fig. 5. Coronal T2-weighted image with endorectal probe demonstrating involvement of the upper part of the right internal anal sphincter (*IAS*). *EAS* external anal sphincter, *PR* puborectalis muscle

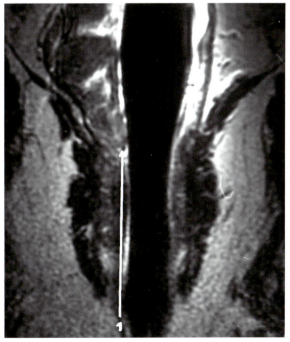

Fig. 6. Coronal T2-weighted image. Same case as in Figure 5. Extensive mid- and lower-rectal tumor (right lateral side) abutting right the levator ani muscle and infiltrating the internal anal sphincter. The distance between the distal border of the tumor to the anal verge is measured (*1*)

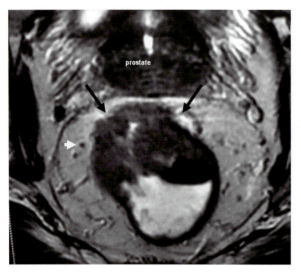

Fig. 7. Axial T2-weighted image. The mesorectal fat is widely invaded close to the prostate and the mesorectum fascia is infiltrated anteriorly (*black arrows*). Lymph nodes in the perirectal fat (*white arrow*)

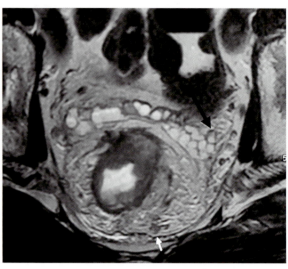

Fig. 8. Axial T2-weighted image. Rectal cancer invading the perirectal fat laterally and extending into the anterior and right lateral side of the mesorectum. Seminal vesicles are intact

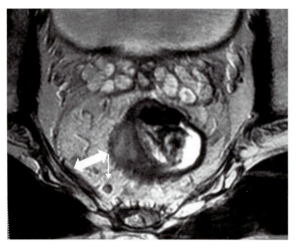

Fig. 9. Axial T2-weighted image. Right lateral tumor and mesorectal lymph node (*thin white arrow*). Distance from the lesion to the mesorectal fascia (*thick white arrow*)

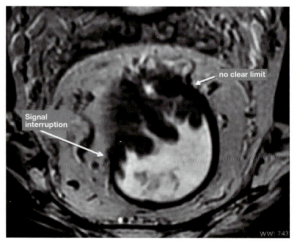

Fig. 10. Axial T2-weighted image. Anterior limit is not well defined. Extensive tumor (anterior left lateral) interrupting the rectal wall signal (*arrows*)

Limitations

A limitation to MRI is the inability to delineate the rectal wall layers involved, decreasing the accuracy to differentiate between pT2 and pT3 tumors (Figs. 10 and 11). However, internal anal sphincter invasion can be clearly identified (Fig. 12). MRI has great ability to distinguish between T3 and T4 lesion (Figs. 13–15).

Lymph Node Involvement

Lymph node status represents a major prognostic factor in colorectal cancer. A positive lymph node significantly reduces the disease-free time and overall 5-year survival. MRI is a valuable tool that identifies enlarged lymph nodes inside the perirectal fat preoperatively and before chemoradiation (Fig. 16), as well as small nodes (Fig. 17).

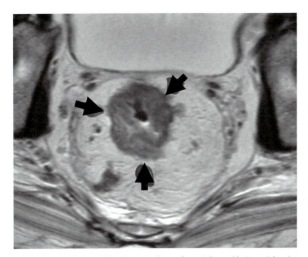

Fig. 11. Axial T2-weighted image. Circumferential rectal lesion with spiculation. Broad circumferential tumor. Nodular fine stranding extending into mesorectal fat (*arrows*)

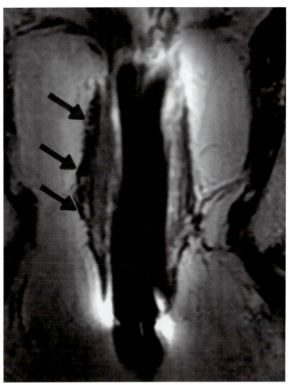

Fig. 12. Coronal T2-weighted image with endorectal probe. Low rectal tumor invading the right side of the internal anal sphincter (*arrows*)

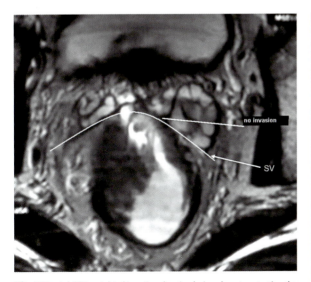

Fig. 13. Axial T2-weighted imaging showing lesion almost contacting the retroprostatic fascia at left side. Minimal space between rectal wall and the mesorectal fascia anteriorly. Seminal vesicles (*SV*) are not invaded, with normal hyperintense signal

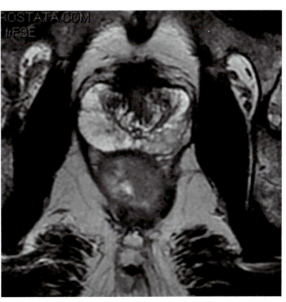

Fig. 14. Axial T2-weighted image with external phased-array probe. Low rectal lesion, close to prostate

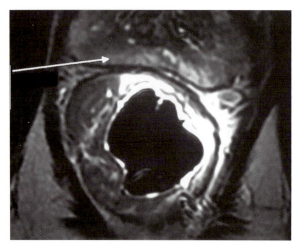

Fig. 15. Axial T2-weighted endorectal probe image. T3 lesion. Clearly visualized is a cleavage plane between tumor and prostate (*arrow*)

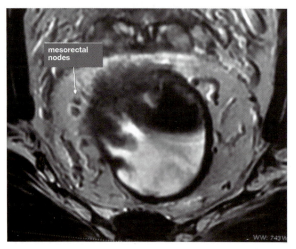

Fig. 16. Axial T2-weighted image. T3 anterior rectal tumor with large perirectal lymph nodes (*arrow*)

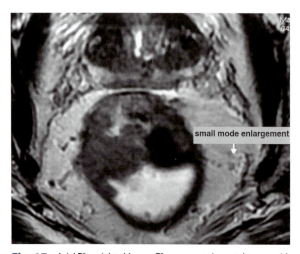

Fig. 17. Axial T2-weighted image. T3 upper anterior rectal tumor with small perirectal nodes (*white arrow*)

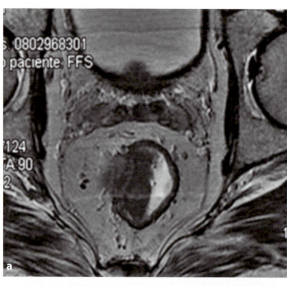

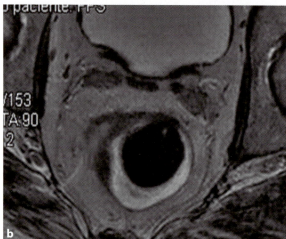

Fig. 18 a, b. **a** Axial T2-weighted image. T3 tumor before chemotherapy with right lateral mesorectal fat infiltration. **b** T3 tumor postchemotherapy. Significant tumor regression

Evaluation of Chemoradiation Response

MRI can demonstrate rectal neoplasm downstaging after chemoradiation. Images are obtained before and after treatment (Fig. 18a, b) in order to demonstrate the significant reduction in primary tumor size. Based on this information, the surgeon can decide whether or not to perform sphincter-saving procedures, associating organ resections, and lateral lymphadenectomy.

Follow-up

Follow-up imaging using MRI can identify postoperative and radiation tissue inflammatory changes that is usually hypointense at T2-weighted imaging, with no enhancement postgadolinium intravenous contrast (Figs. 19 and 20).

Recurrent tumor shows isointense signal enhancing after contrast injection. A large presacral recurrence with no sacral invasion is easily identified (Fig. 21). Conversely, another recurrence is well shown during control imaging (Fig. 22). There are some developing MRI techniques, such as diffusion-weighted imaging, that can be useful in these diagnoses; the tumor usually has restricted diffusion (Fig. 23).

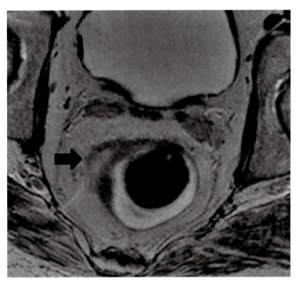

Fig. 19. Sagittal T2-weighted image. Postradiation. Presacral inflammatory tissue (*arrow*). Vaginal stenosis well shown with endovaginal gel

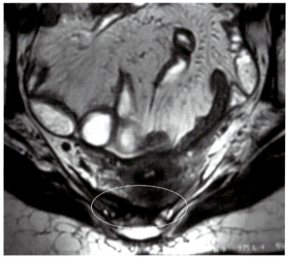

Fig. 20. Axial T2-weighted image. Postradiation. Presacral inflammatory changes. The presacral space with low signal is visualized, associated with uterus dislocation posteriorly (*white circle*)

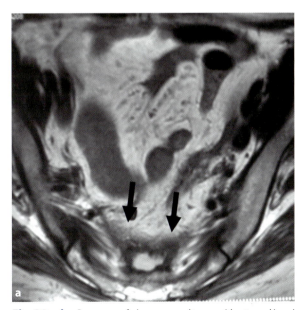

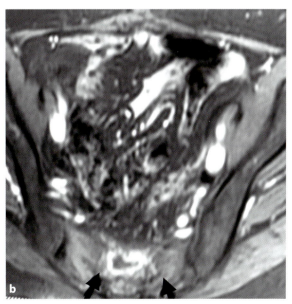

Fig. 21 a, b. Recurrence of a large presacral tumor without sacral invasion (*arrows*). **a** Axial T2-weighted image. Hyperintense lesion. **b** Axial T1-weighted image postcontrast. Peripheral irregular enhancement

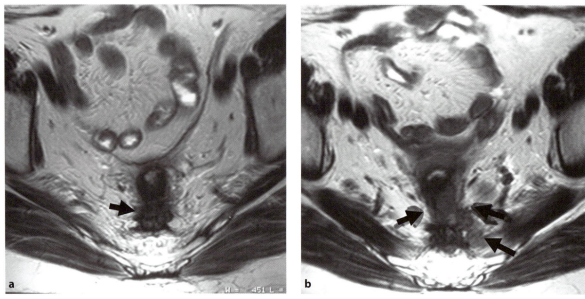

Fig. 22 a, b. **a** Axial T2-weighted image. Postradiation. Presacral inflammatory changes (*arrow*). **b** Axial T2-weighted image. Patient complained of back pain. Presacral recurrence 3 months later. Larger and heterogeneous lesion, mostly with isointense signal (*arrows*)

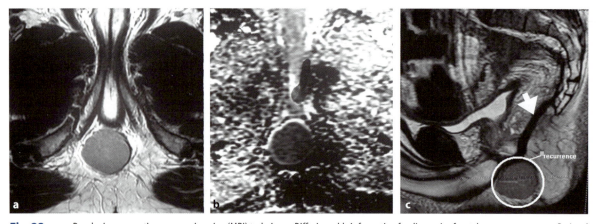

Fig. 23 a-c. Developing magnetic resonance imaging (MRI) techniques. Diffusion adds information for diagnosis of rectal cancer recurrence. **a** Perineal recurrence nodule has isointense signal at T2 weighting and **b** restricted diffusion at apparent diffusion coefficient map. **c** Postsurgical and radiation changes after a rectal excision (Miles operation) (*arrow*) is well seen on sagittal T2-weighted plane

References

1. Ministério da Saúde (2006) Instituto Nacional de Câncer. Estimativa de Câncer no Brasil. www.inca.org.br/estimativa/2006. Cited 23 Sep 2007
2. National Cancer Institute (2007). Estimated new cases and death for rectal cancer 2007. www.cancer.gov/cancertopics/types/colon-and-rectal. Cited 29 Sep 2007
3. Corman ML (1998) Carcinoma of the colon. In: Corman ML (ed). Colon and rectal surgery, 4th edn. Lippincott-Raven, Philadelphia
4. Cohen AM, Winaver SJ Friedman, MA, Gunderson LL (1995) Cancer of the colon rectum and anus. McGraw-Hill, New York
5. Fleming ID, ed (1997) American Joint Committee on Cancer, American Cancer Society, American College of Surgeons. AJCC cancer staging manual, 5th edn. Lippincott-Raven, Philadelphia
6. Wieder HA, Rosenberg R, Lordick F et al (2007) Rectal cancer: MRI before neoadjuvant chemotherapy and radiation for prediction of tumor-free circumferential resection margins and long-term survival. Radiology 243:744-751
7. Klessen C, Rogalla P, Taupitz M (2007) Local staging of rectal cancer: the current role of MRI. Eur Radiol 17(2):379–389

Commentary

Andrew P. Zbar

This chapter expertly outlines the technical factors and outcome-related variables involved in successfully managing patients with low rectal cancers, where magnetic resonance imaging (MRI) is an integral part of the surgical decision-making algorithm. Given the standardization of surgical rectal cancer therapy, the specific advantage of accurate preoperative imaging of this tumour is in the delineation of cases likely to benefit from neoadjuvant therapies designed to provide negative circumferential resection margins (CRMs) in the context of an expertly performed total mesorectal excision (TME) [1–3]. The advantages of this approach, although never subjected to a formal controlled, randomized trial [4], have provided a standard of care that has substantially reduced the incidence of locoregional recurrence in individual units where it has been introduced [5, 6], as well as in units where formal TME training and preoperative staging have been initiated [7]. Along with this surgical gold standard, there has been validation with resected specimens of thin-slice, high spatial resolution MRI that are predictive of the likelihood of successful TME in experienced hands [8–11]. This technique, introduced by Brown and colleagues, provides MRI of high quality with an acceptable signal-to-noise ratio; rapid acquisition speed and high resolution with stronger gradients, which enhance signaling; better image sequencing software (for short-tau inversion recovery and fat saturation T1-weighted images); along with improvements in dedicated multiple-element coil arrays [12]. This technique has supported TME where

the preoperative detection of pelvic side wall and prostate invasion necessitates downstaging therapy to achieve a clear lymphovascular package [13, 14] and where imaging is predictive of close resection margins that extend to within 1 mm of the mesorectal fascia. The imaging also provides insight into selected cases where extended lymphadenectomy with curative intent may be indicated [15, 16]. This view is supplemented by contrast-enhanced semiquantitative recalled sequences that have a moderate sensitivity for detecting locoregional recurrence, particularly when involving the pelvic side wall [17, 18].

The recently reported fused data from 11 separate European centers examining the predictive benefit of preoperative high-resolution MRI – the MagnEtic Resonance Imaging and Rectal Cancer EURopean Equivalence StudY (MERCURY Study) – has defined high-risk cases for locoregional recurrence where extramural spread exceeds 5 mm, where there is demonstrable extramural venous invasion, nodal involvement, and peritoneal infiltration [19] and has prospectively examined the depth of tumour invasion and predicted CRM involvement in low rectal cancers [20]. In these initial analyses, MRI and histopathology agreed on the extramural depth to within 0.5 mm [21]. Given the recent evidence that the technique needs to be modified to widen the perineal extent of resection in abdominoperineal excision [22], it remains to be seen what impact high-resolution MRI will have on local recurrence rates after institution of the "new" cancer surgery [23].

References

1. Heald RJ, Ryall RD (1986) Recurrence and survival after total mesorectal excision for rectal cancer. Lancet i:1479–1482
2. Quirke P, Durdey P, Dixon MF, Williams NS (1986) Local recurrence of rectal adenocarcinoma due to inadequate surgical resection: histopathological study of lateral tumour spread and surgical excision. Lancet ii:996–999
3. Dahlberg M, Stenbourg A, Pahlman L, Glimelius B, Swedish Rectal Cancer Trial (2002) Cost-effectiveness of preoperative radiotherapy in rectal cancer: results for the Swedish Rectal Cancer Trial. Int J Radiat Oncol Biol Phys 54:654–660
4. Polglase AL, McMurrick PJ, Tremayne AP, Bhathal PS (2001) Local recurrence after curative anterior resection with principally blunt dissection for carcinoma of the rectum and rectosigmoid. Dis Colon Rectum 44:947–954
5. Heald RJ, Moran BJ, Ryall RD et al (1998) Rectal cancer: the Basingstoke experience of total mesorectal excision, 1978–1997. Arch Surg 133:894–899
6. Chiappa A, Biffi R, Zbar AP et al (2005) Results of treatment of distal rectal carcinoma since the introduction of total mesorectal excision: a single unit experience, 1994–2003. Int J Colorect Dis 20:221–230

7. Martling AL, Holm T, Rutqvist LE (2000) Effect of a surgical training programme on outcome of rectal cancer in the County of Stockholm. Stockholm Colorectal Cancer Study Group, Basingstoke Bowel Cancer Research Project. Lancet 356:93–96

8. Hermanek P (1999) Impact of surgeon's technique on outcome after treatment of rectal carcinoma. Dis Colon Rectum 42:559–562

9. Beets-Tan RG, Beets GL, Vliegen RF et al (2001) Accuracy of magnetic resonance imaging in prediction of tumour-free resection margin in rectal cancer surgery. Lancet 357(9255):497–504

10. Brown G, Radcliffe AG, Newcombe RG et al (2003) Preoperative assessment of prognostic factors in rectal cancer using high-resolution magnetic resonance imaging. Br J Surg 90:355–64

11. Brown G, Zbar AP (2005) MRI in colorectal surgery: surface magnetic resonance imaging in anorectal practice. In: Complex anorectal disorders: investigation and management. Wexner SD, Zbar AP, Pescatori M (eds) Springer-Verlag, Berlin pp 275–297

12. Kim MJ, Park JS, Park SI et al (2003) Accuracy in differentiation of mucinous and non-mucinous rectal carcinoma on MR imaging. J Comput Assit Tomogr 27:48–55

13. Bissett IP, Fernando CC, Hough DM et al (2001) Identification of the fascia propria by magnetic resonance imaging and its relevance to preoperative assessment of rectal cancer. Dis Colon Rectum 44:259–265

14. Kremser C, Judmaier W, Hein P et al (2003) Preliminary results on the influence of chemoradiation on apparent diffusion coefficients of primary rectal carcinoma measured by magnetic resonance imaging. Strahlenther Onkol 179:641–649

15. Watanabe T, Tsurita G, Muto T et al (2002) Extended lymphadenectomy and preoperative radiotherapy for lower rectal cancers. Surgery 132:27–33

16. Brown G, Richards CJ, Bourne NW et al (2003) Morphologic predictors of lymph node status in rectal cancer with use of high-spatial-resolution MR imaging with histopathologic comparison. Radiology 227:371–377

17. Robinson P, Carrington BM, Swindell R et al (2002) Recurrence or residual pelvic bowel cancer: accuracy of MRI local extent before salvage surgery. Clin Radiol 57:514–522

18. Torricelli P, Pecchi A, Luppi G, Romagnoli R (2003) Gadolinium-enhanced MRI with dynamic evaluation in diagnosing local recurrence of rectal cancer. Abdom Imaging 28:19–27

19. Brown G, Daniels IR (2005) Preoperative staging of rectal cancer: the MERCURY research project. Recent results. Cancer Res 165:58–74

20. Salerno G, Daniels IR, Moran et al (2006) Clarifying margins in the multidisciplinary management of rectal cancer: the MERCURY experience. Clin Radiol 61:916–923

21. MERCURY Study Group (2007) Extramural depth of tumor invasion at thin-section MR in patients with rectal cancer: results of the MERCURY study. Radiology 243:132–139

22. Marr R, Birbeck K, Garvican J et al (2005) The modern abdominoperineal excision. The next challenge after total mesorectal excision. Ann Surg 242:74–82

23. Daniels IR, Strassburg J, Moran BJ (2006) The need for future surgical low rectal cancer studies. Colorectal Dis 8(Suppl 3):25–29

CHAPTER 14

Pelvic Primary and Metastatic Tumors: Computed Tomography Images

Ana Karina Nascimento Borges, Alexandre Cecin, Rafael Darahem, Armando Melani

Abstract

Modern computed tomography (CT), particularly with the now readily available compatible software, is an important imaging technique for diagnosing and evaluating many different types of pelvic neoplasms. Multidetector scanners that permit coronal- and sagittal-plane isotropic image reconstruction, provide a distinct advantage over magnetic resonance imaging, particularly for imaging the rectum and bladder, and may redefine the role of CT imaging of the pelvis. In this chapter, we discuss our routine protocol for single-slice scanners with contrast-enhanced helical acquisition in relation to the specific organ being examined. We also discuss some benign and malignant pelvic tumors encountered in our clinical practice and studied using CT imaging.

Introduction

Computed tomography (CT) is useful in the imaging evaluation of many pelvic tumors. Although we strongly favor magnetic resonance imaging (MRI) in some conditions, such as lower rectal and anal canal neoplasms and uterine cervix tumors, CT still has a role in the diagnosis and staging of many other neoplasms. The development and more widespread availability of multidetector scanners may redefine the role of CT imaging of the pelvis [1], particularly for rectal and bladder imaging, as it allows isotropic image reconstruction in the coronal and sagittal

planes, which is an inherent advantage of MRI. Our routine protocol for a single-slice scanner consists of a contrast-enhanced helical acquisition with 5- to 7-mm collimation after oral administration of contrast medium. Some modifications are made depending on the specific organ to be studied, e.g., rectal contrast medium for intestinal disorders. In this chapter, we depict and discuss some pelvic benign and malignant tumors seen in our clinical practice.

Sacral Meningocele

Anterior sacral meningocele is a rare congenital malformation consisting of a spinal fluid-filled sac in the pelvis communicating by a small neck with the spinal subarachnoid space through a sacral defect (Fig. 1). Anterior meningoceles manifest as asymptomatic or symptomatic pelvic masses and may be associated with partial sacral agenesis. These lesions of the sacrum are optimally imaged with MRI, although plain radiography or CT is used to assess the associated osseous defects [2].

Osteosarcoma

Pelvic osteosarcoma constitutes 4–10% of all osteosarcomas (Fig. 2). The peak incidence is in the second decade of life, and there is a second peak in the eighth decade secondary to Paget's disease. The prognosis is poor for patients with secondary osteosarcomas and for all those with metastases at presentation [3].

M. Pescatori, F.S.P. Regadas, S.M. Murad Regadas, A.P. Zbar (eds.), *Imaging Atlas of the Pelvic Floor and Anorectal Diseases*. ISBN 978-88-470-0808-3. © Springer-Verlag Italia 2008

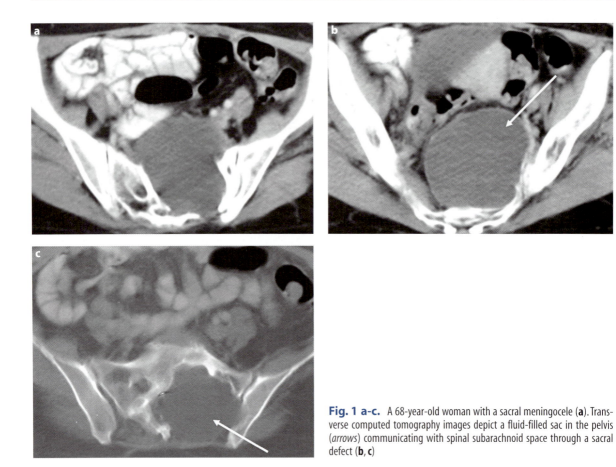

Fig. 1 a-c. A 68-year-old woman with a sacral meningocele (**a**). Transverse computed tomography images depict a fluid-filled sac in the pelvis (*arrows*) communicating with spinal subarachnoid space through a sacral defect (**b**, **c**)

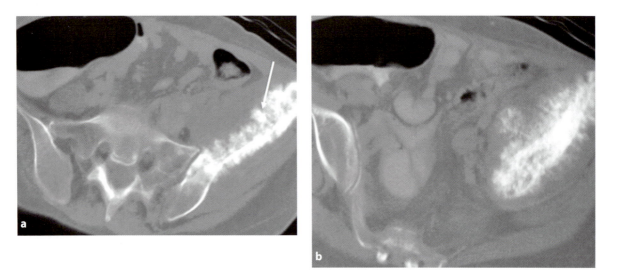

Fig. 2 a, b. A 56-year-old woman with a pelvic osteosarcoma. Axial computed tomography images show an osteoblastic lesion of the left iliac wing with extensive bone destruction (*arrows*)

Bladder Cancer

About 90% of all malignant tumors of the bladders originate from the transitional-cell urothelium (Figs. 3–5); 5% are squamous cell carcinoma, and 2% are adenocarcinomas, the latter of which is associated with cystitis glandularis (Fig. 6). Nonepithelial neoplasms make up less than 5% of malignant bladder tumors. The most common of these tumors is leiomyosarcoma, followed by lymphoma. CT and MRI are used for staging bladder tumors, demonstrating deeper invasion into the perivesical fat or extension to adjacent organs, such as the prostate, seminal vesicles, rectum, and pelvic sidewall [4]. Bladder tumors can be either papillary, sessile, or invasive in growth pattern. The use of intravenous contrast medium is of paramount importance for detecting small tumors.

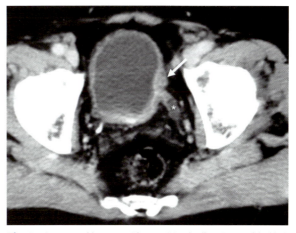

Fig. 3. A 61-year-old woman with a transitional-cell carcinoma of the bladder. Axial computed tomography image shows wall thickening on the left posterolateral aspect of the bladder, with tumor extension to the perivesical fat (*arrow*) and left ureter (*asterisk*), which is dilated

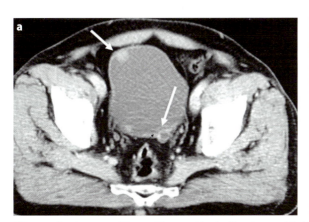
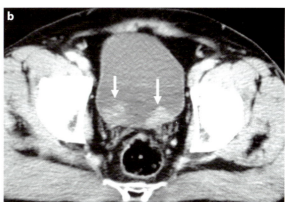

Fig. 4 a, b. A 69-year-old man with a transitional-cell carcinoma of the bladder. Axial contrast-enhanced computed tomography images show multifocal enhancing lesions of the bladder wall (*arrows*)

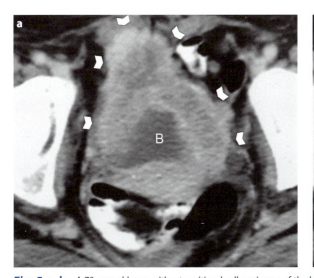
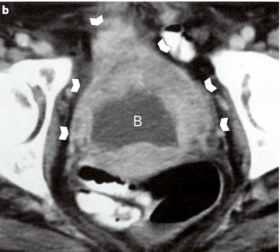

Fig. 5 a, b. A 78-year-old man with a transitional-cell carcinoma of the bladder. Axial contrast-enhanced images show tumor presenting as diffuse bladder-wall thickening (*arrowheads*). There is tumoral invasion of perivesical fat. *B* bladder

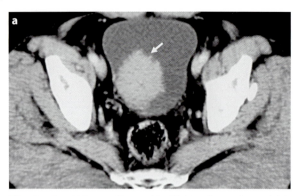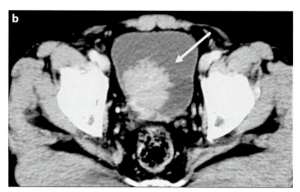

Fig. 6 a, b. A 57-year-old man with a bladder adenocarcinoma. Axial contrast-enhanced computed tomography images show a large polypoid mass arising from the right lateral bladder wall (*arrows*)

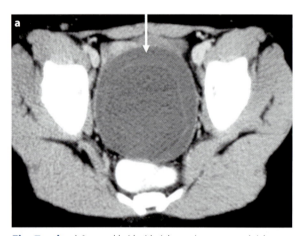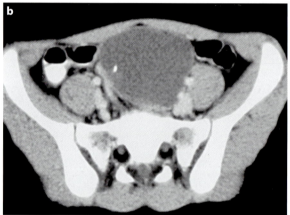

Fig. 7 a, b. A 9-year-old girl with right ovarian teratoma. Axial computed tomography images show a hypodense mass (*arrow*) with no evidence of intralesional fat

Ovarian Germ Cell Tumors

Germ cell tumors of the ovary account for 15–25% of all ovarian tumors [5]. This group includes mature teratoma (Fig. 7), immature teratoma (Fig, 8), dysgerminoma, endodermal sinus tumor (Fig. 9), embryonal carcinoma, and choriocarcinoma [6]. Of these, only mature teratoma is benign. It is by far the most common lesion of this group. Less than 1% of teratomas are malignant. Mature cystic teratomas are composed of well-differentiated derivations from all three germ-cell layers (ectoderm, mesoderm, endoderm). It occurs typically during reproductive age and is easily diagnosed with CT by the presence of fat, fluid, and calcifications. This tumor may be bilateral in 10% of cases. The presence of a fatty component

with or without calcification is diagnostic for a cystic mature teratoma. Fat is reported in 93% of cases, and teeth or calcifications are reported in 56%. A minority of teratomas has no evidence of fat upon imaging [5]. Complications include torsion, rupture, pelvic pain, hydronephrosis, and malignant degeneration.

Dysgerminomas are rare ovarian tumors that occur predominantly in young women. About 20% of cases are diagnosed during pregnancy, and 80% occur in women younger than 30 years of age. Yolk-sac tumors (also known as endodermal sinus tumors) – the second most common germ-cell tumors, accounting for 20% of all cases – are common in girls and young adults (average age 19 years). Less common germ-cell tumors are embryonal carcinoma, choriocarcinoma, polyembryomas, and mixed germ-cell tumors.

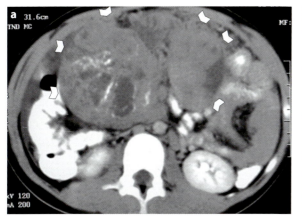
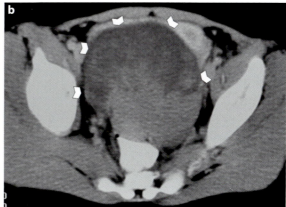
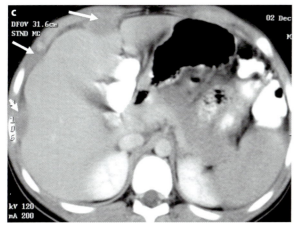

Fig. 8 a-c. An 11-year-old girl with ovarian immature teratoma with areas of dysgerminoma and embryonal carcinoma. **a, b** Axial contrast-enhanced computed tomography (CT) images through the midabdomen and pelvis show a large heterogeneous solid-cystic mass (*arrowheads*) with foci of calcifications. **c** Upper abdomen CT image shows perihepatic tumor implants (*arrows*)

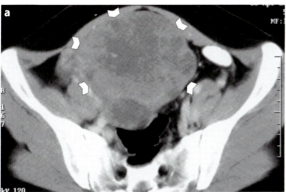
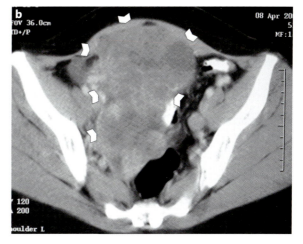
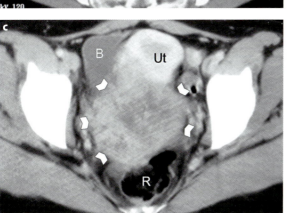

Fig. 9 a-c. A 22-year-old woman with endodermal sinus tumor of the right ovary. Axial contrast-enhanced computed tomography images through the pelvis show a large heterogeneous solid mass (*arrowheads*). The rectum (*R*), bladder (*B*) and uterus (*Ut*) are annotated for anatomical reference. This patient had peritoneal implants upon exploratory laparotomy

Epithelial Ovarian Tumors

Epithelial tumors represent 60% of all ovarian neoplasms and 85% of malignant ovarian neoplasms [6]. Subtypes of epithelial tumors include serous, mucinous, endometrioid, clear-cell, and Brenner tumors (Figs. 10–12). The two most common types are serous and mucinous. They cannot be easily differentiated on the basis of CT, MRI, or sonographic imaging. Benign cystadenomas manifests as a unilocular or multilocular cystic mass with homogeneous CT attenuation and no endocystic or exocystic vegetation. Solid papillary projections, thick septa, thick and irregular walls, and solid component with necrosis are suggestive of a malignant tumor. Ancillary findings of pelvic-organ invasion, implants, ascites, and adenopathy increase diagnostic confidence for malignancy. Most Brenner tumors are benign, accounting for 4–5% of benign surface epithelial–stromal tumors [7]. Brenner tumors have a frequent association with mucinous cystic tumors in the same ovary (Fig. 13). Malignant Brenner tumors are extremely rare. In contrast to benign Brenner tumors, borderline or malignant Brenner tumors have cystic and solid appearances at gross examination (Fig. 14).

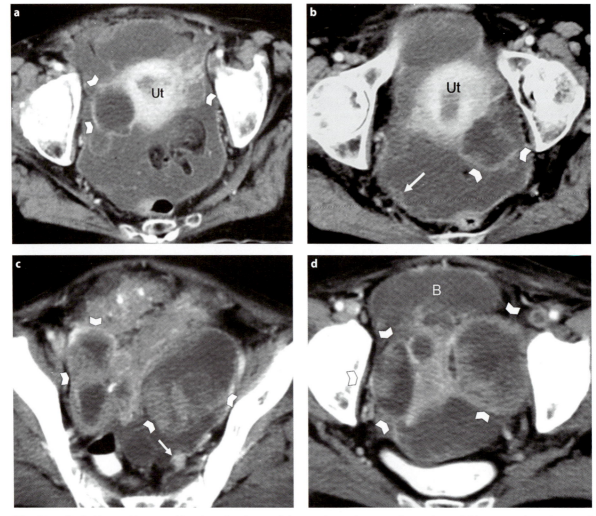

Fig. 10 a-d. An 89-year-old woman with peritoneal carcinomatosis from ovarian mucinous cystadenocarcinoma. Axial contrast-enhanced computed tomography images show bilateral ovarian masses (*arrowheads*) and peritoneal implants (*arrow*). *B* bladder, *Ut* uterus

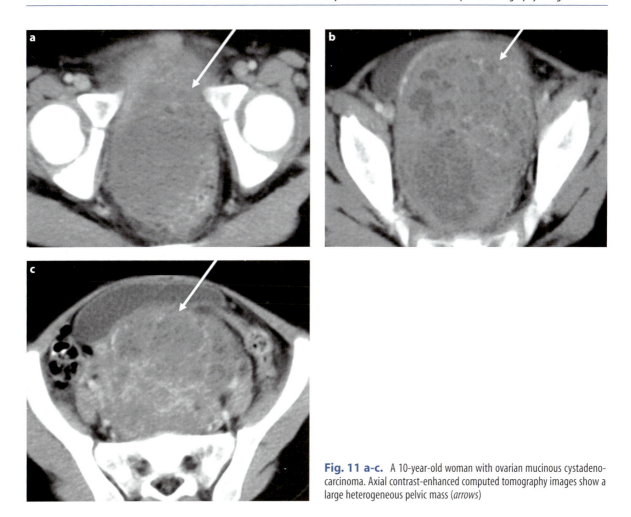

Fig. 11 a-c. A 10-year-old woman with ovarian mucinous cystadeno-carcinoma. Axial contrast-enhanced computed tomography images show a large heterogeneous pelvic mass (*arrows*)

Fig. 12 a, b. A 76-year-woman with peritoneal recurrence of a previously resected ovarian serous cystadenocarcinoma. Axial contrast-enhanced computed tomography images show a large hypodense pelvic mass (*arrows*). *B* bladder, *Ut* uterus

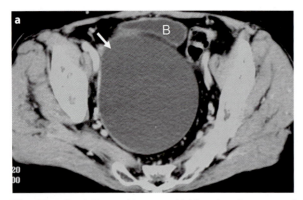
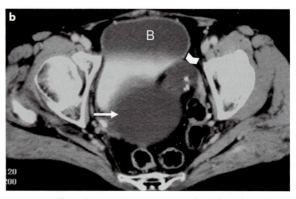

Fig. 13 a, b. A 69-year-old woman with bilateral ovarian tumors, a Brenner tumor with mucinous cystic component on the right and a mucinous cystadenoma on the left. **a** Axial contrast-enhanced computed tomography (CT) image shows a hypodense mass of the right ovary (*arrow*). **b** Axial contrast-enhanced CT image shows a hypodense lesion with internal calcifications on the left ovary (*arrowhead*). *B* bladder

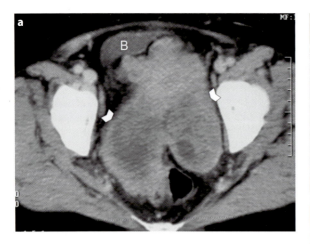
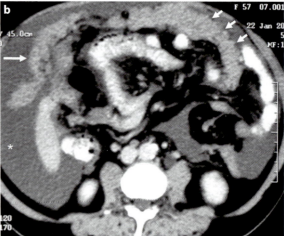

Fig. 14 a, b. A 57-year-old woman with bilateral Brenner tumor and peritoneal metastases. **a** Axial contrast-enhanced computed tomography (CT) image shows bilateral solid-cystic ovarian masses (*arrowheads*). **b** Axial contrast-enhanced CT image though the midabdomen shows omental thickening and nodularity (*arrows*), consistent with tumoral implants, associated with ascites (*asterisk*). *B* bladder

Pelvic Metastatic Peritoneal Disease

Metastatic disease involving the pelvic peritoneum and omentum is commonly seen in patients with primary neoplasms of the ovary, colon, pancreas, and stomach (Fig. 15). Metastases have a varied appearance at CT imaging. They can present as soft tissue nodules varying in size from a few millimeters to several centimeters, as large plaque-like lesions in the peritoneum, and as thickening of the omentum ("omental cake"). Metastases from primary mucinous tumor (ovary and colon adenocarcinoma) can be cystic in appearance. Ascites is a commonly associated finding. Other solid intraperitoneal entities to be considered in the differential diagnosis of peritoneal masses are desmoid tumor, carcinoid tumor, lymphoma, peritoneal mesotheliomas, and tuberculosis.

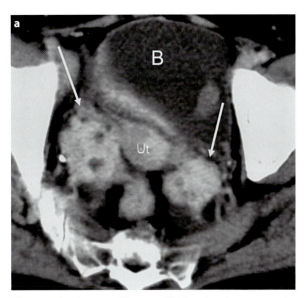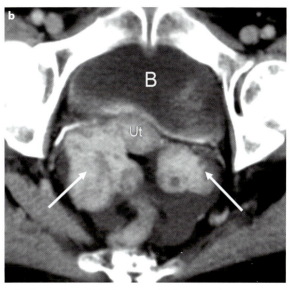

Fig. 15 a, b. A 75-year-old woman with bilateral ovarian metastases from gastric adenocarcinoma Krukenberg tumor. Axial contrast-enhanced computed tomography images show bilateral ovarian enlargement (*arrows*). *B* bladder, *Ut* uterus

References

1. Kulinna C, Eibel R, Matzek W et al (2004) Staging of rectal cancer: diagnostic potential of multiplanar reconstructions with MDCT. AJR Am J Roentgenol 183:421–427
2. Diel J, Ortiz O, Losada RA et al (2001) The sacrum: pathologic spectrum, multimodality imaging, and subspecialty approach. Radiographics 21:83–104
3. Grimer RJ, Carter SR, Tillman RM et al (1999) Osteosarcoma of the pelvis. J Bone Joint Surg Br 81(5):796–802
4. Kim JK, Park SY, Ahn HJ et al (2004) Bladder cancer: analysis of multi-detector row helical CT enhancement pattern and accuracy in tumor detection and perivesical staging. Radiology 231:725–731
5. Outwater KO, Siegelman ES, Hunt JL (2001) Ovarian teratomas: tumor types and imaging characteristics. Radiographics 21:475–490
6. Jung SE, Lee JM, Rha SE et al (2002) CT and MR imaging of ovarian tumors with emphasis on differential diagnosis. Radiographics 22:1305–1325
7. Imaoka I, Wada A, Kaji Y et al (2006) Developing an MR imaging strategy for diagnosis of ovarian masses. Radiographics 26:1431–1448

Commentary

Andrew P. Zbar

In this chapter, Borges and colleagues expertly outline their experience in modern CT scanning for pelvic malignancies, presacral masses, and abdominopelvic pseudotumors. There is no doubt that the recent capacity for sagittal reconstruction in particular, with readily available CT software, has provided great advantage in assessing specific pelvic tumors, most notably in recurrent rectal cancer and presacral tumors, by an ability to define operability and the presence of attendant presacral osseous infiltration [1, 2]. In this group of relatively rare tumors, it also provides sufficient soft tissue contrast, permitting some delineation of histopathogenesis [3] and thereby assisting in overall management and operative decision making concerning the surgical approach [4]. As correctly suggested by the authors, the demonstration of a cystic sacral meningocele is best assessed by MRI because of its better delineation of comorbid sacral agenesis and as part of the Currarino triad of presacral cysts, sacrococcygeal anomalies, and anorectal malformations [5].

CT has been shown to have specific utility in the preoperative staging of colon cancer [6], although it has less sensitivity than MRI in decision making regarding preoperative adjuvant therapy for rectal cancer [7]. As described by the authors, CT scanning is part of the standard algorithm for preoperative staging assessment of non-transitional-cell carcinomas of the urinary tract [8], providing valuable information in both the nephrographic and excretory phases [9], in defining major vascular involvement

by pelvic tumors [10], and important information in volume assessment of peritoneal carcinomatosis as a preliminary to peritonectomy and intraperitoneal chemotherapy [11, 12]. In this respect, standard CT scanning has the lowest sensitivity in the pelvis, particularly when lesions are <5 mm in maximal diameter [13]. The newer-generation scanners now provide submillimeter similarity analysis with digitally reconstructed [14] and sagittal and coronal reformations, particularly in delineating small liver lesions [15]. This new technology has recently shown specific advantage in virtual reconstruction of phantom pelvic masses [16].

The new fluorodeoxyglucose positron emission tomography (FDG-PET) CT fusion images (discussed elsewhere in this book) have specific advantage in the assessment of recurrent pelvic tumors following neoadjuvant therapy, distinguishing between biologically active tumor deposits with semiquantitative FDG uptake and areas of clinical desmoplastic response [17–19]. Recent data suggest distinct advantage in ovarian carcinoma of fusion images when there is a rising cancer antigen 125 (CA-125) and negative conventional imaging [20, 21] as well as in radiotherapeutic planning/simulation for advanced pelvic cancers [22]. These advantages are supplemented by high-resolution reconstructions in pediatric malignancies [23, 24], intra-abdominal desmoids [25], primary and recurrent retroperitoneal sarcoma [26], and various abdominopelvic pseudotumors [27, 28].

References

1. Soye I, Levine E, Banitzky S, Price HI (1982) Computed tomography of sacral and presacral lesions. Neuroradiology 24:71-76
2. Wolpert A, Beer-Gabel M, Lifschitz O, Zbar AP (2002) The management of presacral masses in the adult. Techn Coloprctol 6:43-49
3. Dozois RR (1990) Retrorectal tumors: spectrum of disease, diagnosis and surgical management. Perspect Colon Rectal Surg 3:241-255
4. Bohm B, Milsom JW, Fazio VW et al (1993) Our approach to the management of congenital presacral tumors in adults. Int J Colorect Dis 8:134-138

5. Currarino G, Coln D, Votteler T (1981) Triad of anorectal, sacral and presacral anomalies. AJR Am J Roentgenol 137:395-398
6. Zbar AP, Rambarat C, Shenoy RK (2007) Routine preoperative abdominal computed tomography in colon cancer: a utility study. Techn Coloproctol 11:105-110
7. MERCURY Study Group (2007) Extramural depth of tumor invasion at thin-section MR in patients with rectal cancer: results of the MERCURY study. Radiology 243:132-139
8. Yeoman LJ, Mason MD, Olliff JF (1991) Non-

Hodgkin's lymphoma of the bladder – CT and MRI appearances. Clin Radiol 44:389-392

9. Chow LC, Kwan SW, Olcott EW, Sommer G (2007) Split-bolus MDCT urography with synchronous nephrographic and excretory phase enhancement. AJR Am J Roentgenol 189:314-322

10. Umeoka S, Koyama T, Togashi K et al (2004) Vascular dilatation in the pelvis: identification with CT and MR imaging. RadioGraphics 24:193-208

11. Petsieau SR, Jelinek JS, Sugarbaker PH (2002) Abdominal and pelvic CT for detection and volume assessment of peritoneal sarcomatosis. Tumori 88:209-214

12. Inniss M, Sandiford N, Shenoy RK et al (2005) Carcinoma of the jejunum with multideposit peritoneal seeding. Resection and intraperitoneal chemotherapy. West Indian Med J 54:242-246

13. Jacquet P, Jelinek JS, Steves MA, Sugarbaker PH (1993) Evaluation of computed tomography in patients with peritoneal carcinomatosis. Cancer 72:1631-1636

14. Kim J, Li S, Pradhan D et al (2007) Comparison of similarity measures for rigid-body CT/dual X-ray image registrations. Technol Cancer Res Treat 6:337-346

15. Sandrasegaran K, Rydberg J, Tann M et al (2007) Benefits of routine use of coronal and sagittal reformations in multi-slice CT examination of the abdomen and pelvis. Clin Radiol 62:340-347

16. Russell ST, Kawashima A, Vrtiska TJ et al (2005) Three-dimensional CT virtual endoscopy in the detection of simulated tumors in a novel phantom bladder and ureter model. J Endourol 19:188-192

17. Schaffler GJ, Groell R, Schoellnast H et al (2000) Digital image fusion of CT and PET data sets – clinical value in abdominal/pelvic malignancies. J Comput Assist Tomogr 24:644–647

18. Schaefer O, Langer M (2007) Detection of recurrent rectal cancer with CT, MRI and PET/CT. Eur Radiol 17:2044-2054

19. Capirci C, Rampin L, Erba PA et al (2007) Sequential FDG-PET/CT reliably predicts response of locally advanced rectal cancer to neo-adjuvant chemoradiation therapy. Eur J Nucl Med Mol Imaging 34:1583–1593

20. Kubik-Huch RA, Dorffler W, von Schulthess GK et al (2000) Value of (18F)-FDG positron emission tomography, computed tomography and magnetic resonance imaging in diagnosing primary and recurrent ovarian carcinoma. Eur Radiol 10:761-767

21. Thrall MM, DeLoia JA, Gallion H, Avril N (2007) Clinical use of combined positron emission tomography and computed tomography (FDG PET/CT) in recurrent ovarian cancer. Gynecol Oncol 105:17–22

22. Li XA, Qi XS, Pitterle M et al (2007) Interfractional variations in patient setup and anatomic change assessed by daily computed tomography. Int Radiat Oncol Biol Phys 68:581–591

23. Tannous WN, Azouz EM, Homsy YL et al (1989) CT and ultrasound imaging of pelvic rhabdomyosarcoma in children. A review of 56 patients. Pediatr Radiol 19:530-534

24. Rice HE, Frush DP, Harker MJ et al (2007) APSA Education Committee. Peer assessment of pediatric surgeons for potential risks of radiation exposure from computed tomography scans. J Pediatr Surg 42:1157-1564

25. Kreuzberg B, Koudelova J, Ferda et al (2007) Diagnostic problems of abdominal desmoid tumors in various locations. Eur J Radiol 62:180-185

26. Chiappa A, Zbar AP, Biffi R et al (2004) Primary and recurrent retroperitoneal sarcoma: factors affecting survival and long-term outcome. Hepatogastroenterology 51:1304–1309

27. Bercovich A, Guy M, Karayiannakis AJ (2003) Ureteral obstruction and reconstruction in pelvic actinomycosis. Urology 61:224 (iv–vii)

28. Li Y, Yang ZG, Guo YK et al (2007) Distribution and characteristics of hematogenous disseminated tuberculosis within the abdomen on contrast-enhanced CT. Abdom Imaging 32:484-488

CHAPTER 15

Magnetic Resonance Imaging of Pelvic Primary and Metastatic Tumors

Rafael Darahem, Alexandre Cecin, Ana Karina Nascimento Borges, Armando Melani

Abstract

The excellent anatomic details and soft-tissue contrast obtained on magnetic resonance imaging (MRI) makes the technique extremely useful for diagnosing and staging pelvic tumors. MRI allows determination of the neoplasm's origin and aids in the extensive differential diagnosis of pelvic tumors, which may develop in the genitourinary or gastrointestinal systems, peritoneum, retroperitoneum, soft tissues, bone, and lymph nodes, as well as from metastases. MRI is a valuable tool for preoperative evaluation, imaging and characterizing lesions, estimating their extent and the risk of malignancy, distinguishing organ-confined disease from tumor spread into adjacent pelvic structures and inguinal lymph node involvement, and deciding upon the most appropriate intervention strategies and imaging follow-up requirements. It is also the most effective imaging technique for determining the extent of bone marrow involvement by conventional chondrosarcoma. In this chapter, we discuss the use of MRI imaging in several types of pelvic tumors.

Introduction

Magnetic resonance imaging (MRI) is often used in diagnosing and staging pelvic tumors, as it provides excellent anatomic detail and soft-tissue contrast. Pelvic tumors may arise from the genitourinary system (uterus, ovaries, fallopian tubes, vagina, bladder, prostate), gastrointestinal system, peritoneum, retroperitoneum, soft tissues, bone, and lymph nodes, or from metastases [1]. Therefore, we face a very extensive differential diagnosis when studying pelvic tumors. The first issue is determining the organ of origin of the mass. Even though this topographic diagnosis is usually straightforward, one may encounter problems when evaluating large tumors (in excess of 5 cm) [1]. The next step is estimating the risk of malignancy of the mass, as this will aid in indicating intervention or imaging follow-up. A third issue is defining the extent of the lesion, i.e. staging, as this may define the subsequent method of therapy. A useful approach to characterizing pelvic tumors is to topographically sort out the various lesions, some of which are briefly discussed and illustrated here.

Genitourinary Neoplasms

The most frequent uterine neoplasm is the leiomyoma, which is of mesenchymal origin (Fig. 1). Leiomyomas are benign tumors classified as intramural, submucosal, or subserosal depending on their location. A subserosal leiomyoma may cause some diagnostic difficulty, as it can be mistaken for an adnexal mass on imaging. Submucosal leiomyomas may prolapse through the uterine cervix, becoming clinically evident at vaginal inspection (Fig. 2). The differential diagnosis for this type of presentation is a giant endometrial polyp, another benign neoplasm (Fig. 3). Endometrial cancer is the most common cancer of the female genital tract in developed countries. MRI plays a role in preoperative evaluation of theses patients, allowing assessment of myometrial invasion, metastases, and adenopathy (Fig. 4). It may be also be useful in de-

M. Pescatori, F.S.P. Regadas, S.M. Murad Regadas, A.P. Zbar (eds.), *Imaging Atlas of the Pelvic Floor and Anorectal Diseases*.
ISBN 978-88-470-0808-3. © Springer-Verlag Italia 2008

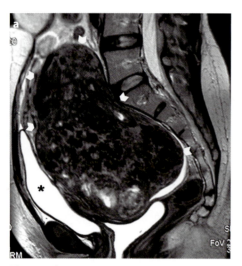
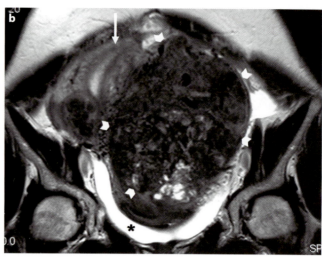

Fig. 1 a, b. A 46-year-old woman with uterine leiomyomas. **a** Sagittal and **b** coronal fast spin-echo T2-weighted images show massive uterine enlargement (*arrowheads*) due to multiple heterogeneous myometrial fibroids. Uterine cavity is displaced to the right in **b** (*arrow*), and the bladder is compressed anteriorly (*)

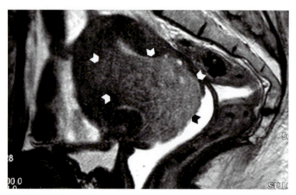

Fig. 2. A 41-year-old woman with a prolapsed uterine leiomyoma. Sagittal fast spin-echo T2-weighted image shows a moderately hyperintense lesion (*arrowheads*) originating from the anterior uterine wall and protruding though the endocervical canal into the vagina

tecting and staging local recurrences after treatment. Other less frequent uterine neoplasms are endometrial stromal sarcoma (Fig. 5), carcinosarcoma, and adenosarcoma [1].

Uterine cervix neoplasms are frequent malignancies in developing countries, most of which are of squamous cell type and related to herpes papilloma virus (HPV) infection. MRI is extremely valuable in tumor staging, particularly in evaluating parametrial and adjacent organ invasion, lymph node metastasis, and ureteral obstruction [2] (Figs. 6 and 7). A possible complication of treatment is genitourinary fistula (Fig. 6).

Vulvar neoplasms are generally squamous cell carcinomas and are easily assessed by clinical ex-

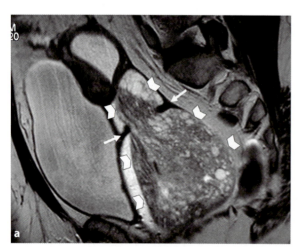
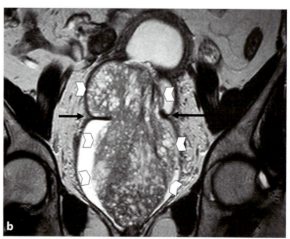

Fig. 3 a, b. A 53-year-old woman with a giant endometrial polyp. **a** Sagittal and **b** coronal fast spin-echo T2-weighted images after administration of intravaginal gel show a large heterogeneous pedunculated mass (*arrowheads*) originating from the uterine cavity and protruding through the cervix (*arrows*) into the vagina, which is markedly distended

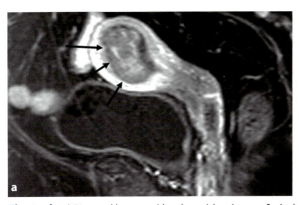

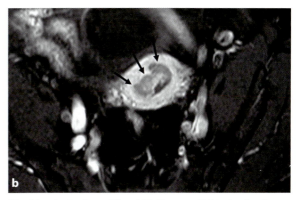

Fig. 4 a, b. A 71-year-old woman with endometrial carcinoma. **a** Sagittal and **b** axial contrast-enhanced T1-weighted images with fat saturation demonstrate a polypoid lesion (*arrows*) arising from the anterior endometrial lining, with marked enhancement

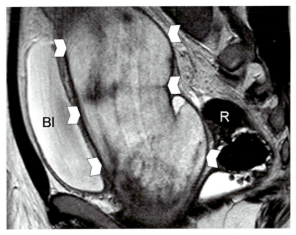

Fig. 5. A 29 year-old woman with high-grade endometrial stromal sarcoma. Sagittal fast spin-echo T2-weighted image shows a large tumor in the endocervical canal and vaginal cavity (*arrowheads*). Rectum (*R*) and bladder (*Bl*) are marked for anatomical reference

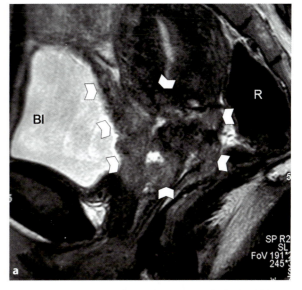

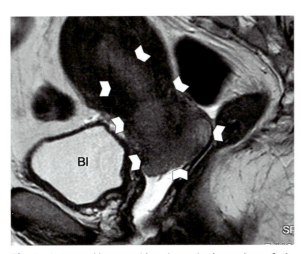

Fig. 7. A 49-year-old woman with uterine cervix adenocarcinoma. Sagittal fast spin-echo T2-weighted image after administration of intravaginal gel depicts a moderately hyperintense lesion (*arrowheads*) involving the endocervical canal, with upward extension to the uterine cavity and downward protrusion to the vagina. The bladder (*Bl*) is not involved

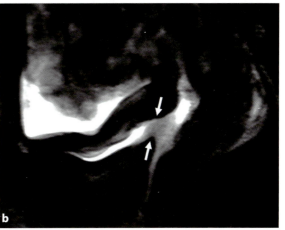

Fig. 6 a, b. A 41-year-old woman with uterine cervix squamous cell carcinoma treated with radiotherapy and studied with magnetic resonance imaging at two different times. **a** Pretreatment sagittal fast spin-echo T2-weighted image shows a large tumor with posterior bladder (*Bl*) wall invasion (*arrowheads*). The rectum (*R*) is not involved by the tumor. **b** Sagittal half-Fourier acquisition single-shot turbo spin-echo image 30 months later shows a large vesicovaginal fistula (*arrows*)

amination when they are small. MRI is suitable for evaluating more locally advanced tumors and assessing the depth of invasion and involvement of adjacent pelvic structures (e.g., anal sphincters) [3] (Fig. 8). A further potential and important role for MRI may lie in assessing tumor spread to the inguinal lymph nodes.

Primary vaginal neoplasms are much less frequent than secondary involvement from neoplasms of the uterus, cervix, bladder, and rectum. Squamous cell carcinomas comprise the majority of primary vaginal neoplasms. Among the rare primary tumors are sarcoma botryoides (Fig. 9) and malignant mixed Müllerian-type tumor (Fig. 10).

Evaluating ovarian masses is a well-established indication of MRI [4]. Its use in these cases includes evaluating morphologic characteristics and signal intensity characteristics on T1- and T2-weighted images [5]. In general, cystic masses represent benign tumors, whereas cystic and solid masses are strongly associated with malignancy (Fig. 11). Predominantly solid masses include benign and malignant tumors. T1-weighted images provide useful information because hemorrhagic adnexal masses (e.g., endometriotic cyst) and cystic teratomas can be correctly diagnosed when the mass has high signal intensity [6] (Fig. 12). Significant low signal intensity in solid masses on T2-weighted images is indicative of fibrothecomas and Brenner tumors because of extensive fibrous tissue in these lesions (Fig. 13). The ovaries are also a frequent site of metastases, particularly from the breast, stomach, and intestines [7] (Fig. 14).

The role of MRI in evaluating and staging prostate cancer is somewhat controversial and is evolving as new techniques, such as MR spectroscopy, come into clinical use. MRI can aid in detecting the presence and location of extracapsular extension (ECE) and seminal-vesicle invasion (SVI), with 13–95% sensitivity and 49–97% specificity for detecting ECE and 23–80% sensitivity and 81–99% specificity for detecting SVI [8]. The combination of tumor at the base of the prostate that extends beyond the capsule and low signal intensity within a seminal vesicle is highly predictive of SVI (Fig. 15).

The most frequent bladder neoplasm is transitional cell carcinoma. Whereas MRI can be useful for diagnosing challenging cases, it is more frequently used for staging (Fig. 16). Preoperative imaging is important in distinguishing organ-confined disease from tumor that has spread outside the bladder [9]. This distinction is relevant because patients with extravesical disease have higher recurrence rates and worse survival rates than patients with organ-confined disease. Patients with urothelial carcinoma may develop recurrences anywhere along the urinary tract (Fig. 17). Rhabdomyosarcoma is the most common bladder tumor in the pediatric age group [10]. These tumors often involve the bladder base. At MRI, rhabdomyosarcoma has low signal intensity on T1-weighted images and high signal intensity on T2-weighted images, with heterogeneous enhancement (Fig. 18).

Urethral tumor is a rare entity. Overall, 80% of male urethral carcinomas are squamous cell carcinoma, 15% are transitional cell carcinoma, and 5% are adenocarcinoma or undifferentiated carcinoma [11]. At MRI, urethral carcinoma is a mass with decreased signal intensity relative to the normal cor-

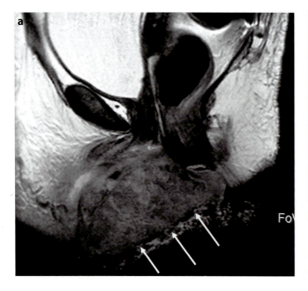
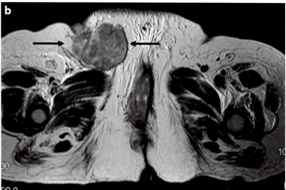

Fig. 8 a, b. A 66-year-old woman with vulvar squamous cell carcinoma. **a** Sagittal fast spin-echo T2-weighted image shows an infiltrative right-sided vulvar lesion (*arrows*) with characteristic moderate to high signal intensity. **b** Axial T2-weighted image shows ipsilateral inguinal metastatic lymphadenopathy (*arrows*)

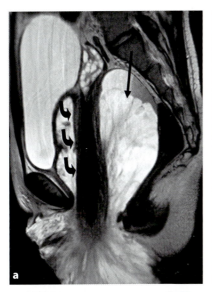

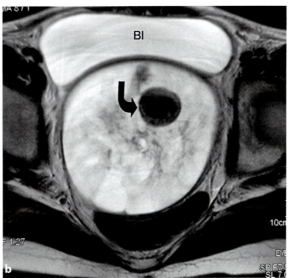

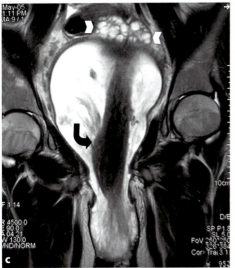

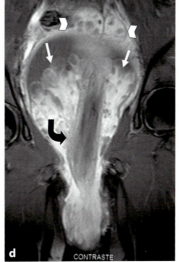

Fig. 9 a-d. A 15-year-old girl with vaginal sarcoma botryoides. **a** Sagittal fast spin-echo T2-weighted image shows vaginal distension from a large heterogeneous mass containing vesicles (*straight arrows*), with vaginal extrusion of its lower portion. The uterus is everted (*curved arrows*) and completely surrounded by the lesion, as confirmed in the **b** axial image. The bladder (*Bl*) is uninvolved by the mass. **c** In the coronal plane , there is retraction and midline displacement of the ovaries (*arrowheads*). **d** Coronal contrast-enhanced T1-weighted image with fat saturation shows intense heterogeneous enhancement of the lesion

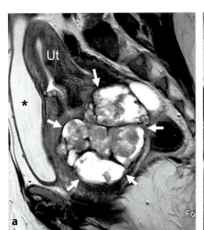

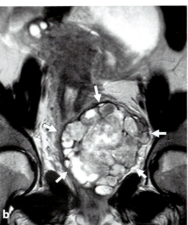

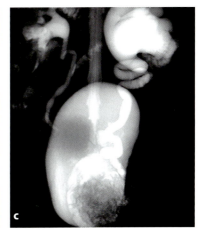

Fig. 10 a-c. A 33-year-old woman with malignant mixed Müllerian tumor of the vagina. **a** Sagittal and **b** coronal fast spin-echo T2-weighted images show a large heterogeneous mass with cystic and solid components occupying the vaginal cavity (*arrows*). The uterus (*Ut*) and bladder (*) are not involved by the mass. **c** Thick-slab half-Fourier acquisition single-shot turbo spin-echo image with fat suppression shows associated bilateral hydronephrosis

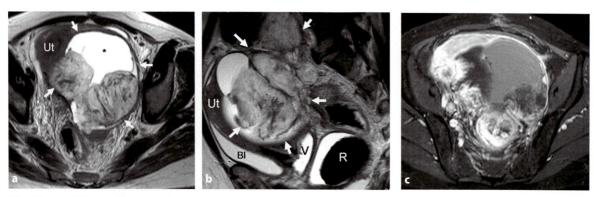

Fig. 11 a-c. A 45-year-old woman with mucinous adenocarcinoma of the left ovary. **a** Axial and **b** sagittal fast spin-echo T2-weighted images show a large left adnexal mass (*arrows*) with cystic (*) and solid components. The uterus (*Ut*) is displaced forward and to the right. The rectum (*R*), vagina (*V*), and bladder (*Bl*) are annotated for anatomical reference. **c** Axial fat-saturated T1-weighted gradient-echo image demonstrates intense heterogeneous enhancement of the solid portions of the tumor

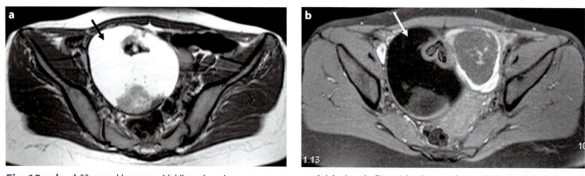

Fig. 12 a, b. A 22-year-old woman with bilateral ovarian mature teratomas. **a** Axial spin-echo T1-weighted image shows a high-signal-intensity mass in the right ovary (*arrow*). **b** Axial fat-saturated T1-weighted gradient-echo image demonstrates saturation of the cyst contents (*arrow*). There is an adjacent left ovarian mass without demonstrable lipid content, which also was proven to be a teratoma

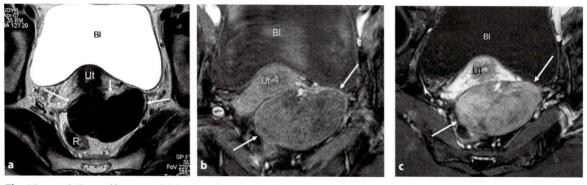

Fig. 13 a-c. A 47-year-old woman with right ovarian fibroma. **a** Axial fast spin-echo T2-weighted image shows a characteristically hypointense retrouterine mass (*arrows*). Axial T1-weighted images with fat saturation **b** before and **c** after contrast administration show weak contrast enhancement of the tumor (*arrows*) compared with that of the myometrium. The rectum (*R*), bladder (*Bl*), and uterus (*Ut*) are annotated for anatomical reference

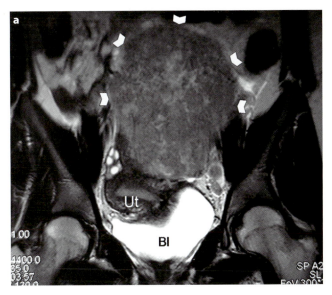
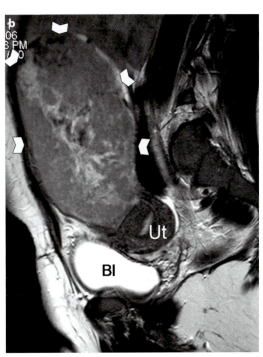

Fig. 14 a, b. An 18-year-old woman with ovarian metastasis from synovial sarcoma. **a** Coronal and **b** sagittal fast spin-echo T2-weighted images demonstrate a large solid left adnexal mass (*arrowheads*). The uterus (*Ut*) is displaced inferiorly and to the right. The bladder (*Bl*) is uninvolved

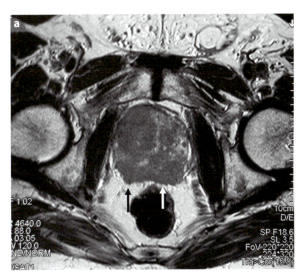
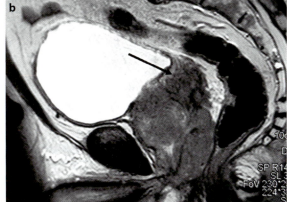
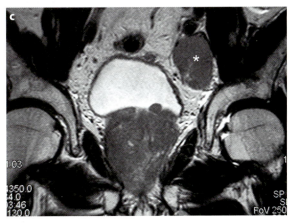

Fig. 15 a-c. A 72-year-old man with prostate adenocarcinoma. **a** Axial fast spin-echo T2-weighted image shows a breech of the capsule with evidence of periprostatic tumor extension (*arrows*). **b** Sagittal image shows seminal vesicle infiltration (*arrow*) and **c** coronal image shows left iliac lymph node metastasis (*)

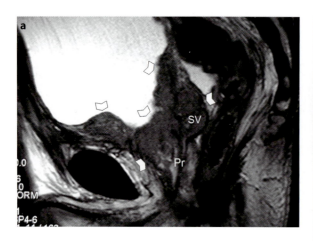
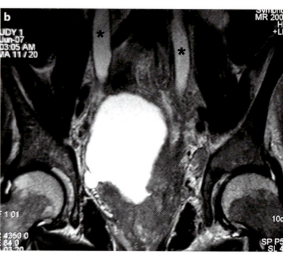

Fig. 16 a, b. A 53-year-old man with transitional-cell carcinoma of the bladder. **a** Sagittal fast spin-echo T2-weighted image shows a large infiltrative mass (*arrowheads*) involving the bladder floor and extending to the prostate (*Pr*) and seminal vesicles (*SV*). **b** Coronal fast spin-echo T2-weighted image demonstrates bilateral ureteral dilatation (*asterisks*)

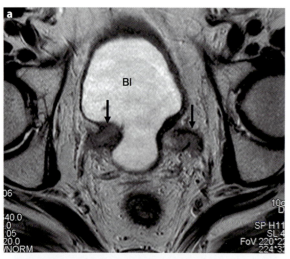
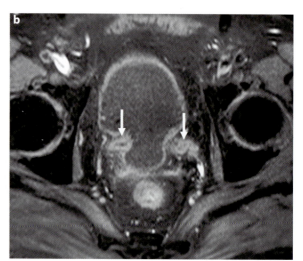

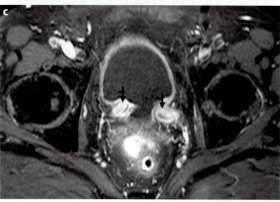

Fig. 17 a-c. A 76-year-old man with bilateral ureteral transitional-cell carcinoma. **a** Axial fast spin-echo T2-weighted image shows bilateral ureteral-wall thickening near the ureterovesical junction (*arrows*). *Bl* bladder. Axial T1-weighted images with fat saturation **b** before and **c** after contrast administration show intense enhancement of the thickened ureteral walls (*arrows*)

poral tissue at both T1- and T2-weighted imaging. MRI can depict corpora cavernosa invasion and is useful for demonstrating tumor location, size, and lo-cal staging. Secondary urethral involvement can occur in bladder, penile, vaginal, and cervix carcinomas, among others (Fig. 19).

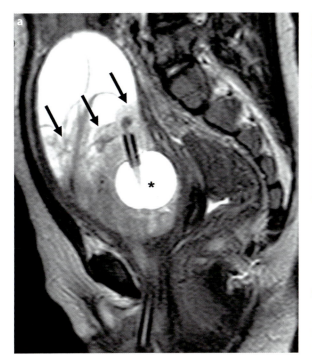

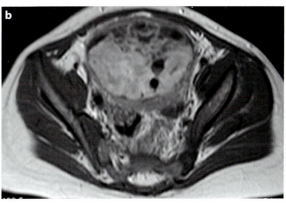

Fig. 18 a, b. A 2-year-old girl with embryonal rhabdomyosarcoma. **a** Sagittal fast spin-echo T2-weighted image depicts a large intraluminal mass arising from the bladder floor (*arrows*) and surrounding a Foley catheter (***). **b** Axial contrast-enhanced spin-echo T1-weighted image demonstrates intense enhancement of the bladder neoplasm

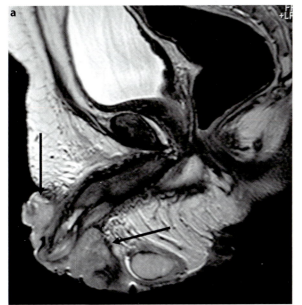

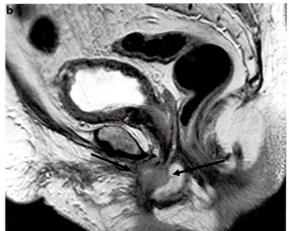

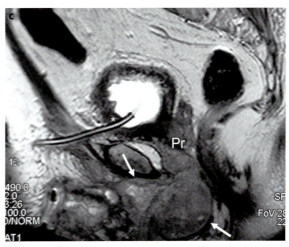

Fig. 19 a-c. A 69-year-old man with multiple recurrences after surgery for penile squamous-cell carcinoma, with ultimate urethral involvement. **a** Sagittal fast spin-echo T2-weighted image shows an infiltrating tumor involving the penile gland (*arrows*). **b** Four months after penile resection, there is tumor recurrence at the lower urethral margin (*arrows*). **c** Three months later, there is upward progression of the tumor with prostatic (*Pr*) involvement and the need for suprapubic cystostomy (***)

Lymph Node Tumors

Lymph node metastases and lymphoma are the diseases to be considered when pelvic neoplastic lymph node enlargement is suspected (Figs. 20 and 21). Whereas MRI is very useful for detecting enlarged lymph nodes, it lacks specificity for malignancy in borderline enlarged nodes and also for histological determination of the primary tumor when it is not obvious on the same examination.

Bone Tumors

A wide variety of primary and metastatic neoplasms can affect the lower spine and pelvic bones and present as pelvic masses. Common primary tumors of the lower spine include chordoma (Fig. 22), giant cell tumor, and aneurysmal bone cysts [12]. Ewing's sarcoma and primitive neuroectodermal tumors of the spine are the most common nonlymphoproliferative primary malignant tumors of the spine in children

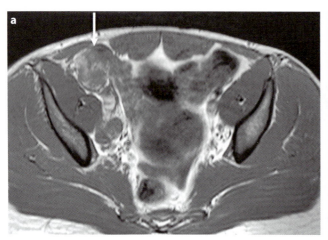
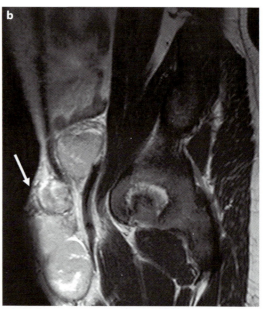

Fig. 20 a, b. A 23-year-old man with lymph node metastases from melanoma. **a** Axial spin-echo T1-weighted image shows right iliac lymphadenopathy (*arrow*) with internal hyperintense foci, probably representing melanin or hemorrhage. **b** Sagittal fast spin-echo T2-weighted image depicts extensive right iliac-inguinal lymphadenopathy (*arrow*)

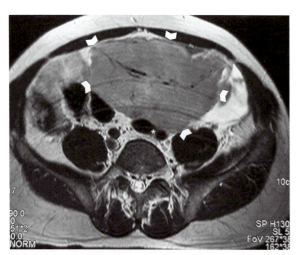
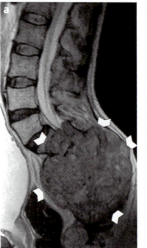
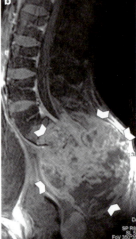

Fig. 21. A 44-year-old man with non-Hodgkin's lymphoma. Axial fast spin-echo T2-weighted image shows a large abdominopelvic mass (*arrowheads*) along the left common iliac vessels (*)

Fig. 22 a, b. A 48-year-old man with sacral chordoma. **a** Sagittal fast spin-echo T2-weighted image reveals a bulky heterogeneous sacral mass (*arrowheads*). **b** Sagittal T1-weighted image with fat saturation after contrast administration reveals marked heterogeneous enhancement of the tumor (*arrowheads*)

[13] (Fig. 23). Common tumors of the pelvic bones include metastases, plasmocytoma, and chondrosarcoma (Fig. 24). MRI provides the best method for depicting the extent of marrow involvement by conventional chondrosarcoma. The nonmineralized components of chondrosarcoma have high signal intensity on T2-weighted MRI, reflecting the high water content of hyaline cartilage [14].

Peritoneal and Soft-Tissue Tumors

Peritoneal diseases that present as masses include mesothelial tumors, pseudomyxoma peritonei, secondary lesions (Fig. 25), and less frequent entities such as desmoplastic small-cell tumor [15] (Fig. 26). Soft-tissue masses include smooth and skeletal muscle tumors (rhabdomyosarcoma and leiomyosarcoma), neural tumors, vascular tumors (angiosarcoma, hemangiopericytoma), lipid tumors (liposarcoma), and fibromatoses (Fig. 27). Neurogenic tumors are frequently encountered in the pelvis. Common subtypes include neurofibromas, neurilemoma, and peripheral malignant nerve-sheath tumors (Fig. 28). On MRI, neurogenic neoplasm signal intensity is relatively nonspecific and is similar to that of muscle on T1-weighted images and higher than that of fat on T2-weighted images. Contrast enhancement is variable in both benign and malignant nerve-sheath tumors. Generally, more contrast enhancement is apparent in malignant tumors [16].

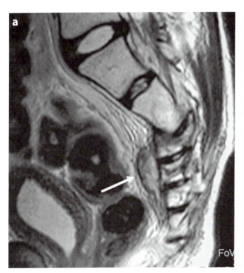
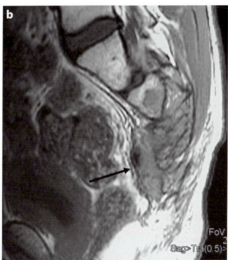

Fig. 23 a, b. A 17-year-old man with sacral Ewing's sarcoma. **a** Sagittal fast spin-echo T2-weighted and **b** right parasagittal spin-echo T1-weighted images depict sacral fracture at the S2 level with associated soft-tissue mass in the presacral space (*arrow*)

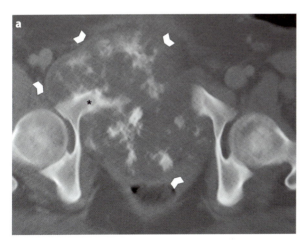
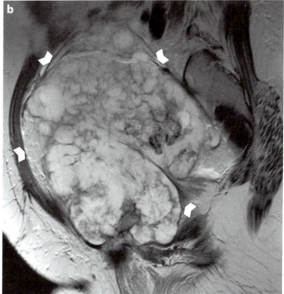

Fig. 24 a, b. A 34-year-old woman with pubic chondrosarcoma. **a** Axial computed tomography image shows a large mass (*arrowheads*) originating from the pubis (*) with chondroid-type calcifications. **b** Right parasagittal fast spin-echo T2-weighted image shows a predominantly hyperintense tumor (*arrowheads*) protruding into the pelvic cavity

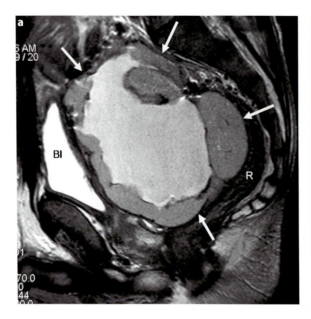

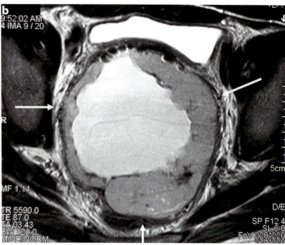

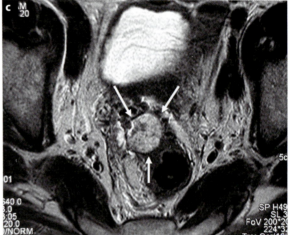

Fig. 25 a-c. A 57-year-old man with ileal gastrointestinal stromal tumor resected 2 years earlier and partial resection of peritoneal metastases 8 months earlier. **a** Sagittal and **b** axial fast spin-echo T2-weighted images demonstrate a pelvic cul-de-sac mass (*arrows*) displacing the bladder (*Bl*) anteriorly and the rectum (*R*) posteriorly. Peripheral artifacts from surgical clips are also seen. **c** After 22 months of treatment with imatinib mesylate, axial fast spin-echo T2-weighted image show marked reduction of the lesion (*arrows*)

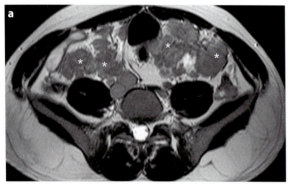

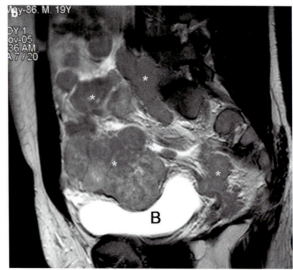

Fig. 26 a, b. A 19-year-old man with abdominal desmoplastic small-round-cell tumor. **a** Axial and **b** sagittal fast spin-echo T2-weighted images show multiple intraperitoneal and retroperitoneal solid masses (*) *B* bladder. Bulky peritoneal soft-tissue masses without an apparent organ-based primary site are characteristic of intra-abdominal desmoplastic small-round-cell tumor, although nonspecific

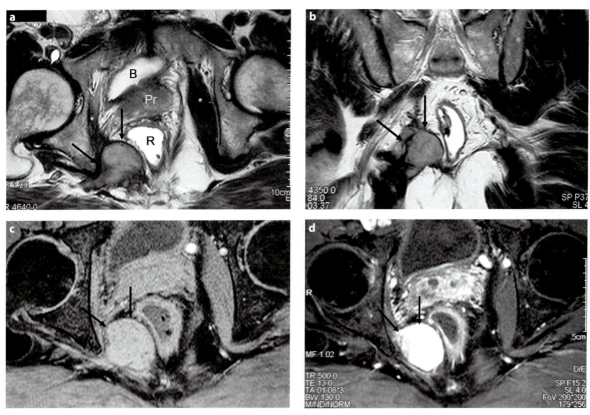

Fig. 27 a-d. A 40-year-old man with retroperitoneal desmoid tumor. **a** Axial and **b** coronal fast spin-echo T2-weighted images depict a right ischiorectal fossa tumor adjacent to the ischial tuberosity and levator ani (*arrows*). There is asymmetry of the obturator internus muscles (*), with right hypotrophy. The rectum (*R*), bladder (*B*), and prostate (*Pr*) are annotated for anatomical reference. Axial T1-weighted image with fat saturation **c** before and **d** after contrast administration reveal marked homogeneous enhancement of the tumor (*arrows*)

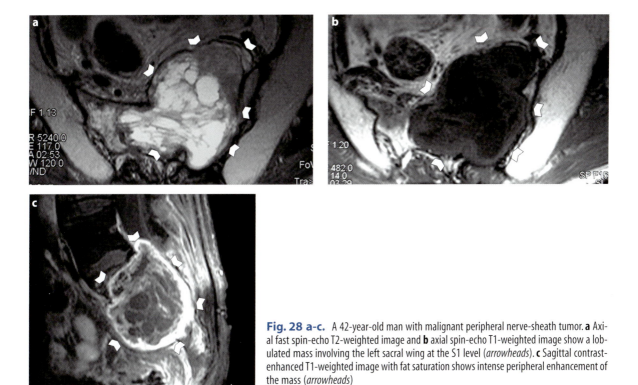

Fig. 28 a-c. A 42-year-old man with malignant peripheral nerve-sheath tumor. **a** Axial fast spin-echo T2-weighted image and **b** axial spin-echo T1-weighted image show a lobulated mass involving the left sacral wing at the S1 level (*arrowheads*). **c** Sagittal contrast-enhanced T1-weighted image with fat saturation shows intense peripheral enhancement of the mass (*arrowheads*)

References

1. Szklaruk J, Tamm EP, Choi H et al (2003) MRI of common and uncommon large pelvic masses. RadioGraphics 23:403–424
2. Okamoto Y, Tanaka YO, Nishida M et al (2003) MRI of the uterine cervix: imaging – pathologic correlation. RadioGraphics 23:425–445
3. Sohaib SAS, Richards PS, Ind T et al (2002) MRI of carcinoma of the vulva. AJR Am J Roentgenol 178:373–377
4. Riesber A, Nüssle K, Stöhr I et al (2001) Preoperative diagnosis of ovarian tumors with MR imaging: comparison with transvaginal sonography, positron emission tomography, and histologic findings. AJR Am J Roentgenol 177:123–129
5. Imaoka I, Wada A, Kaji Y et al (2006) Developing an MRI strategy for diagnosis of ovarian masses. RadioGraphics 26:1431–1448
6. Outwater EK, Siegelman ES, Hunt JL (2001) Ovarian teratomas: tumor types and imaging characteristics. RadioGraphics 21:475–490
7. Chang WC, Meux MD, Yeh BM et al (2006) CT and MRI of adnexal masses in patients with primary nonovarian malignancy. AJR Am J Roentgenol 186:1039–1045
8. Hricak H, Choyke PL, Eberhardt SC et al (2007) Imaging prostate cancer: a multidisciplinary perspective. Radiology 243:28–53
9. Tekes AK, Kamel I, Imam K et al (2005) Dynamic MRI of bladder cancer: evaluation of staging accuracy. AJR Am J Roentgenol 184:121–127
10. Wong-You-Cheong JJ, Woodward PJ, Mannin M et al (2006) Neoplasms of the urinary bladder: radiologic-pathologic correlation. RadioGraphics 26:553–580
11. Kawashima A, Sandler CM, Wasserman NF et al (2004) Imaging of urethral disease: a pictorial review. Radiographics 24:S195–S216
12. Llauger J, Palmer J, Amores S et al (2000) Primary tumors of the sacrum. AJR Am J Roentgenol 174:417–424
13. Murphey MD, Andrews CL, Flemming DJ et al (1996) From the archives of the AFIP. Primary tumors of the spine: radiologic pathologic correlation. RadioGraphics 16:1131–1158
14. Murphey MD, Walker EA, Wilson AJ et al (2003) Imaging of primary chondrosarcoma: radiologic-pathologic correlation. RadioGraphics 23:1245–1278
15. Pickhardt PJ, Fisher AJ, Balfe DM et al (1999) Desmoplastic small round cell tumor of the abdomen: radiologic-histopathologic correlation. Radiology 210:633–638
16. Murphey MD, Smith WS, Smith Se et al (1999) Imaging of musculoskeletal neurogenic tumors: radiologic-pathologic correlation. RadioGraphics 19:1253–1280

CHAPTER 16

The use of PET/PET CT in the Management of Colorectal Cancer

Sergio Carlos Nahas, Jose G. Guillem, Caio Sergio R. Nahas,
Manoel de Souza Rocha

Abstract

Positron emission tomography (PET) is considered a potentially useful diagnostic tool in the management of a variety of malignancies. It has been used for staging, evaluating recurrent and metastatic disease and tumoral response to neoadjuvant therapy, and providing prognostic information. However, some data are available about its definitive role in the colorectal cancer (CRC) population. In this chapter, the most recent evidence and future perspectives are presented for $[^{18}F]$fluorodeoxyglucose PET in managing patients with CRC.

Introduction

Positron emission tomography (PET) is an imaging modality based on the acquisition of functional images of the body after intravenous injection of a positron-emitter radiopharmaceutical [1]. $[^{18}F]$fluorodeoxyglucose ($[^{18}F]$FDG), a positron-emitter glucose analog, is the most commonly used radiotracer [2]. After infusion, $[^{18}F]$FDG enters the cells and is phosphorylated to $[^{18}F]$FDG-6-phosphate, which is not a substrate for glycolysis and, therefore, stays trapped intracellularly. The radiotracer decays through positron emission, generating two gamma rays per positron emitted. The PET scanner detects the released gamma photons and displays an image of their biodistribution [2–5]. The rationale for using $[^{18}F]$FDG PET in malignancies is based in the increased tumoral uptake of $[^{18}F]$FDG, as tumoral cells have enhanced glycolysis and a higher number of glucose transporters at their membranes [3, 4].

The importance of $[^{18}F]$FDG PET in managing colorectal cancer (CRC) is increasing. It can be used for staging, evaluating recurrent and metastatic disease, evaluating tumoral response to neoadjuvant therapy, and as a prognostic tool. More recently, development of the integrated PET computed tomography (PET-CT) equipment, which allows simultaneous acquisition of functional and anatomical images, has made the exam even more effective.

Staging Newly Diagnosed Colorectal Cancer

Although there are many studies based on series of patients with already known or highly suspicious liver metastases or recurrent CRC, there are only a few studies that evaluate the ability of PET scan for staging newly diagnosed CRC [6–10].

Abdel-Nabi et al. [6], in 1998, compared the diagnostic utility of $[^{18}F]$FDG PET and nonhelicoidal CT in the initial staging of 48 patients with CRC. The sensitivities to depict lymph node metastases were similar (29%), but PET had superior specificity (96% vs. 85%). With respect to detection of hepatic metastases, PET had a higher sensitivity (88% vs. 38%) with similar specificity (100% vs. 97%, respectively).

Mukai et al. [7] submitted 24 patients with CRC to preoperative $[^{18}F]$FDG PET. They reported a sensitivity of 96% for detecting the primary lesion, whereas the sensitivity for lymph node metastases was 22%. The authors attributed the low detection rate of lymph node metastases to the inability of PET imaging to distinguish lymph nodes in close proximity to the primary tumor.

M. Pescatori, F.S.P. Regadas, S.M. Murad Regadas, A.P. Zbar (eds.), *Imaging Atlas of the Pelvic Floor and Anorectal Diseases*.
ISBN 978-88-470-0808-3. © Springer-Verlag Italia 2008

Kantorova et al. [8] compared the use of [^{18}F]FDG PET, CT, and abdominal ultrasound (US) for staging 38 consecutive patients with CRC. [^{18}F]FDG PET was superior for detecting both lymph node metastases (29%, 0%, and 0%, respectively) and hepatic metastases (78%, 67%, and 25%, respectively). PET also changed the treatment plan in 16% of the cases.

Heriot et al. [10] submitted 46 patients with locally advanced primary rectal cancer being considered for neoadjuvant therapy to [^{18}F]FDG PET scan. Tumor staging changed in 39% of the cases, whereas patients' treatment modality was modified in 17% (six patients had their operation canceled, whereas two had their radiotherapy field changed). They suggested that PET scan should be considered part of the standard workup for patients with advanced primary rectal cancer. In a recent study, Gearhart et al. [9] analyzed the use of [^{18}F]FDG PET-CT in staging newly diagnosed rectal cancer. Thirty-seven patients with primary adenocarcinoma of the rectum underwent PET-CT scan. The images were compared with conventional spiral CT images and demonstrated discordant findings in 14 patients (38%). These findings resulted in change of the initial treatment plan in ten patients (27%) as a result of detection of pelvic or extrapelvic lymph node metastases, liver metastases, or additional colonic mass.

Cohade et al. [11] compared [^{18}F]FDG PET with [^{18}F]FDG PET-CT in the staging of 45 patients with primary or recurrent CRC and observed that PET-CT reduced the frequency of equivocal and probable lesion characterization by 50%, increased the frequency of definite lesion characterization by 30%, and increased the number of definite locations by 25%. Correct staging increased from 78% to 89%.

A study with 98 patients compared [^{18}F]FDG PET-CT and magnetic resonance imaging (MRI) for staging different malignant diseases. [^{18}F]FDG PET-CT was superior in correctly determining tumor staging (77% vs. 54%) and the lymph node staging (93% vs. 79%). Both imaging procedures showed a similar performance in detecting distant metastases. [^{18}F]FDG PET-CT superiority led the authors to suggest its use as a possible first-line modality for whole-body tumor staging [12].

More recently, Nahas et al. [13] prospectively evaluated the ability of [^{18}F]FDG PET to detect distant disease in 93 patients with locally advanced rectal cancer who were otherwise eligible for combined modality therapy. At a median follow-up of 34 months, the overall accuracy, sensitivity, and specificity of PET in detecting distant disease were 93.7%, 77.8%, and 98.7%, respectively. Greatest accuracy was demonstrated in detecting liver (accuracy 99.9%, sensitivi-

ty 100%, specificity 98.8%) and lung (accuracy 99.9%, sensitivity 80%, specificity 100%) disease; however, the same accuracy was not observed in relation to the remaining distant sites. PET detected 11/12 confirmed malignant sites in the liver and lung. Ten patients were confirmed to have M1 stage disease: all were correctly staged by pre-combined-modality-therapy (CMT) PET, whereas abdominopelvic CT scans were able to detect nine of them.

An additional advantage of PET when compared with conventional staging workup in any cancer population is the increased detection of unsuspected second primary tumors. Choi et al. [14] diagnosed a second primary cancer in 4.8% of 547 consecutive patients scanned with [^{18}F]FDG PET-CT for any kind of known primary tumor.

Finally, considering that 19% of the CRC population presents distant metastases by the time of initial diagnosis [15], PET/PET-CT may become an important routine exam in initial staging of CRC patients. Unfortunately, at this moment, there is a lack of studies about the cost-effectiveness of [^{18}F]FDG PET/PET-CT as part of the routine workup in the initial staging of CRC. Therefore, the use of [^{18}F]FDG PET/PET-CT in the initial staging of CRC population seems economically inconceivable, but we look forward to studies that address this issue, as it can be performed as the only imaging tool and might also avoid unnecessary surgery (Figs. 1 and 2).

Detection of Metastatic Disease

Hepatectomy is a potentially curative therapy for hepatic colorectal metastases. However, up to two thirds of patients explored for resection are found to have unsuspected disease. Based on this, Fong et al. [16] used [^{18}F]FDG PET to scan 40 patients with colorectal metastatic disease. They observed an influence in the clinical management in 40% of the patients and a direct change in managing nine patients (23%). Sensitivity was related to lesion size. Whereas 85% of hepatic metastases larger than 1 cm were detected, only 25% of lesions smaller than 1 cm were identified. Kalff et al. [17] also reported a low sensitivity of the exam for hepatic lesions smaller than 1 cm. Despite the fact that [^{18}F]FDG PET scan has high specificity for hepatic colorectal metastases, all suspected lesions must be further investigated if they can change the proposed therapy.

With respect to changing the therapy plan by the use of [^{18}F]FDG PET scan in patients with colorectal metastatic disease, a meta-analysis of the most recent literature studies showed that this oc-

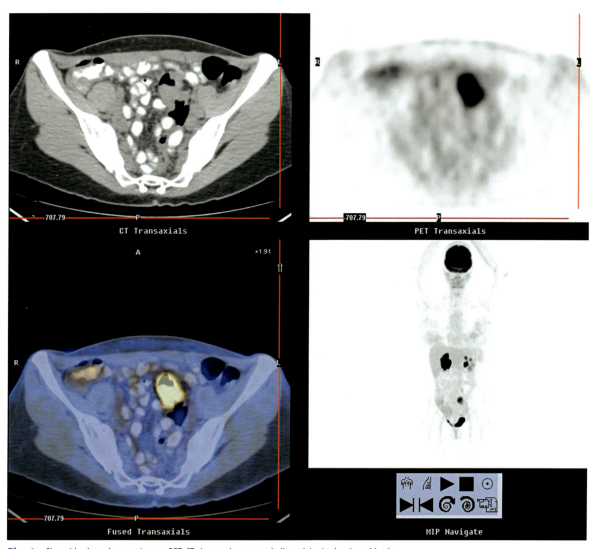

Fig. 1. Sigmoid colon adenocarcinoma. PET-CT shows a hypermetabolic activity in the sigmoid colon

curs in 31.6% of cases (range 20–58%) [18]. Selzner et al. [19] compared helicoidal CT to [^{18}F]FDG PET-CT in 66 patients with hepatic colorectal metastases. Although they had similar efficiency in detecting metastatic liver disease, PET-CT was superior for detecting both recurrent liver disease following hepatic resection (similar sensitivity and specificity of 100% vs. 50%, P 0.04) and local recurrence of the primary CRC lesion after resection (sensitivity of 93% vs. 53%, P 0.03). PET-CT failed to detect extrahepatic disease in only 11% of cases (sensitivity of 89% vs. 64%, P 0.02) and altered the therapy plan in 21% of patients. The authors recommended performing routine [^{18}F]FDG PET-CT on all patients being considered for liver resection of metastatic CRC.

Kahn et al. [20] studied a group of 23 patients, 14 with hepatic colorectal metastases and nine with previous liver resection for colorectal metastases, with [^{18}F]FDG PET-CT. They observed a major impact on managing seven patients due to unexpected findings such as the presence of extrahepatic disease or even the absence of metastatic disease. A clinical decision, based on the PET-CT report alone, could be undertaken in 21 of the 23 patients.

Few studies report the cost-effectiveness of the PET-CT in patients with CRC and metachronic hepatic metastases. Lejeune et al. [21] compared CT with [^{18}F]FDG PET-CT and concluded that although the use of the PET-CT for diagnosis and staging did not generate additional survival, it was associated with a cost saving of US $3,213.00 per patient as a

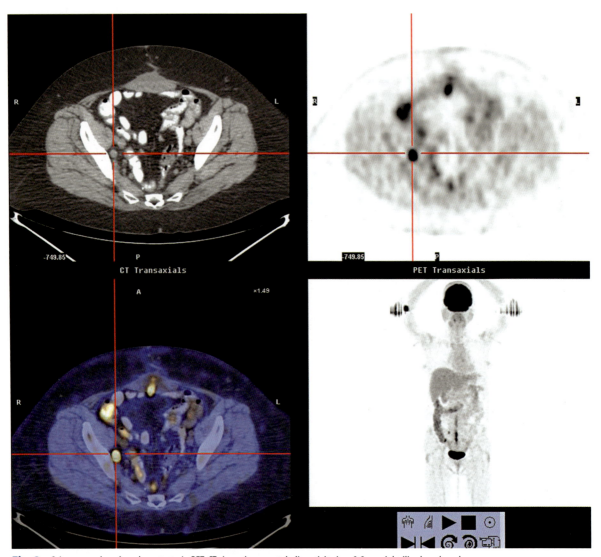

Fig. 2. Colon cancer lymph node metastasis. PET-CT shows hypermetabolic activity in a 0.8-cm right iliac lymph node

result of improvement in the therapeutic plan (for example, it avoided unnecessary laparotomies in 6.1% of patients). As [^{18}F]FDG PET-CT was cost effective, the authors concluded that its general use in clinical practice is justified in similar cases. Zubeldia et al. [22] compared the use of CT with [^{18}F]FDG PET-CT for evaluating patients with hepatic colorectal metastases being considered for surgery. They concluded that the inclusion of the PET-CT in the presurgical evaluation of these patients substantially reduced the cost and morbidity of their treatment as a result of its ability to detect extrahepatic disease and, therefore, to avoid unnecessary surgical procedures.

As chemotherapy is cytotoxic, it impairs tumoral metabolic activity, leading to a decrease in FDG uptake by the neoplastic cells. Based on this, Akhurst

et al. [23] studied the ability of [^{18}F]FDG PET to identify colorectal metastases after preoperative chemoradiation. Forty-two patients with colorectal liver metastases were studied. Thirteen of those patients received preoperative chemotherapy, and 42 were submitted to liver resection. PET findings were compared with the pathologic analysis of the specimens. [^{18}F]FDG PET did not identified 23% of liver metastases present in those patients who did not receive neoadjuvant treatment, whereas in the group treated with preoperative chemotherapy, 37% of the lesions were missed. They concluded that [^{18}F]FDG PET scanning during the course of chemotherapy or early after a session is less efficient in detecting colorectal liver metastases and, therefore, the images should be interpreted with caution (Figs. 3–5).

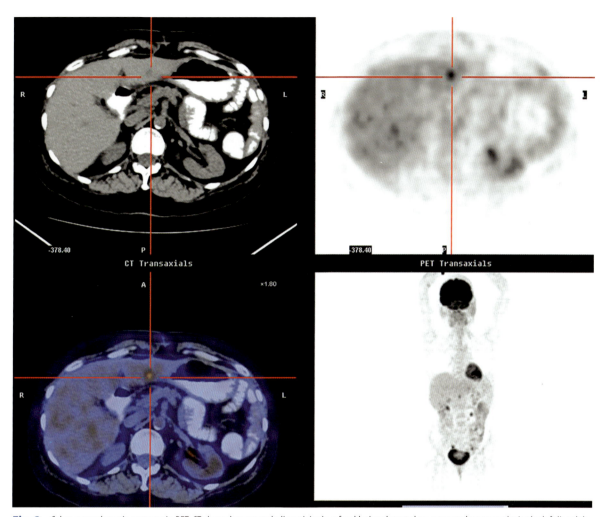

Fig. 3. Colon cancer hepatic metastasis. PET-CT shows hypermetabolic activity in a focal lesion detected on computed tomography in the left liver lobe

Recurrence Assessment

Perhaps the most promising use of the PET scan in CRC is for detecting recurrent disease either locally or systemically. This is even enhanced with PET-CT. Whereas the diagnostic tools usually used in suspected recurrent CRC are imprecise and quite frequently inconclusive, [18F]FDG PET-CT has high accuracy. It has great value in cases of high tumor marker measurement despite normal conventional imaging, cases with anatomic changes that might be due to postoperative fibrosis, and patients with inexplicable symptoms [24].

[18F]FDG PET has high sensitivity for detecting and staging CRC local recurrence and allows the se-

lection of patients for appropriate treatment. False positives rarely occur and have been credited to granulomas, abscess, and even sarcoidosis [17, 25, 26]. There is concern about PET identifying posttreatment inflammatory changes as recurrence. Zervos et al. [27], in a study with 277 patients suspected for recurrent CRC [increasing carcinoembryonic antigen (CEA) levels and nondiagnostic imaging or symptoms with normal CEA level and nondiagnostic imaging] demonstrated that [18F]FDG PET is accurate in both localizing the occult source of recurrence and selecting patients for potential curative laparotomy. Conversely, the authors observed that false positives were common in symptomatic patients with normal CEA levels (only one of four PET-positive patients had CRC recurrence).

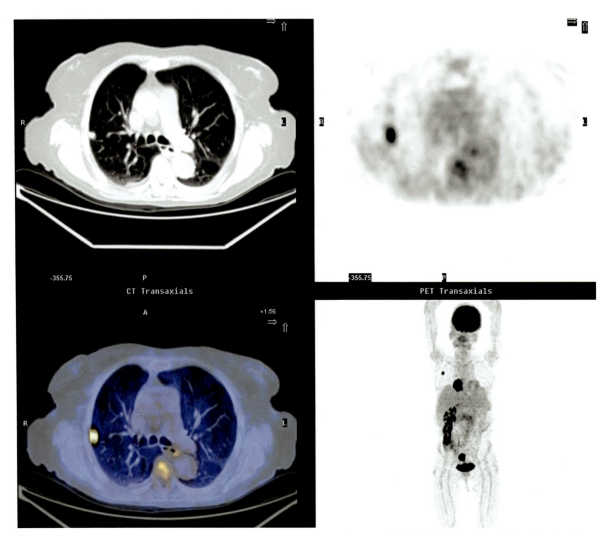

Fig. 4. Colon cancer pulmonary metastasis. Positron emission tomography computed tomography (PET-CT) shows hypermetabolic activity in a 1.0 cm pulmonary nodule seen on the CT image. Coronal PET image also shows metabolic hyperactivity metastasis situated in peridiaphragmatic lymph nodes and in the pelvis

Moore et al. [28] studied the accuracy of [^{18}F]FDG PET for detecting rectal cancer recurrence in the irradiated pelvis of patients with surgically resected rectal cancer. PET was performed at least 6 months after external-beam radiation therapy (EBRT) in two groups of patients, one with confirmed pelvic recurrence (19 cases) and the other without clinical or radiologic evidence of pelvic recurrence (41 cases). They observed a sensitivity of 84%, specificity of 88%, positive predictive value of 76%, and negative predictive value of 92%. The authors also observed that both positive predictive value and accuracy improved in scans performed more than 12 months after EBRT, concluding that the reliability of [^{18}F]FDG PET scan appears to improve with time, perhaps because of resolution of early postradiation inflamma-

tion. We look forward to similar studies addressing postoperative inflammation.

Whiteford et al. [29], in a study including 105 patients with suspected metastatic or recurrent CRC, observed a superior sensitivity of [^{18}F]FDG PET in detecting locoregional recurrence when compared with CT plus colonoscopy (90% vs. 71%, respectively).

Simo et al. [30] prospectively evaluated with [^{18}F]FDG PET 120 patients with suspected CRC recurrence. Patients with elevated tumor markers, inconclusive imaging exams, confirmed recurrence, or abdominal pain were included. PET contributed with drastic changes in the proposed therapy in 48% of cases, thanks to its ability to confirm or exclude recurrence.

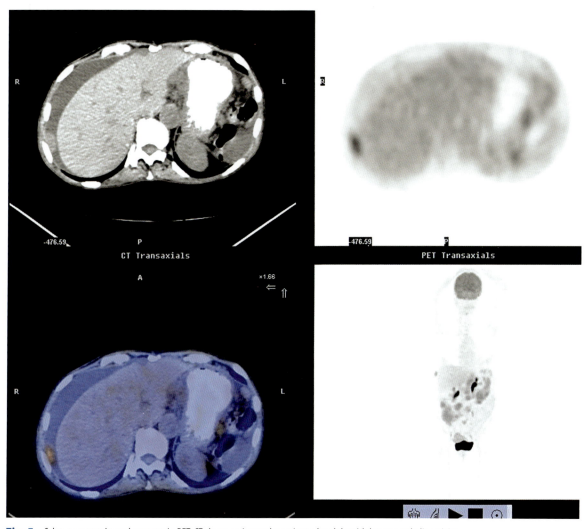

Fig. 5. Colon cancer peritoneal metastasis. PET-CT shows ascites and a peritoneal nodule with hypermetabolic activity

Desai et al. [31] reported that [¹⁸F]FDG PET affected the surgical management in patients with recurrent or metastatic CRC. From a total of 114 patients, CT scan referred 42 patients for surgical resection. In this group, PET altered the proposed therapy in 17 cases (40%) due to the finding of unsuspected disease. In another group including 25 patients with isolated liver metastases, PET showed more extensive disease, preventing surgical resection in 18 patients (72%). The ability of PET to change the proposed therapy, thus avoiding improper treatments due to the recognition of advanced disease, is considered by some authors as its major benefit [17].

In a study designed to compare the capacity of [¹⁸F]FDG PET scan, ⁹⁹ᵐTc-labeled arcitumomab (CEA scan), and blind laparotomy to locate recurrent CRC in 28 patients with increasing CEA levels, Libutti et al. [32] observed that PET was capable of identifying which patients with recurrent CRC would benefit from surgery. It correctly predicted as resectable 81% of lesions and 90% of unresectable lesions. The authors concluded that laparotomy can be considered if PET indicates resectable disease, and other therapies should be considered if the image predicts unresectable disease.

Concerning the difficult task of accurately distinguishing benign and malignant presacral abnormalities after rectal cancer resection, Even-Sapir et al. [33] compared [¹⁸F]FDG PET with [¹⁸F]FDG PET-CT in 62 patients. They observed that PET-CT had a higher sensitivity (98% vs. 82%), specificity

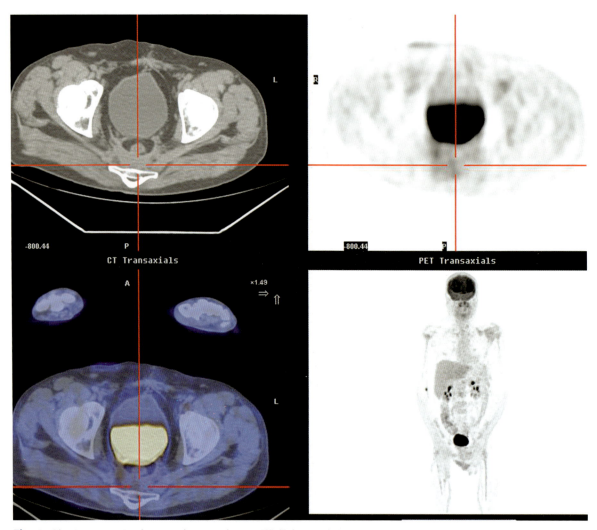

Fig. 6. Fibrotic postoperative changes in the presacral region. PET-CT shows no hypermetabolic activity in the dense fibrous tissue that occupies the presacral space 4 months after a rectal resection

(96% vs. 65%), and accuracy (93% vs. 74%). The authors concluded that PET-CT is an accurate technique in detecting pelvic recurrence after surgical removal of rectal cancer (Figs. 6 and 7).

Assessing Rectal Cancer Response to Neoadjuvant Therapy

Preoperative chemoradiation (CMT) followed by radical resection is a well-established therapy for locally advanced rectal cancer [34]. Accurate assessment of neoplasm response to CMT is a desirable achievement, allowing early and more efficient alterations in the management plan. As there is no test that accurately esti-

mates this response, PET scan became an option.

Guillem et al. [35], in a study of 15 patients with rectal cancer treated with preoperative CMT, compared the ability of [^{18}F]FDG PET and CT to estimate tumor response to the neoadjuvant regimen. Evidence of response was detected by [^{18}F]FDG PET and CT in 100% and 78% of patients, respectively. PET also accurately estimated the extent of response in 60% of patients, whereas the accuracy of the CT was 22%.

In another study, 22 patients with locally advanced rectal cancer were submitted to [^{18}F]FDG PET scan before and after CMT. FDG uptake reduction was considered as evidence of tumoral response, and this data was compared with endorectal ultrasound (EUS) and histopathological findings [36]. [^{18}F]FDG PET was superior to EUS in evaluating tumoral response

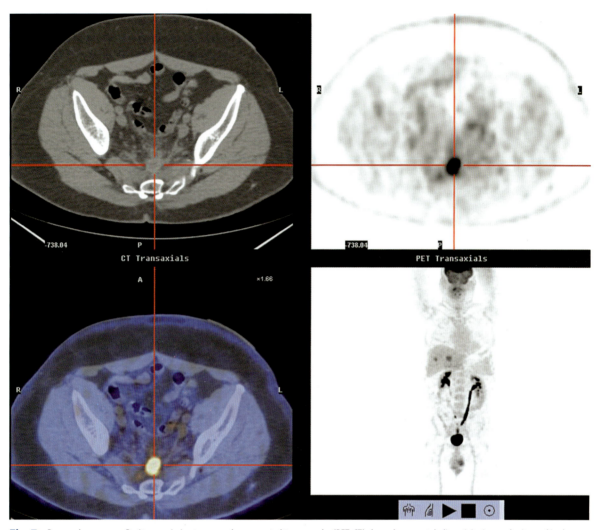

Fig. 7. Presacral recurrence. Positron emission tomography-computed tomography (PET-CT) shows hypermetabolic activity in a node situated in the presacral space. Coronal PET-CT image also shows hypermetabolic activity in two hepatic metastases

to chemoradiation. Sensitivity was 100% (against 33% for EUS), with a specificity of 86% (80% EUS). PET positive and negative predictive values were 93% and 100%, respectively, whereas EUS values were 89% and 33%, respectively [36].

Patients who have minimal response to CMT might benefit from alternative therapy, but identifying them in an early phase is a challenge. Based on that, Chessin et al. [37] submitted 21 patients with rectal carcinoma to [18F]FDG PET 10–12 days after the first session of chemoradiation and compared this findings with the histopathological specimen. PET identified complete or partial response in 20 of 21 pathologic responders (95%). The authors concluded that PET might allow identification of those patients who would benefit from the proposed scheme.

[18F]FDG PET has also been evaluated in its capacity to predict long-term oncologic outcomes in patients with rectal cancer submitted to CMT. Guillem et al. [38] demonstrated that two PET parameters (standard uptake value and total lesion glycolysis) were significant predictors of overall survival and recurrence-free survival. Calvo et al. [39], in a similar study, observed that the maximum standardized uptake value correlated with 3-year survival rate (Fig. 8).

Conclusion

The role of [18F]FDG PET in CRC is still being established. Recent evidence points to its usefulness and accuracy in detecting metastatic or recurrent dis-

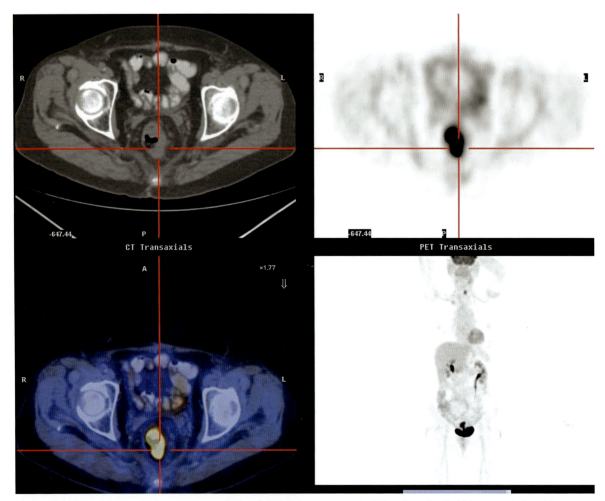

Fig. 8. Rectal cancer not completely responsive to radiotherapy. PET-CT shows asymmetric, thickened rectal wall with hypermetabolic activity

ease and staging newly diagnosed CRC in patients with inconclusive routine workup. It might also have a role in evaluating tumoral response to chemoradiation and in predicting long-term outcome in patients with rectal adenocarcinoma.

PET-CT has been shown to be superior to PET alone, as the combination of anatomical and functional alterations diminishes the frequency of equivocal lesions and increases the accuracy of the exam. These advantages largely expand the role of this imaging tool and will probably lead PET-CT to substitute for the PET scan in the near future.

References

1. Rosenbaum SJ, Stergar H, Antoch G et al (2006) Staging and follow-up of gastrointestinal tumors with PET/CT. Abdom Imaging 31(1):25–35
2. Kumar R, Nadig MR, Chauhan A (2005) Positron emission tomography: clinical applications in oncology. Part 1. Expert Rev Anticancer Ther 5(6):1079–1094
3. Pauwels EK, Ribeiro MJ, Stoot JH et al (1998) FDG accumulation and tumor biology. Nucl Med Biol 25(4):317–322
4. Chung JK, Lee YJ, Kim C et al (1999) Mechanisms related to [18F]fluorodeoxyglucose uptake of human colon cancers transplanted in nude mice. J Nucl Med 40(2):339–346
5. Young H, Baum R, Cremerius U (1999) Measurement of clinical and subclinical tumour response using [18F]-fluorodeoxyglucose and positron emission tomography: review and 1999 EORTC recommendations. European Organization for Research and Treatment of

Cancer (EORTC) PET Study Group. Eur J Cancer 35(13):1773–1782

6. Abdel-Nabi H, Doerr RJ, Lamonica DM et al (1998) Staging of primary colorectal carcinomas with fluorine-18 fluorodeoxyglucose whole-body PET: correlation with histopathologic and CT findings. Radiology 206(3):755–760

7. Mukai M, Sadahiro S, Yasuda S et al (2000) Preoperative evaluation by whole-body 18F-fluorodeoxyglucose positron emission tomography in patients with primary colorectal cancer. Oncol Rep 7(1):85–87

8. Kantorova I, Lipska L, Belohlavek O et al (2003) Routine (18)F-FDG PET preoperative staging of colorectal cancer: comparison with conventional staging and its impact on treatment decision making. J Nucl Med 44(11):1784–1788

9. Gearhart SL, Frassica D, Rosen R et al (2006) Improved staging with pretreatment positron emission tomography/computed tomography in low rectal cancer. Ann Surg Oncol 13(3):397–404

10. Heriot AG, Hicks RJ, Drummond EG et al (2004) Does positron emission tomography change management in primary rectal cancer? A prospective assessment. Dis Colon Rectum 47(4):451–458

11. Cohade C, Osman M, Leal J, Wahl RL (2003) Direct comparison of (18)F-FDG PET and PET/CT in patients with colorectal carcinoma. J Nucl Med 44(11):1797–1803

12. Antoch G, Vogt FM, Freudenberg LS et al (2003) Whole-body dual-modality PET/CT and whole-body MRI for tumor staging in oncology. JAMA 290(24):3199–3206

13. Nahas CS, Akhurst T, Yeung H et al (2008) Positron emission tomography detection of distant metastatic or synchronous disease in patients with locally advanced rectal cancer receiving preoperative chemoradiation. Ann Surg Oncol 15:704–711

14. Choi JY, Lee KS, Kwon OJ et al (2005) Improved detection of second primary cancer using integrated [18F] fluorodeoxyglucose positron emission tomography and computed tomography for initial tumor staging. J Clin Oncol 23(30):7654–7659

15. Jemal A, Siegel R, Ward E et al (2006) Cancer statistics, 2006. CA Cancer J Clin 56(2):106–130

16. Fong Y, Saldinger PF, Akhurst T et al (1999) Utility of 18F-FDG positron emission tomography scanning on selection of patients for resection of hepatic colorectal metastases. Am J Surg 178(4):282–287

17. Kalff V, Hicks RJ, Ware RE et al (2002) The clinical impact of (18)F-FDG PET in patients with suspected or confirmed recurrence of colorectal cancer: a prospective study. J Nucl Med 43(4):492–499

18. Wiering B, Krabbe PF, Jager GJ et al (2005) The impact of fluor-18-deoxyglucose-positron emission tomography in the management of colorectal liver metastases. Cancer 104(12):2658–2670

19. Selzner M, Hany TF, Wildbrett P et al (2004) Does the novel PET/CT imaging modality impact on the treatment of patients with metastatic colorectal cancer of the liver? Ann Surg 240(6):1027–1034; discussion 1035–1036

20. Khan S, Tan YM, John A et al (2006) An audit of fusion CT-PET in the management of colorectal liver metastases. Eur J Surg Oncol 32(5):564–567

21. Lejeune C, Bismuth MJ, Conroy T et al (2005) Use of a decision analysis model to assess the cost-effectiveness of 18F-FDG PET in the management of metachronous liver metastases of colorectal cancer. J Nucl Med 46(12):2020–2028

22. Zubeldia JM, Bednarczyk EM, Baker JG, Nabi HA (2005) The economic impact of 18FDG positron emission tomography in the surgical management of colorectal cancer with hepatic metastases. Cancer Biother Radiopharm 20(4):450–456

23. Akhurst T, Kates TJ, Mazumdar M et al (2005) Recent chemotherapy reduces the sensitivity of [18F]fluorodeoxyglucose positron emission tomography in the detection of colorectal metastases. J Clin Oncol 23(34):8713–8716

24. Flanagan FL, Dehdashti F, Ogunbiyi OA (1998) Utility of FDGPET for investigating unexplained plasma CEA elevation in patients with colorectal cancer. Ann Surg 227(3):319–323

25. Lim JW, Tang CL, Keng GH (2005) False positive F-18 fluorodeoxyglucose combined PET/CT scans from suture granuloma and chronic inflammation: report of two cases and review of literature. Ann Acad Med Singapore 34(7):457–460

26. Ogunbiyi OA, Flanagan FL, Dehdashti F et al (1997) Detection of recurrent and metastatic colorectal cancer: comparison of positron emission tomography and computed tomography. Ann Surg Oncol 4(8):613–620

27. Zervos EE, Badgwell BD, Burak WE Jr et al (2001) Fluorodeoxyglucose positron emission tomography as an adjunct to carcinoembryonic antigen in the management of patients with presumed recurrent colorectal cancer and nondiagnostic radiologic workup. Surgery 130:636–644

28. Moore HG, Akhurst T, Larson SM et al (2003) A case-controlled study of 18-fluorodeoxyglucose positron emission tomography in the detection of pelvic recurrence in previously irradiated rectal cancer patients. J Am Coll Surg 197(1):22–28

29. Whiteford MH, Whiteford HM, Yee LF et al (2000) Usefulness of FDG-PET scan in the assessment of suspected metastatic or recurrent adenocarcinoma of the colon and rectum. Dis Colon Rectum 43(6):759–767; discussion 767–770

30. Simo M, Lomena F, Setoain J et al (2002) FDG-PET improves the management of patients with suspected recurrence of colorectal cancer. Nucl Med Commun 23(10):975–982

31. Desai DC, Zervos EE, Arnold MW et al (2003) Positron emission tomography affects surgical management in recurrent colorectal cancer patients. Ann Surg Oncol 10(1):59–64

32. Libutti SK, Alexander HR Jr et al (2001) A prospective study of 2-[18F] fluoro-2-deoxy-D-glucose/positron

emission tomography scan, 99mTc-labeled arcitumomab (CEA scan), and blind second-look laparotomy for detecting colon cancer recurrence in patients
with increasing carcinoembryonic antigen levels. Ann
Surg Oncol 8(10):779–786

33. Even-Sapir E, Parag Y, Lerman H et al (2004) Detec-
tion of recurrence in patients with rectal cancer:
PET/CT after abdominoperineal or anterior resection.
Radiology 232(3):815–822

34. Sauer R, Becker H, Hohenberger W et al (2004) Preoperative versus postoperative chemoradiotherapy for
rectal cancer. N Engl J Med 351(17):1731–1740

35. Guillem JG, Puig-La Calle J Jr et al (20000 Prospective assessment of primary rectal cancer response to
preoperative radiation and chemotherapy using 18-flu-
orodeoxyglucose positron emission tomography. Dis
Colon Rectum 43(1):18–24

36. Amthauer H, Denecke T, Rau B et al (2004) Response
prediction by FDG-PET after neoadjuvant radiochemotherapy and combined regional hyperthermia of
rectal cancer: correlation with endorectal ultrasound
and histopathology. Eur J Nucl Med Mol Imaging
31(6):811–819

37. Chessin DB, Yeung H, Shia J et al (2005) Positron
emission tomography during preoperative combined
modality therapy for rectal cancer may predict ultimate
pathologic response. A prospective analysis. Am Soc
Clin Oncol 165:3612 (abstract)

38. Guillem JG, Moore HG, Akhurst T et al (2004) Sequential preoperative fluorodeoxyglucose-positron
emission tomography assessment of response to preoperative chemoradiation: a means for determining
long-term outcomes of rectal cancer. J Am Coll Surg
199(1):1–7

39. Calvo FA, Domper M, Matute R et al (2004) 18F-FDG
positron emission tomography staging and restaging
in rectal cancer treated with preoperative chemoradiation. Int J Radiat Oncol Biol Phys 58(2):528–535

Commentary

Andrew P. Zbar

This excellent chapter outlines the controversies in the utilization (given its limited availability) of PET scanning and PET-CT fusion images in managing colorectal cancer (CRC). Consensus decisions regarding its role and cost benefits are as yet unproven [1]. The advantages of PET-CT recently confirmed in non-small-cell lung cancer (NSCLC) can provide some special lessons on its potential use in rectal cancer, where in the former disease, integrated PET-CT has permitted a functional/morphological acquisition of data concerning tumor volume and contouring, which is proving critical in radiotherapy planning with a specific benefit, particularly when there is attendant atelectasis and an advantage over CT imaging alone in node-negative cases [2, 3]. In NSCLC, this has provided a marked improvement in therapeutic ratio for radiotherapeutic simulation with an enhanced tumor coverage while at the same time reducing irradiated volumes and allowing the potential for local dose escalation. Such issues, in theory, could exist in part in relation to some rectal cancers; however, data pertaining to radiotherapy protocols for rectal cancer are not yet incorporated to suggest PET-based survival benefit in the same way that it is for NSCLC [4]. Moreover, there is some recent evidence that PET functional analysis of FDG kinetics in NSCLC can identify patients in whom chemotherapy may offer some survival advantage, which may also lead to reduced radiation toxicity when there is a policy to avoid elective nodal irradiation [5]. This finding has been coupled with the fact that regional lymph node involvement in the mediastinum can identify those cases requiring mediastinoscopy [6]. Such issues clearly have limited, if any, relevance for managing rectal cancers.

However, there are lessons to be learned from this "cross-cultural cancer talk" regarding the role of PET-CT in CRC. First, there is a distinct advantage in fusion imagery for attenuation correction and acquisition speed, effectively eliminating some artifacts generated with contrast agents in PET scanning and some motion-generated CT artifacts when each modality is used alone [7]. The recent trend is toward neoadjuvant chemotherapy (and more recently chemoimmunotherapy) in patients presenting with hepatic metastatic disease while the primary tumor

is in situ so that patients may be treated with formal hepatectomy, although improving progression-free survival [8–11] has not shown a proven economic benefit for PET-CT introduced early into the management algorithm [12]. The poor histological response to such aggressive first-line therapy (often despite conventional imaging showing complete tumor response) suggests a specific place for the biological advantages of PET-CT fusion [13, 14], as does the demonstration of potentially resectable extrahepatic disease that, in selected cases, can be removed with curative intent [15]. Further controversy exists for the initial role of PET-CT in primary colonic cancer, where it is likely that its impact will be limited. In rectal cancer, its use is still also likely to be fairly selective, perhaps being advisable in tumors that are predictably more likely to have nodal involvement that is neither detected by CT nor MRI. This is a small group of cases, as estimates suggest that approximately 10% of cases with bulkier tumors have nodes located outside conventional radiotherapy fields, namely, in the lateral iliac nodes [16]. Further, because up to one third of nodal metastases in rectal cancer are microscopic and one quarter of lymph nodes are < 5 mm in maximal diameter, even if uninvolved with tumor, this implies that the possible tumor-specific advantages of greater nodal diagnosis are likely to be small [17, 18]. Given that the current locoregional recurrence rates after total mesorectal excision are < 5% in experienced hands in the absence of more extended lymphadenectomy and in the absence of primary PET diagnosis, decisions regarding more routine PET-CT scanning as a first-line part of rectal cancer workup must at this time remain circumspect. This view would currently also not be supportive of the early use of "all-in-one" PET colonography for the primary diagnosis of this tumor, despite its many theoretical advantages [19, 20].

There is a distinct value in using PET-CT fusion images for detecting recurrent CRC, particularly following radiotherapy, as pointed out in this chapter by Nahas and colleagues, where there is difficulty in distinguishing recurrence from postradiotherapy desmoplasia, particularly in the presence of a near-normal CEA level [21–23]. The recent advances in more conventional imaging modalities, such as superparamagnetic iron oxide (SPIO)-enhanced MRI or the new multidetector CT (MDCT), for detecting potentially operable isolated liver metastases, given that there are now liver-specific contrast agents, modern sequences, and high-performance gradients, may selectively define the place for more advanced specialized imaging such as PET-CT in managing recurrent colorectal cancer [24]. New therapy modalities also hold promise for specific use and relative contraindications of PET in CRC management. Although many hepatic metastatic cases are now being treated by radiofrequency ablation (RFA), other imaging techniques are still required for correct probe positioning to institute RFA. This is particularly true where there is some evidence that better morphological imaging than can be provided by PET may define those perivascular hepatic metastatic lesions that are less well suited to primary RFA treatment [25]. Against this, the introduction of newer forms of immunotherapy, such as the antiepidermal growth factor receptor (anti-EGFR) monoclonal antibody cetuximab, have created a new role for PET usage, which is perhaps predictive of biologic responsiveness [26], although it is well known that EGFR-negative tumors may still respond to such therapy [27]. The place of PET and PET-CT in CRC is going to remain specialized in the foreseeable future.

References

1. Sheehan JJ, Ridge CA, Ward EV et al (2007) FDG PET in preoperative assessment of colorectal liver metastases combining "evidence-based practice" and "technology assessment" methods to develop departmental imaging protocols: should FDG PET be routinely used in the preoperative assessment of patients with colorectal liver metastases? Acad Radiol 14:389–397
2. De Wever W, Stroobants S, Verschakelen JA (2007) Integrated PET/CT in lung cancer imaging: history and technical aspects. JBR-BTR 90:112–119
3. Greco C, Rosenzweig K, Cascini GL, Tamburrini O (2007) Current status of PET/CT for tumour volume definition in radiotherapy treatment planning for non-small cell lung cancer (NSCLC). Lung Cancer 57:125–134
4. Shin SS, Jeong YY, Min JJ et al (2007) Preoperative staging of colorectal cancer: CT vs. integrated FDG PET/CT. Abdom Imaging [Epub ahead of print]
5. Schimmer C, Neukam K, Elert O (2006) Staging of non-small cell lung cancer: clinical value of positron emission tomography and mediastinoscopy. Interact Cardiovasc Thorac Surg 5:418–423
6. Ceresoli GL, Cattaneo GM, Castellone P et al (2007) Role of computed tomography and [^{18}F] fluorodeoxyglucose positron emission tomography image fusion in conformal radiotherapy of non-small-cell lung cancer: a comparison with standard techniques with and without elective nodal irradiation. Tumori 93:88–96
7. Hicks RJ, Ware RE, Lau EW (2006) PET/CT: will it change the way that we use CT in cancer imaging? Cancer Imaging 6:S52–S62
8. Louvet C, de Gramont A, Tournigand C et al (2001) Correlation between progression free survival and response rate in patients with metastatic colorectal cancer. Cancer 91:2033–2038
9. Yoo PS, Lopez-Soler RI, Longo WE, Cha CH (2006) Liver resection for metastatic colorectal cancer in the age of neoadjuvant chemotherapy and bevacizumab. Clin Colorectal Cancer 6:202–207
10. Kemeny N (2006) Management of liver metastases from colorectal cancer. Oncology 20:1161–1176
11. Mentha G, Majno PE, Andres A et al (2006) Neoadjuvant chemotherapy and resection of advanced synchronous liver metastases before treatment of the colorectal primary. Br J Surg 93:872–878
12. Takahashi S, Kuroki Y, Nasu K et al (2006) Positron emission tomography with F-18 fluorodeoxyglucose in evaluating colorectal hepatic metastasis down-staged by chemotherapy. Anticancer Res 26:4705–4711
13. Benoist S, Brouquet A, Penna C et al (2006) Complete response of colorectal liver metastases after chemotherapy – does it mean cure? J Clin Oncol 24:3939–3945
14. Riedl CC, Akhurst T, Larson S et al (2007) 18F-FDG PET scanning correlates with tissue markers of poor prognosis and predicts mortality for patients after liver resection for colorectal metastases. J Nucl Med 48:771–775
15. Elias D, Liberale G, Vernerey D et al (2005) Hepatic and extrahepatic colorectal metastases: when resectable their localization does not matter, but their total number has a prognostic effect. Ann Surg Oncol 12:900–909
16. Watanabe T, Tsurita G, Muto T et al (2002) Extended lymphadenectomy and preoperative radiotherapy for lower rectal cancers. Surgery 132:27–33
17. Herrera-Ornelas L, Justiniano J, Castillo N et al (1987) Metastases in small lymph nodes from colon cancer. 122:1253–1256
18. Dworak O (1989) Number and size of lymph nodes and node metastases in rectal carcinomas. Surg Endosc 3:96–99
19. Veit-Haibach P, Kuehle CA, Beyer T et al (2006) Diagnostic accuracy of colorectal cancer staging with whole-body PET/CT colonography. JAMA 296:2590–2600
20. Kinner S, Antoch G, Bockisch A, Veit-Haibach P (2007) Whole-body PET/CT-colonography: a possible new concept for colorectal cancer staging. Abdom Imaging 32(5):606–612

21. Schaefer O, Langer M (2007) Detection of recurrent rectal cancer with CT, MRI and PET/CT. Eur Radiol 17:2044–2054

22. Nakamoto Y, Sakamoto S, Okada T et al (2007) Clinical value of manual fusion of PET and CT images in patients with suspected recurrent colorectal cancer. AJR Am J Roentgenol 188:257–267

23. Sarikaya I, Bloomston M, Povoski SP et al (2007) FDG-PET scan in patients with clinically and/or radiologically suspicious colorectal cancer recurrence but normal CEA. World J Surg Oncol 5:64

24. Rappeport ED, Loft A (2007) Liver metastases from colorectal cancer: imaging with superparamagnetic iron oxide (SPIO)-enhanced MR imaging, computed tomography and positron emission tomography. Abdom Imaging 32(5):624–634

25. Prior JO, Kosinski M, Delaloye AB, Denys A (2007) Initial report of PET/CT-guided radiofrequency ablation of liver metastases. J Vasc Interv Radiol 18:801–803

26. Pantaleo MA, Fanti S, Lollini PL et al (2007) PET detection of epidermal growth factor receptor in colorectal cancer: a real predictor of response to cetuximab treatment? Eur J Nucl Med Mol Imaging 34:1510–1511

27. Scartozzi M, Bearzi I, Berardi R et al (2004) Epidermal growth factor receptor (EGFR) status in primary colorectal tumors does not correlate with EGFR expression in related metastatic sites: implications for treatment with EGFR-targeted monoclonal antibodies. J Clin Oncol 22:4720–4726

CHAPTER 17

2- and 3-D Ultrasonography of Endometriosis, Pelvic Cyst, Rectal Solitary Ulcer, Muscle Hypertrophy, Rare Neoplasms

Sthela M. Murad Regadas, F. Sérgio P. Regadas

Abstract

Here we discuss the role of the anorectal two- and three-dimensional ultrasonography in evaluating rarer benign and malignant anorectal and pelvic diseases. This is a useful exam to stage such lesions, identifying their relationship with the rectal wall and sphincter muscles and helping choose the best treatment option.

Introduction

Two- and three-dimensional ultrasonography is beneficial for evaluating anorectal disorders such as endometriosis, presacral neoplasias, solitary rectal ulcer, and rare neoplasias, as well as helping determine optimal treatment modalities for such disorders.

Endometriosis

Anorectal ultrasound scanning provides the most detailed view of endometriosis infiltration in the rectal wall. The three-dimensional mode allows accurate longitudinal measurements of the lesion and the distance to sphincter muscles, thus providing crucial information for choosing the most appropriate therapeutic approach [1]. Lesions appear as heterogeneous hypoechoic images, mostly located in the perirectal fat and infiltrating the layers of the rectal wall extending to the muscle layer or sphincter muscles (Fig. 1) or even as far as the mucosa (Fig. 2). Whereas proctological examination allows a diagnosis of perianal endometriosis to be established,

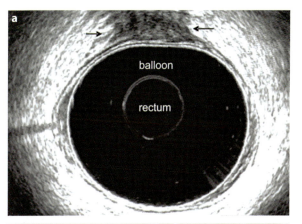

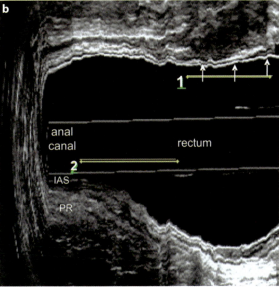

Fig. 1 a, b. Endometriosis lesion infiltrating the rectal wall as far as the muscle layer. **a** Axial plane. Heterogeneous image compromising 20% of the rectal circumference (*arrows*). **b** Sagittal plane. Lesion length is 2.1 cm (*1*) and is located 2.5 cm from the internal anal sphincter (*IAS*) and puborectalis (*PR*) muscle posteriorly (*2*) (*arrows*)

M. Pescatori, F.S.P. Regadas, S.M. Murad Regadas, A.P. Zbar (eds.), *Imaging Atlas of the Pelvic Floor and Anorectal Diseases*.
ISBN 978-88-470-0808-3. © Springer-Verlag Italia 2008

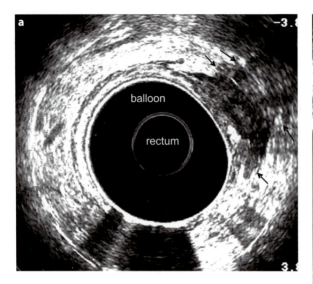
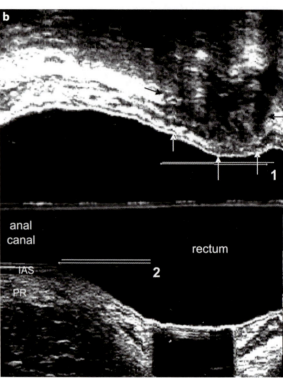

Fig. 2 a, b. Endometriosis lesion infiltrating the rectal wall as far as the mucosal layer. **a** Heterogeneous image compromising 30% of the rectal circumference (*arrows*). **b** Lesion length is 2.2 cm (*1*) and is located 1.9 cm from the internal anal sphincter (*IAS*) and puborectalis (*PR*) muscle posteriorly (*2*) (*arrows*)

three-dimensional ultrasound scanning makes it possible to determine the exact circumferential and longitudinal extent of infiltration into the sphincter muscles and the rectovaginal septum (Fig. 3).

Presacral Neoplasm

Perirectal neoplasm is most often located in the retrorectal space and may be of varied etiology. Half the cases are congenital, and two thirds are cystic in nature [2, 3]. It tends to affect young female adults but is uncommon in infants. Teratoma is the most frequently observed form in pediatric patients [3, 4]. Anorectal ultrasound scanning is useful in evaluating lesion size, type, and relationship with the rectal wall and sphincter muscles. Perirectal neoplasm appears as a hypoechoic area (cyst) or as an area of mixed echogenicity, usually with regular outline and not adhering to the rectal wall (Figs. 4 and 5).

Solitary Rectal Ulcer

A solitary rectal ulcer is located in the lower rectum and is most common in young adults. On ultrasound, the muscle layer of the rectal wall is thicker

than normal, and the injury appears as a hypoechoic area in one of the quadrants, although it may occasionally involve the entire rectal circumference. The internal anal sphincter also appears thickened [5] (Fig. 6).

Rare Neoplasms

Schwannoma, or neurilennoma, is a rare neoplasm originally referred to as malignant schwannoma, now known as malignant peripheral nerve-sheath tumor. Although a definitive diagnosis requires anatomical and pathological examination, endorectal ultrasound scanning shows the exact extent of tumor infiltration into the layers of the rectal wall and sphincter muscles (Fig. 7).

Peculiar Ultrasound Images

In order to choose the best treatment approach, endorectal three-dimensional ultrasound is very useful in evaluating some other rare types of diseases, such as posttraumatic urinary fistula (Fig. 8), granuloma in the rectovaginal septum (Fig. 9), perineal recurrent sarcoma (Fig. 10), and pelvic sarcoma (Fig. 11).

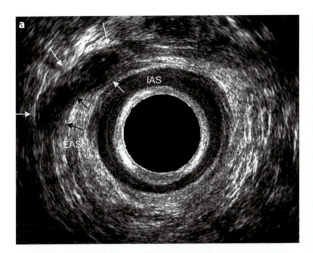

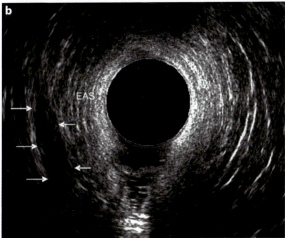

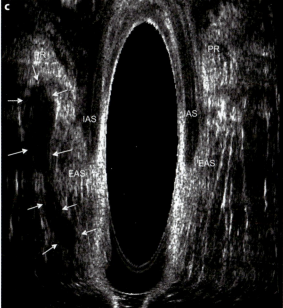

Fig. 3 a-c. Endometriosis lesion infiltrating the external anal sphincter (*EAS*)/puborectalis muscle and perianal fat. **a** Mid anal canal and **b** lower anal canal; heterogeneous images (*arrows*). **c** Coronal with diagonal planes. Lesion length is 3.1 cm (*arrows*). *PR* puborectalis muscle, *IAS* internal anal sphincter

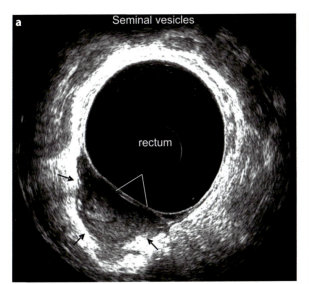

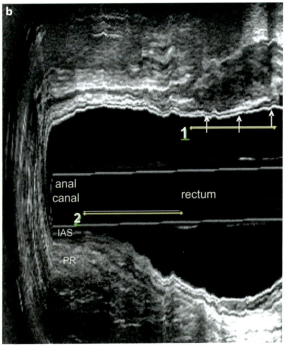

Fig. 4 a, b. Presacral neoplasm with regular outline and without adherence to the rectal wall. **a** Mixed echogenicity (*arrows*). **b** Sagittal with diagonal planes. Lesion size is 2.5 cm × 2.1 cm (*1*) and is located 2.2 cm from the posterior internal anal sphincter (*IAS*) and puborectalis (*PR*) muscle (*2*) (*arrows*)

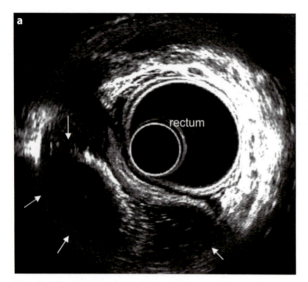

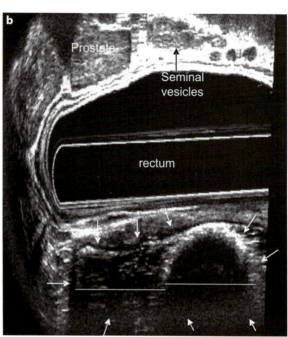

Fig. 5 a, b. Bilobulated presacral neoplasm, regular outline, without adherence to the rectal wall. **a** Hypoechoic echogenicity (*arrows*). **b** Sagittal with diagonal planes. Lesion length is 5.0 cm, located at the anorectal junction and lower rectum (*arrows*)

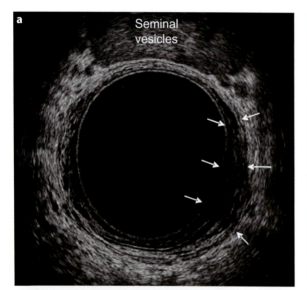

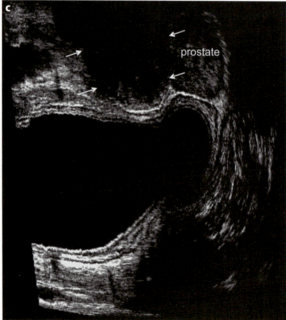

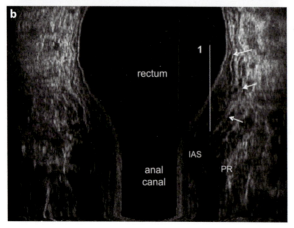

Fig. 6 a-c. Solitary rectal ulcer. **a** Hypoechoic area involving the left quadrant of the rectal wall (*arrows*). **b** Coronal plane. **c** Sagittal with diagonal plane. Lesion length is 2.2 cm, compromising the anorectal junction and lower rectum (*1*) (*arrows*). *IAS* internal anal sphincter, *PR* puborectalis muscle

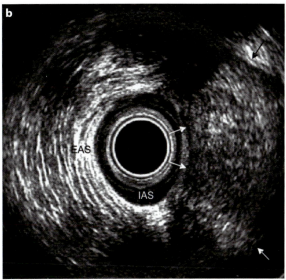

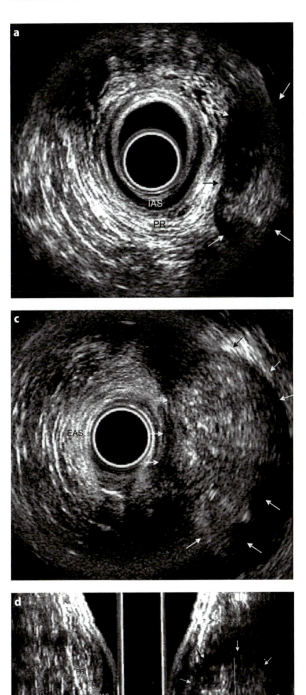

Fig. 7 a-d. Schwannoma. Heterogeneous image compromising 50% of the anal circumference, the entire anal canal length, and the anorectal junction (*arrows*). **a** Upper anal canal. Puborectalis (*PR*) muscle and perianal fat involvement (*arrows*). **b** Mid and **c** lower anal canal. External anal sphincter (*EAS*) and perianal fat compromised (*arrows*). **d** Lesion length is 4.2 cm, involving the anal canal and the anorectal junction (*arrows*). *IAS* internal anal sphincter

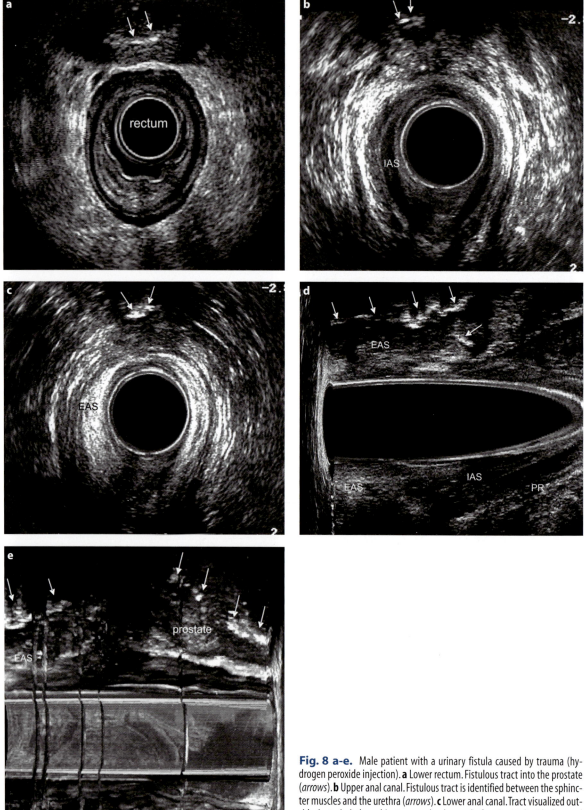

Fig. 8 a-e. Male patient with a urinary fistula caused by trauma (hydrogen peroxide injection). **a** Lower rectum. Fistulous tract into the prostate (*arrows*). **b** Upper anal canal. Fistulous tract is identified between the sphincter muscles and the urethra (*arrows*). **c** Lower anal canal. Tract visualized outside (anterior) the sphincter muscles (*arrows*). **d, e** Sagittal with diagonal planes. Fistulous tract is visualized outside the sphincter muscles and into the prostate (*arrows*). *EAS* external anal sphincter, *IAS* internal anal sphincter, *PR* puborectalis muscle

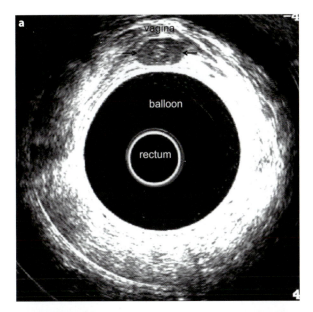

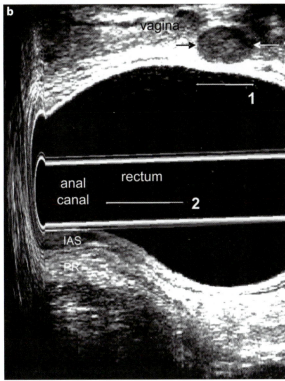

Fig. 9 a, b. Female patient. Granulomatous lesion in the rectovaginal septum after hysterectomy. **a** Heterogeneous image located in the rectovaginal septum without adherence to the rectal wall (*arrows*). **b** Lesion length is 1.1 cm (*1*) and is located 2.2 cm from the posterior internal anal sphincter (*IAS*) and puborectalis (*PR*) muscle (*2*) (*arrows*)

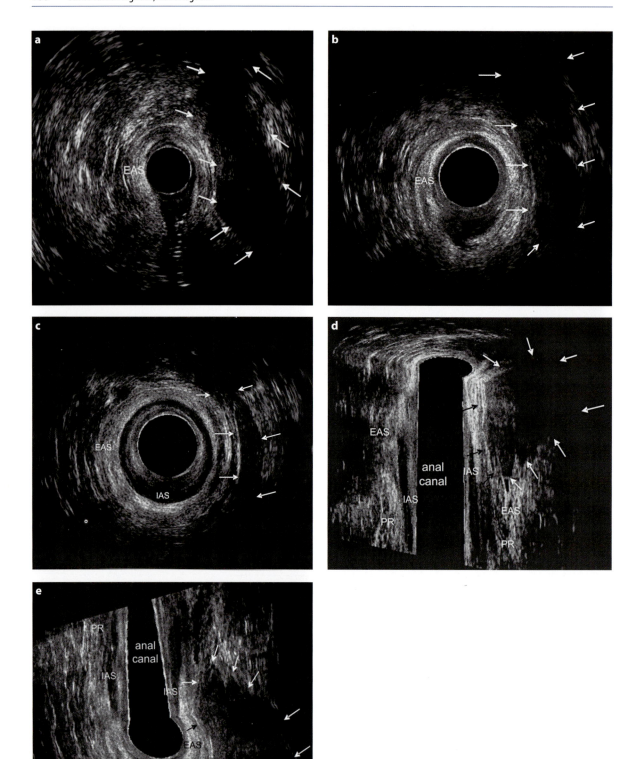

Fig. 10 a-e. Recurrent sarcoma. Perianal and perineal bilobulated heterogeneous image compromising the perianal fat and the external anal sphincter (*EAE*). **a**, **b** Lower anal canal and **c** mid anal canal. Involvement of perianal fat and external anal sphincter (*EAS*), with anterior perineum infiltration (*arrows*). **d**, **e** Coronal with diagonal planes (*arrows*). *PR* puborectalis muscle

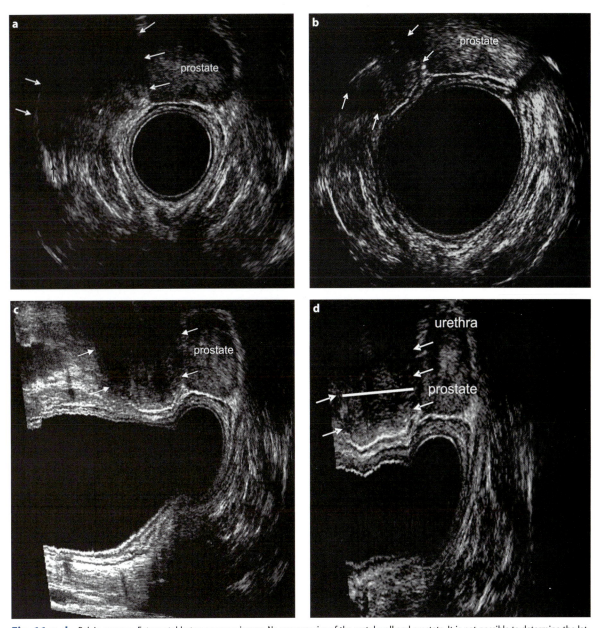

Fig. 11 a-d. Pelvic sarcoma. Extrarectal heterogeneous image. No compromise of the rectal wall and prostate. It is not possible to determine the lateral boundaries. **a, b** Lower rectum. Lesion is visualized at the prostate level (*arrows*). **c, d** Sagittal with diagonal planes. Lesion length is 2.7 cm (*arrows*)

References

1. Regadas SMM, Regadas FSP, Rodrigues LV et al (2005) Importância do ultra-som tridimensional na avaliação anorretal. Arq Gastroenterol 42:226–232
2. Dozois RR, Chiu LKM (1997) Retrorectal tumours in surgery of the colon and rectum. Nicholls RJ, Dozeis RR (eds) Surgery of the colon and rectum. Churchill Livingston, New York, pp 533–545
3. Gordon PH (1999) Retrorectal tumours. In: Gordon PH, Nivatvongs S (eds) Principles and practice of surgery for the colon, rectum and anus. Quality Medical Publishers Inc, St Louis, pp 427–445
4. Hjemslad BM, Helwin EB (1988) Tailgut cysts. Report of 53 cases. Am J Clin Pathol 89:139–147
5. Marshall M, Halligan S, Fotheringham T et al (2002) Predictive value of internal anal sphincter thickness for diagnosis of rectal intussusception in patients with solitary rectal ulcer. Br J Surg 89:1281–1285

SECTION IV

Large Bowel and Pelvic Floor Functional Assessment: Imaging Indications and Technical Principles

CHAPTER 18

Radiography and Radiopaque Markers in Colonic Transit-Time Studies

Angelita Habr-Gama, José Marcio Neves Jorge

Abstract

Although considered an indirect test to evaluate colonic motility, colonic transit-time assessment provides a definition for constipation by converting an otherwise hopelessly subjective symptom to an objective part of the medical record. Its most important role lies in excluding factitious constipation; however, its association with video defecography is crucial. Additionally, colonic transit times can help uncover causative diagnoses by stratifying motility disorders into two main patterns: colonic inertia and outlet obstruction. Several factors, including diet, physical activity, and psychological and hormonal factors may affect digestive transit-time results; therefore, some variation is expected. The most commonly used technique to measure colonic transit time involves two abdominal radiographs taken on days 3 and 5 after a single-day ingestion of 24 solid radiopaque markers.

Introduction

Chronic constipation is a common condition and affects about 3% of the adult population and 20% of the elderly population. It is more common in women than in men. The diagnostic criteria for definition of constipation have been recently revised in the Rome II classification as the presence during the precedent year, for at least 12 weeks not necessarily consecutive and in more than one fourth of defecations, of two or more of the following complaints: straining, lumpy or hard stools, sensation of incomplete evacuation, sensation of anorectal obstruction/blockage, manual maneuvers (digital evacuation, support of the pelvic floor, etc.) to facilitate defecation, and/or less than three defecations per week. Loose stools are not present, and there are insufficient criteria for the diagnosis of irritable bowel syndrome. Although very common, its pathophysiology is not well understood.

Two major pathophysiologic subtypes of constipation may be identified, with a third being the coexistence of both in the same patient. The most frequent subtype is represented by pelvic floor dysfunction (also known as outlet obstruction, obstructed defecation, dyschezia, animus, pelvic dyssynergia), which features normal or slightly slowed colonic transit with residual storage in the rectum or rectosigmoid area. The main pathophysiologic mechanism is due to an inability to adequately evacuate contents from the rectum. The other subtype is slow-transit constipation (STC), a clinical syndrome usually affecting women and characterized by often intractable constipation and heavily delayed colonic transit. This condition is usually attributed to a disorder in colonic motor function.

The colon, through segmentation, mass, and retrograde movements, accounts for approximately 90% of the total digestive transit time. Since 1907, colonic transit time has been primarily evaluated as the total digestive transit through the elimination of different markers in the feces: contrast medium (barium sulphate), dyes (carmine, charcoal), particles (seeds, colored glass beads), chemical substances (copper thiocyanate) [1–6]. In fact, because patient complaints of stool frequency are subjective, an objective method for measuring colonic transit time is desirable. These methods, however, have been abandoned due to lack of practicality, difficulty in interpretation, or inaccuracy.

In 1969, Hinton et al. [7] described a method using markers initially prepared by cutting radiopaque Levine tubes in circular or cylindrical shapes. Lat-

M. Pescatori, F.S.P. Regadas, S.M. Murad Regadas, A.P. Zbar (eds.), *Imaging Atlas of the Pelvic Floor and Anorectal Diseases*. ISBN 978-88-470-0808-3. © Springer-Verlag Italia 2008

er, these markers became commercially available, enclosed in gelatin capsules that ensure their arrival *in bolus* into the gastric lumen (Fig. 1). The simplest and most practical method of evaluating colonic transit requires ingestion of 24 radiopaque markers and quantification of these markers on abdominal radiographs. Normal total intestinal transit time involves elimination of at least 80% of markers on the fifth day of study (Fig. 2).

Subsequently, segmental colonic transit-times study was proposed as the ideal assessment of colonic transit [8, 9]. Rather than measuring the elimination or clearance of markers, the index of transit time of this method was the actual number of retained markers in each colonic segment. The spinal processes and imaginary lines from the fifth lumbar vertebra to the pelvic outlet have been used to recognize the three segments of the large bowel (right colon, left colon, and rectosigmoid) on radiographs (Fig. 3) [10]. The classical technique of measuring segmental transit time consisted of a single ingestion of 20 or 24 markers followed by serial radiographs taken at 24-h intervals until total elimination of markers occurred. When using 24 markers, the sum of the retained markers in each colonic segment on the successive radiographs represents the value, in hours, for each segmental transit time [11, 12]. To reduce radiation exposure and achieve more practicality, subsequent technical modifications included multiple ingestion of markers rather than multiple ra-

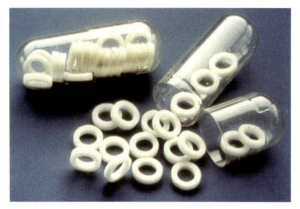

Fig. 1. Colonic transit-time markers

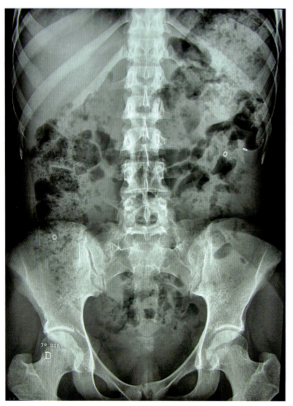

Fig. 2. Colonic transit-time study showing normal elimination (≥ 80%) of markers

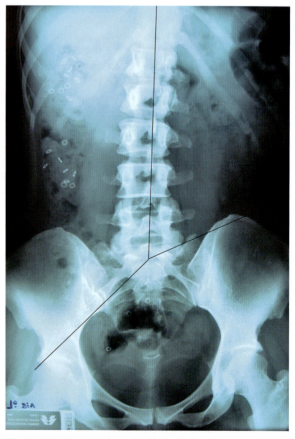

Fig. 3. Colonic transit-time study with distribution of markers on the first abdominal radiograph after ingestion. The landmarks shown are required for segmental colonic transit-time assessment and divide the large intestinal segment into right colon, left colon, and rectosigmoid

diographs, and the use of markers of different shapes. The rationale behind segmental colonic transit-time study is that embryological, anatomical, and functional differences exist among the right colon, left colon, and rectosigmoid. Therefore, all three segments may be affected independently in motility disorders. In fact, with the advent of this method of study, the motility patterns of colonic inertia, outlet obstruction, and left-colon delay could be demonstrated [12]. However, although proven useful, the value of this assessment remains a controversial issue. Accurate assessment of segmental transit times still involves either multiple ingestion of markers or multiple abdominal radiographs.

For practicality, however, the technique involving two radiographs, taken on days 3 and 5 after a single-day ingestion of 24 radiopaque markers, may suffice. Prior to testing, a digital examination and, if necessary, a simple abdominal radiograph are indicated to ensure that the colon is cleared of any contrast material from previous studies and that there is no fecal impaction in the rectum. The use of enemas, laxatives, or any other medication known to affect gastrointestinal motility should be discontinued for 3 days prior to ingestion of the markers until study completion. Markers should be taken at a specified time, usually at 8 a.m. Patients are oriented to maintain their normal diet; however, supplemental fiber such as bran or psyllium can be helpful to exclude dietary causes. The use of a diary of bowel frequency and related symptoms during the study period is also helpful, as symptoms can be better evaluated. The study may be repeated if the patient reports that defecation frequency during the study is not representative of his or her usual bowel habits. The abdominal radiograph should include the diaphragm and the pubis to yield identification of all markers in the colon.

In normal individuals, markers reach the cecum within 8 h after ingestion. The mean and maximal values for normal individuals for total colonic transit time are 36 and 55 h, respectively [11]. The mean segmental transit times are 12, 14, and 11 h for right colon, left colon, and rectosigmoid, respectively; the maximal values for segmental transit times are 22, 34, and 27 h for right colon, left colon, and rectosigmoid, respectively [11]. The mean value of normal total colonic transit time is about 32 h for men and 41 h for women. This difference for gender is even greater when the right colon transit time is analyzed separately. Age, however, does not seem to affect total colonic transit times. In children, although the rectosigmoid transit time is more prolonged, the total colonic transit time is similar to that in the adult, probably due to the proportional reduction of segmental transit times for the right and left colon [9].

Colonic transit-time assessment provides a definition for constipation by converting an otherwise hopelessly subjective symptom to an objective part of the medical record. Therefore, its most important role lies in excluding factitious constipation. Additionally, segmental transit times can help to uncover causative diagnoses by stratifying motility disorders into two main patterns: colonic inertia and outlet obstruction (Figs. 4 and 5).

Colonic inertia is characterized by diffuse stasis of markers throughout the colon, usually more markedly in the right colon. This condition typically affects young women as a severe and incapacitating symptom. The etiopathogeny of colonic inertia remains unclear. Lesions of the myenteric plexus have been demonstrated in patients with colonic inertia; however, these lesions can be either primary or related to chronic use of laxatives. Colonic inertia can be also associated with other symptoms of visceral stasis, and a hypothesis of a systemic disorder has been proposed. Its treatment, however, has been less controversial; total colectomy with ileorectal anastomosis may alleviate

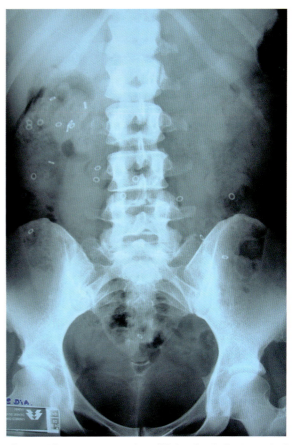

Fig. 4. Colonic transit-time study on fifth day of study showing stasis of colonic markers in right colon

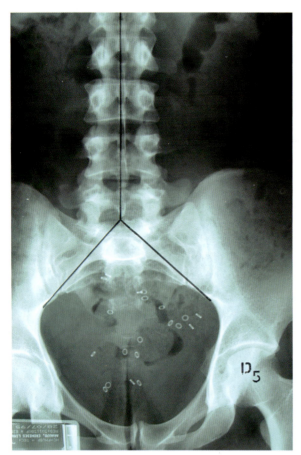

Fig. 5. Colonic transit-time study on fifth day of study showing retention of markers in the rectosigmoid colon

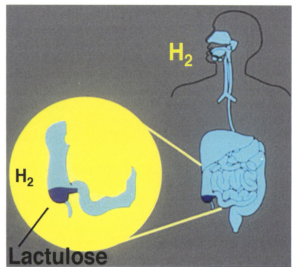

Fig. 6. Small-bowel transit-time study [hydrogen (H_2) breath-test equipment]

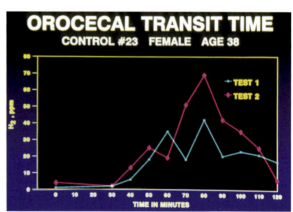

Fig. 7. Curves showing normal elimination of hydrogen (H_2) breath test

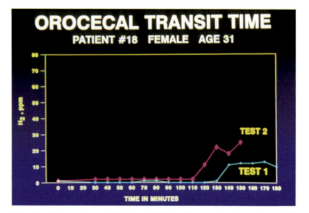

Fig. 8. Slow, prolonged hydrogen (H_2) breath excretion in a patient with colonic inertia

symptoms in 80–96% of cases, yet careful patient selection is mandatory. Selection criteria include assessing symptom severity (history, transit times, and response to trials of therapy with laxatives and prokinetics) and exclusion of both pelvic-floor dysfunction and small-bowel dysmotility [lactulose, hydrogen (H_2) breath test] (Figs. 6–8) [13]. If dyspeptic symptoms such as nausea, vomiting, heartburn, and bloating are present, gastric emptying studies are indicated to exclude a generalized gastrointestinal stasis.

Outlet obstruction is characterized when the stasis of markers is limited to the rectosigmoid. In this condition, the association of other tests, particularly cinedefecography, anorectal manometry, and anal electromyography, is of paramount importance to diagnose the causative disorder. A third abnormal pattern found during segmental colonic transit-time assessment is the isolated delay of markers in the left colon (Fig. 9). Although some controversy exists concerning the physiopathology explaining this pattern, this is the most representative pattern in patients with chagasic megacolon (Fig. 10) [14].

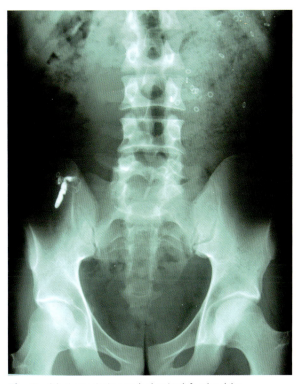

Fig. 9. Colonic transit-time study showing left-colon delay

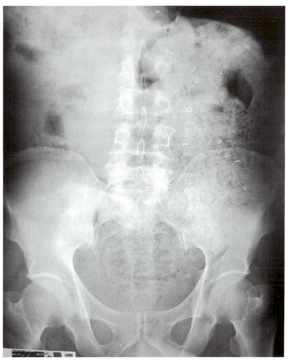

Fig. 10. Colonic transit-time study showing left-colon-delay pattern in a patient with chagasic megacolon

Several factors, including diet, physical activity, and psychological and hormonal factors, may affect digestive transit-time results; therefore, significant variation is expected. However, segmental colonic transit-time study using radiopaque markers has proven reproducible when analyzed in the same individual within a mean interval of 3 months [15]. When colonic transit times are evaluated using two different methods – specifically, single and multiple ingestion of markers – the mean difference between the two measurements are 2.1, 0.34, and 1.54 h for the right colon, left colon, and rectosigmoid, respectively [15]. Recently, in a study of reproducibility of colonic transit time in patients with chronic constipation, Nam et al. [16] have shown the method is best for patients with idiopathic constipation and worst for colonic inertia; therefore, according to these authors, consideration should be given to repeat colonic transit-time studies before colectomy to secure the diagnosis and improve outcome.

Another way to assess colonic transit time is the radionuclear scintigraphic technique: with this method, the colon is easier to outline, and it is con-sequently easier to identify the different colon segments. Furthermore, multiple images can be obtained without adding excessive radiation. However, the scintigraphic technique is not widely used in clinical practice.

Suspected gastrointestinal tract motility disorders are among the most frequently encountered diseases in clinical gastroenterology. However, the pathophysiology of these conditions is yet to be elucidated; one reason for this obscurity is inadequacy of the technical approach to these diseases.

More recently, a novel approach for measuring segmental transit time through the gut using the biomagnetic method was proposed [17]. This method features the unique ability to identify magnetic-field source in the body either generated by the electrical activity of specific organs and tissues or by magnetic marker particles. The magnetic method offers the possibility of simultaneously studying small and large intestinal transit times in groups of patients with suspected motility disorders who cannot be investigated for safety reasons, such as children and pregnant women.

References

1. Hertz AF, Morton CJ, Cook F et al (1907) The passage of food along the human alimentary canal. Guy's Hospital Reports 61:389–427
2. Labayle D, Modigliani R, Matuchansky C et al (1977) Diarrhee avec acceleration du transit intestinal. Gastroenterol Clin Biol 1:231–242
3. Alvarez WC, Freedlander BL (1924) The rate of progress of food residues through the bowel. JAMA 23:576–580
4. Dick M (1969) Use of cuprous thiocyanate as a short-term continuous marker for faeces. Gut 10:408–412
5. Kirwan WO, Smith AN (1974) Gastrointestinal transit estimated by an isotope capsule. Scand J Gastroenterol 9:763–766
6. Krevsky B, Malmud LS, D'ercole et al (1986) Colonic transit scintigraphy. A physiologic approach to the quantitative measurement of colonic transit in humans. Gastroenterology 91:1102–1112
7. Hinton JM, Lennard-Jones JE, Young AC (1969) A new method for studying gut transit times using radiopaque markers. Gut 10:842–847
8. Martelli H, Devroede G, Arhan P et al (1978) Some parameters of large bowel motility in normal man. Gastroenterology 75:612–618
9. Arhan P, Devroede G, Jehannin B et al (1981) Segmental colonic transit time. Dis Colon Rectum 24:625–629
10. Martelli H, Devroede G, Arhan P, Duguay C (1978) Mechanisms of idiopathic constipation: outlet obstruction. Gastroenterology 75:623–631
11. Jorge JMN, Habr-Gama A (1991) Tempo de transito colonico total e segmentar: analise critica dos metodos e estudo em individuos normais com marcadores radiopacos. Rev Bras Colo Proct 11:55–60
12. Cohen S, Vaccaro C, Kaye M, Wexner S (1994) Can segmental colonic transit times be reproduced with reliable results? (Presented as a poster) In: 93rd Annual Meeting of the American Society of Colon & Rectal Surgeons, Orlando, 1994
13. Jorge JMN, Wexner SD, Ehrenpreis E (1994) The lactulose H2 breath test as a measure of orocecal transit time (OCTT) Eur J Surg 160:409–416
14. Jorge JMN, Habr-Gama A, Yusuf AS et al (2001) Physiologic investigation of constipated patients with Chagas disease. Colorectal Dis 3(1):86
15. Bouchoucha M, Devroede G, Arhan P (1992) What is the meaning of colorectal transit time measurement? Dis Colon Rectum 35:773–782
16. Nam Y-S, Pikarsky AJ, Wexner SD (2001) Reproducibility of colonic transit study in patients with chronic constipation. Dis Colon Rectum 44:86–92
17. Basile M, Neri M, Carriero A et al (1992) Measurement of segmental transit through the gut in man. A novel approach by the biomagnetic method. Dig Dis Sciences 37:1537–1543

Commentary

Mario Pescatori

This chapter is very well written, and the authors are to be commended for their expertise. There are just a few things to add, which concern the most difficult cases of chronic constipation in patients with an important psychosomatic component. Such patients are likely to be women, dressed in dark clothing, not remembering their dreams, reporting sexual abuse in adolescence, preferring the color blue to the color red, with a weak handshake to the doctor. In the mid-1990s, Devroede [1] demonstrated in his chapter on Psychopathology and Physiopathology in the book *Constipation*, edited by Wexner and Bartolo, that transit times may change in the same patient according to progression of both psychotherapy and pelvic floor rehabilitation and the patient's improved symptoms. Simultaneously, normalization of rectal sensation may also be recorded at anal manometry, thus showing the close connections between the myenteric plexus, the extrinsic nerves, and the brain. Therefore, the crucial point is that transit times may vary with variation of conservative treatment, and therefore, the value of such treatment should not be taken as absolute by the clinician. A draw-the-family test or a self portrait carried out by the patient may be helpful to show a nonverbalized comment to the doctor, allowing him or her to understand hidden family events that might have influenced the patient's pathology. This may represent a useful indirect psychological test, taking in account that most patients, if invited to consult a psychologist, would refuse and would go and see another doctor, being afraid to "be considered mad". Instead, the drawings are carried out by the majority of patients without

any difficulty and may be evaluated both by the doctor and the psychologist in a further stage.

In case of slow transit and colonic inertia not responding to conservative treatment, colectomy and ileorectal anastomosis may be the last option. However, patients must be aware that constipation is likely to be relieved after surgery, whereas other troublesome symptoms, such as abdominal pain and bloating or headache or dysmenorrhea will persist in 50% of cases. Moreover, up to 70% of cases, as reported by the Wexner group [2], may have either diarrhea or incontinence, which may affect their quality of life.

Finally, after colectomy and ileorectal anastomosis, gross hypokalemia due to frequent diarrhea, leading to profound asthenia and incontinence, may be due to an unrecognized plasma loss of the hormone peptide tyrosine (PYY), which is also called "ileal brake". The hormone is produced mainly by the large bowel and is aimed at slowing the output of the terminal ileum into the caecum. A patient with chronic, severe slow-transit constipation may well have a decreased production of this hormone after meals. Therefore, the peristaltic drive of the terminal ileum is not counteracted and, in absence of the removed colon, the rectal reservoir is unable to antagonize the ileal effluent, with the consequence of bowel dysfunction. Such postoperative dysfunction may be prevented by the study of small-bowel transit time, either with a barium meal or by breath test.

The construction of an ileal reservoir above the ileorectal anastomosis possibly associated with a sphincteroplasty may help normalize the patient's disturbances, as reported by Pescatori et al. [3].

References

1. Devroede G (1994) Psychological considerations in subjects with chronic idiophatic constipation. In: Wexner SD and Bartolo DCC (eds) Constipation: etiology, evaluation and management. Butterworth Heinemann, London

2. Thaler K, Dinnerwitzer A, Oberwalder M et al (2005) Quality of life after colectomy for colonic inertia. Tech Coloproctol 5:133–138
3. Pescatori M, Pietroletti R, Anastasio G, Rossi Z (1992) Endocrine pathogenesis and surgical treatment of postcolectomy diarrhoea. Coloproctology 4:244–247

CHAPTER 19

Cinedefecography in Functional Pelvic Floor Disorders

Bianca Santoni, Steven D. Wexner

Abstract

Cinedefecography is one of the most important exams to be performed in patients with pelvic floor dysfunction. Its popularity has rapidly increased compared with other routine studies for evaluating anorectal disorders, as it is inexpensive and relatively easy to perform. Additionally, it provides dynamic and static images of pelvic-floor structures during rest, squeeze, and evacuation.

Introduction

Cinedefecography, also named fluoroscopic evacuation proctography, is a well-known radiologic exam used to evaluate patients with functional pelvic-floor disorders [obstructed defecation syndrome (ODS)]. It was first used by Walldén in 1952 [1], when he initiated a study that was timed to correlate between deep rectovaginal pouches, enterocele, and obstructed defecation. However, it was not until the 1980s that Mahieu et al. [2, 3] developed a technique that became standardized by the modification of performing opacification of the pelvic anatomy landmarks.

As this exam is a combination of dynamic and static images taken during rest, squeeze, and evacuation [4], it is very helpful in diagnosing evacuatory problems. Cinedefecography allows a closer physiologic evaluation of the evacuation process compared with other diagnostic tools. It also provides measurements in the resting, squeezing, and pushing positions to show both anatomical and physiological abnormalities.

As defecography is an image-based study, it does not evoke any physiologic responses. Physiologic response is based on rectal fullness leading to distension of the rectal wall to accommodate stool, causing reflex internal anal sphincter (IAS) relaxation and external anal sphincter (EAS) contraction. When a person is in an adequate environment to allow evacuation, the EAS and pelvic floor muscles relax, and the anal canal opens for the stool to pass. The exam depends only on voluntary control of the pelvic floor and passive emptying of the rectum [5].

Technique

Knowledge of both anorectal anatomy and physiology are fundamental to perform cinedefecography, which is an otherwise relatively simple examination. Challenges are more closely related to interpretation rather than performance of the evaluation.

The patient self-administers a Fleet enema at home 1–2 h prior to the scheduled test. The patient is usually placed on the X-ray table in the left lateral side position with the legs flexed. A digital rectal exam is performed, and explanations are given to the patient regarding the instructions that will be given during the exam to rest, squeeze, and push. After the explanation, the lubricated injector is carefully positioned into the rectum, and barium suspension is gradually administered until it reaches the sigmoid colon. A mixture of 150 cc of barium paste, oatmeal, and a sufficient quantity of water is used to give a very hard and thick appearance to the mixture, because this paste should mimic stool. This preparation was commercially available as a paste (Evacu-Paste™, E-Z-EM Inc., Westbury, NY, USA) but is

M. Pescatori, F.S.P. Regadas, S.M. Murad Regadas, A.P. Zbar (eds.), *Imaging Atlas of the Pelvic Floor and Anorectal Diseases.*
ISBN 978-88-470-0808-3. © Springer-Verlag Italia 2008

no longer marketed [5]. At Cleveland Clinic Florida (CCF), vaginal opacification is also performed in which a mixture of iodine and ultrasound gel is inserted into the vagina with a rubber catheter or a syringe. This allows differentiation from the anal canal and visualization of enterocele (image of widening of the space between the anal canal and the vaginal canal). Neither oral barium contrast nor intraperitoneal instillation of nonionic contrast medium is used to identify enterocele, as has been described by other centers. An alternative to vaginal-gel contrast medium is to insert a tampon soaked in iodine contrast medium to assess the depth of the rectogenital fossa and visualize the interposition any of intra-abdominal content between the rectum and vagina [6].

After the insertion of the contrasts, the patient is asked to step off of the X-ray table and sit on a commode placed parallel to the X-ray table to allow lateral visualization of the rectum. This commode should be made of a material that can capture radiation filtrate equivalent to 4 mCi to obtain good radiographic results at the anal canal level while allowing visualization of the bony landmarks [7, 8]. A sequence of images is taken in the rest, squeeze, and push positions, all of which are recorded on a tape DVD. The position adopted at CCF is to perform the exam after insertion of the contrast medium while the patient is seated on a commode. However, the radiologists considered this position to provide poor-quality images for static films [9] and may predispose to overdiagnosis [10]. Accordingly, the left lateral decubitus position is more acceptable to the radiologists.

The radiation dose for defecography is 3–7 mSv, a little lower than that used for barium enema studies (10–17 mSv) [11]. This radiation dosage is considered higher in comparison with the barium enema because the area in which the beam acts is smaller, and thus more radiation per unit is used. The radiation dose for 100 s of videofluoroscopy is five times higher for a barium enema (750 mrad) than for a cinedefecogram (270 mrad) [9].

Lines

Before analyzing the three stages of the defecogram, it is very important to identify some structures (Fig. 1). The coccyx, sacrum, head of the femur, posterior wall of the rectum, and anal canal should be identified. A line is drawn in the middle of the anal canal, described as the anorectal line. The pubococcygeal line is drawn from the tip of the coccyx to the head of the femur, because it is very difficult to

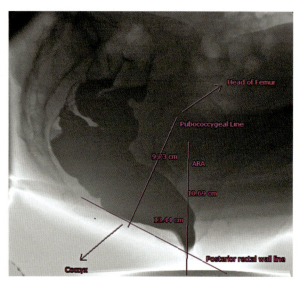

Fig. 1. Main lines on defecography. *ARA* anorectal angle

identify the pubis, as it is almost at the same level as the head of the femur. At the posterior wall of the rectum, a third line is drawn.

After all these lines are drawn, measurements are taken of the anorectal angle (ARA), perineal descent (PD), and puborectalis length (PRL). The ARA is the angle between the anal canal line and one third of the posterior rectal wall line [2, 12]. The PD is the measurement of the vertical distance between the position of the ARA and the pubococcygeal line [13], forming an angle of 90°. The PRL is the distance between the ARA and the pubic symphysis that will be substituted by the head of the femur. ARA, PRL, and PD values are shown in Table 1.

Positions

On a normal defecogram, in the rest stage (Fig. 2a), the rectum is posteriorly angled, parallel to the presacral space [14]. The anal canal is closed, and the anorectal junction is identified. The position of the rectum is due to the puborectalis (PR) muscle that forms a sling posterior to the rectum at the junction of the rectal ampulla and the anal canal.

Table 1. Static values in the different positions. From [9]

Measures	Rest	Squeeze	Push
Anorectal angle	70–140°	75–90°	100–180°
Puborectalis length	14–16 cm	12–15 cm	15–18 cm
Perineal descent	3–4 cm	–	6–8 cm

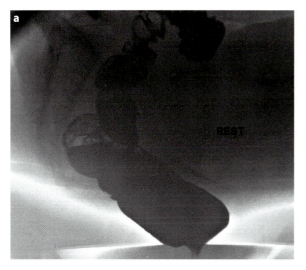
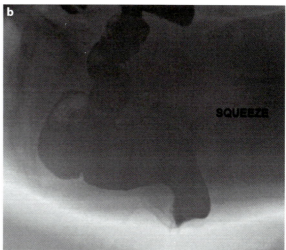
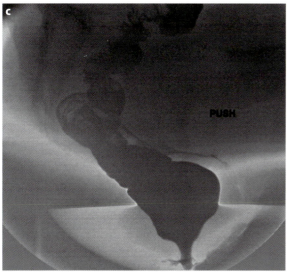

Fig. 2 a-c. a Rest position. **b** Squeeze position. Notice the sling of the puborectalis muscle pushing upward the anorectal junction. **c** Push position. Notice the straightening of the posterior rectal wall (puborectalis muscle relaxation)

In the resting position, the inferior part of the ischial tuberosity defines the pelvic floor and the anorectal junction. When defecography was first used, the anorectal angle was considered a very important tool to maintain continence, but further studies have shown that normal patients and those with anorectal disturbances have common characteristics [7, 15, 16]. The normal pelvic floor is 1.8 cm below the pubococcygeal line; an increase in this value at rest on the dynamic image reveals increased perineal descent.

During the squeeze stage (Fig. 2b), the anorectal junction is anteriorly pulled together with the pelvic floor due to contraction of the PR muscle. In this position, the ARA and the length of the anal canal should decrease.

During the push stage (Fig. 2c), the anorectal junction increases as the anal canal opens completely, and the distal rectum should empty in less than 30 s.

The normal pelvic floor is 3.0 cm below the pubococcygeal line. Intussusception, sigmoidocele, and enterocele are best identified in the push position.

Indications

Cinedefecography maybe indicated in patients with chronic constipation to evaluate the obstructed defecation, which is normally produced by rectocele, sigmoidocele and/or enterocele, internal rectal intussusception, and increased perineal descent.

Rectocele

This bulge or herniation of the rectal wall can be anterior or, less commonly, posterior (Fig. 3). A recto-

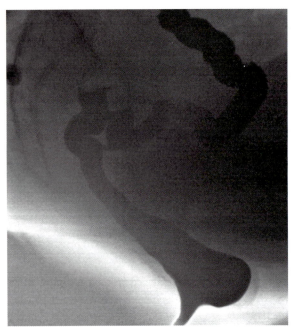

Fig. 3. Anterior rectocele. Presence on anterior bulging of the rectal wall

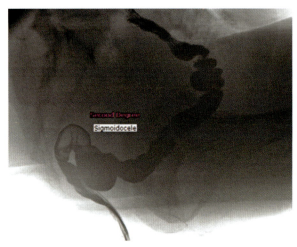

Fig. 4. Second-degree sigmoidocele. The sigmoid loop is below the pubococcygeal line

cele is localized posterolateral to the rectum can be associated with levator ani damage during childbirth, and some rare rectoceles, >4.0 cm, may be associated with an ischiorectal hernia [17]. This condition is more common in women, and the few cases diagnosed in men occur following prostatectomy [18]. Rectoceles are clinically characterized by straining during evacuation and the need to digitate, the function of pushing the anterior vaginal wall toward the posterior vaginal wall to assist evacuation.

Although rectoceles can be found in approximately 70% of women, they tend to be symptomatic only when they are >4 cm and are associated with prolonged or failed rectal emptying [9, 19].

Sigmoidocele or Enterocele

Sigmoidocele is defined as a laxity of the pelvic floor due to weakened tissues that support the vagina and the pelvic diaphragm. It is classified based on the position of the sigmoid loop during evacuation or during defecographic push. First-degree sigmoidocele is when the sigmoid loop does not cross the pubococcygeal line; second-degree sigmoidocele is when the sigmoid loop is between the pubococcygeal line and the ischiococcygeal line; third-degree sigmoidocele is when the sigmoid loop is below the ischiococcygeal line (Fig. 4). The main complaint is usually incomplete evacuation, straining, sensation of rectal pressure, and fullness [20].

Internal Rectal Intussusception

Intussusception is a circular infolding of the rectal wall which can occur during pushing. It can be intrarectal (limited to the rectum) or intra-anal (when it enters the anal canal) (Fig. 5) and may include mucosa and submucosa or even the full thickness of the rectal wall (procidentia). In most instances, this finding is not clinically significant. The classic complaint is constipation, presenting as difficult evacuation, and in more severe cases rectal pain with or without a solitary rectal ulcer.

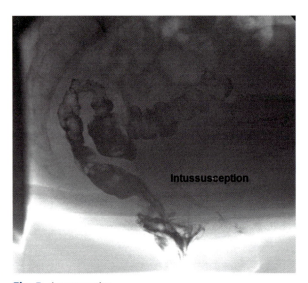

Fig. 5. Intussusception

Perineal Descent

This syndrome was first noticed by Porter [21] in 1962 and described by Parks et al. [22] in 1966. It is caused by a viscous cycle that is a combination of repeated, prolonged forceful straining, theoretically causing pelvic-floor muscle weakness and therefore causing protrusion of the anterior rectal wall into the anal canal. Multiple vaginal childbirths and chronic evacuatory difficulty may lead to pudendal nerve injury and the development of defecatory disturbances [20].

The seated position is more sensitive for diagnosing increased perineal disease due to the fact that this position is more physiologic and patients prefer it. It is classified in increased dynamic when the measurement during push is >3.0 cm from the measurement at rest (PD rest – PD push), and increased when the distance is >4.0 cm at rest [9].

Puborectalis Nonrelaxation

This syndrome is also called anismus or spastic pelvic-floor syndrome [5]. It is characterized by constant contraction of the PR muscle during push to evacuate (Fig. 6). There are several theories that attempt to explain this muscle dysfunction, such as muscular dystonia, abuse of cathartic laxatives, voluntary suppression of the normal inhibitory reflex, inflammation of the perianal area leading to spastic contraction, partial denervation of the pelvic floor,

and psychological factors [23]. The main complaint is usually constipation, straining, tenesmus, and incomplete evacuation. In 75–92% of patients, outlet obstruction is associated with PR nonrelaxation confirmed during cinedefecography [24].

To diagnose this syndrome, it is important to measure the PRL and the ARA [20]. Associated findings on cinedefecography include megarectum, failure of anal canal opening, and the presence of an anterior and/or posterior rectocele. A false positive result can occur secondary to patient embarrassment at the expulsion of stool in front of the physician and technicians in the radiology room. In such cases, the patient can be asked to go the bathroom to try to evacuate in privacy, following which a fluoroscopy is performed. A good predictor of relaxation of the PR is absence of excessive PD and relaxation of the muscle [7].

Conclusion

Cinedefecography is a dynamic and static radiologic exam based upon as reasonable a regulation of defecation physiology as possible. It is an inexpensive, simple, and fast exam, but as with any other diagnostic tool, it has its limitations. It is a very good exam to diagnose anismus, intussusception, rectocele, and sigmoidocele and enterocele. However, the treatment decision should be based on the association of clinical symptoms and radiologic images rather than solely on images, because, as mentioned, some findings are not clinically relevant if considered in isolation from clinical symptoms.

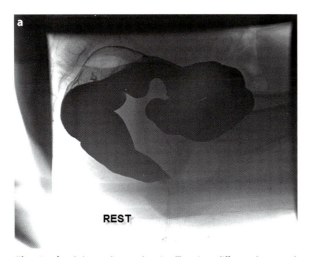 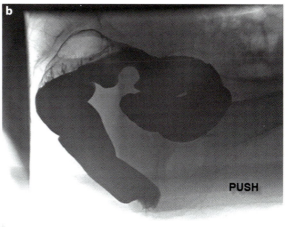

Fig. 6 a, b. Puborectalis nonrelaxation. There is no difference between the rest (**a**) and the push (**b**) position. The posterior rectal wall does not straighten

References

1. Walldén L (1952) Defecation block in cases of deep rectogenital pouch; a surgical roentgenological and embryological study with special reference to morphological conditions. Acta Chir Scand 165 (Suppl):1–122
2. Mahieu P, Pringot J, Bodart (1984) Defecography: I. Description of a new procedure and results in normal patients. Gastrointest Radiol 9(3):247–251
3. Mahieu P, Pringot J, Bodart (1984) Defecography: II. Contribution to the diagnosis of defecation disorders. Gastrointest Radiol 9(3):253–261
4. Bartram C (2003) Dynamic evaluation of the anorectum. Radiol Clin North Am 41(2):425–441
5. Maglinte DD, Bartram C (2007) Dynamic imaging of posterior compartment pelvic floor dysfunction by evacuation proctography: techniques, indications, results and limitations. Eur J Radiol 61(3):454–461
6. Hock D, Lombard R, Jehaes C et al (1993) Colpocystodefecography. Dis Colon Rectum 36(11):1015–1021
7. Bartram CI, Turnbull GK, Lennard-Jones JE (1988) Evacuation proctography: an investigation of rectal expulsion in 20 subjects without defecatory disturbance. Gastrointest Radiol 13(1):72–80
8. Ginai AZ (1990) Evacuation proctography (defecography). A new seat and method of examination. Clin Radiol 42(3):214–216
9. Bartolo DC, Bartram CI, Ekberg O et al (1988) Symposium. Proctography. Int J Colorectal Dis 3(2):67–89
10. Poon FW, Lauder JC, Finlay IG (1991) Technical report: evacuating proctography – a simplified technique. Clin Radiol 44(2):113–116
11. Goei R, Kemerink G (1990) Radiation dose in defecography. Radiology 176(1):137–139
12. Jorge JM, Wexner SD, Marchetti F et al (1992) How reliable are currently available methods of measuring the anorectal angle? Dis Colon Rectum 35(4):332–338
13. Hardcastle JD, Parks AG (1970) A study of anal incontinence and some principles of surgical treatment. Proc R Soc Med 63 (Suppl):116–118
14. Burhenne HJ (1964) Intestinal evacuation study: a new roentgenologic technique. Radiol Clin 33:79–84
15. Shorvon PJ, McHugh S, Diamant NE et al (1989) Defecography in normal volunteers: results and implications. Gut 30(12):1737–1749
16. Selvaggi F, Pesce G, Scotto Di Carlo E et al (1990) Evaluation of normal subjects by defecographic technique. Dis Colon Rectum 33(8):698–702
17. Grassi R, Pommeri F (1995) Defecography study of outpouchings of the external wall of the rectum: posterior rectocele and ischio-rectal hernia. Radiol Med (Torino) 90(1–2):44–48
18. Chen HH, Iroatulam A, Alabaz O et al (2001) Associations of defecography and physiologic findings in male patients with rectocele. Tech Coloproctol 5(3):157–161
19. Yoshioka K, Matsui Y, Yamada O et al (1991) Physiologic and anatomic assessment of patients with rectocele. Dis Colon Rectum 34(8):704–708
20. Jorge JM, Habr-Gama A, Wexner SD (2001) Clinical applications and techniques of cinedefecography. Am J Surg 182(1):93–101
21. Porter NH (1962) A physiological study of the pelvic floor in rectal prolapse. Ann R Coll Surg Engl 31:379–404
22. Parks AG, Porter NH, Hardcastle J (1966) The syndrome of the descending perineum. Proc R Soc Med 59(6):477–482
23. MacDonald A, Shearer M, Paterson PJ et al (1991) Relationship between outlet obstruction constipation and obstructed urinary flow. Br J Surg 78(6):693–695
24. Kuijpers HC, Bleijenberg G (1985) The spastic pelvic floor syndrome. A cause of constipation. Dis Colon Rectum 28(9):669–672

Commentary

Roberto Misici

When combined, diagnostic imaging techniques provide useful information for detecting and understanding pelvic-floor dysfunctions. Despite the apparent inconvenience associated with some of these techniques, as well as uncertainties regarding sensitivity, specificity, prediction ability, knowledge of natural history, and the result of surgical intervention, there is no better way to obtain objective information on coloanal function [1]. Investigations and images of coloproctological function provide objective information that can help confirm clinical findings, make adjustments to therapy, and produce important legal medical records [2].

Defecography is the dynamic study of evacuation. In 1952, Walldén [3] was the first to investigate the relationship between changes in pelvic dynamics, rectocele, enterocele, and symptoms of obstructed evacuation. After a number of adaptations, defecography was eventually perfected and made a standard examination in cases of evacuation disorders [4–6]. The method was first described by Burhennè [7] in 1964 but became more widespread after 1984 due to studies published by Mahieu et al. [5, 8] and due to the extensive knowledge acquired with the development of new investigation methods [9].

To perform a defecographic examination, the rectosigmoid is filled with a viscous barium sulphate solution, and the patient is asked to defecate while a series of radiographs are taken in lateral projection. Originally, defecography employed a simple X-ray device to register isolated moments of evacuation, but the technique is actually more dynamic with the addition of video technology (videodefecography) and digital or analogical image storage. Moreover, the latest computer software makes it possible to measure and represent the scanned structures directly on the screen. Videodefecography may give rise to more doubts than answers when performed alone [10], as many findings, such as rectocele, intussusception, perineal descent, and anismus, may be present in up to two thirds of asymptomatic subjects [11].

Harvey et al. [12] carried out a study at St. Mark's Hospital in London analyzing the impact of videodefecography on diagnosis and patient management. Forty-seven physicians examined 50 patients with regard to clinical findings and confidence level in diagnosis and proposed treatment. The first results showed an increase in diagnostic credibility, with 18% of diagnoses changed. Originally, surgical management became conservative in 14% of cases, whereas conservative approaches were replaced by surgical interventions in 4% of cases. In 10% of patients, the surgical approach was maintained but with a different technique. Also, in 10% of cases, ambiguous diagnoses were clarified. Eighteen percent of physicians stated that videodefecography revealed unsuspected changes. The addition of videodefecography was considered a major advantage by 40% of physicians and a moderate advantage by 40%. Overall, 43% of physicians found the technique very useful and 51% found it moderately useful. As with any medical examination, the usefulness of videodefecography depends on careful indication.

Although the physical anorectal examination may be an efficient way of diagnosing changes in pelvic anatomy and in the rectal wall, in one study, 46% and 73% of patients with negative physical examination were found to have enterocele and rectocele, respectively, when scanned with videodefecography [13]. In patients with surgical indication to treat pelvic functional disorders, videodefecography may help guide or even completely change surgical planning [14].

Videodefecography is simple and quick to perform, although a great deal of time and research went into standardizing the technique. Many difficulties had to be overcome [4], such as developing a contrast with fecal consistency, designing a chair allowing the reproduction of evacuation under near-physiological conditions without compromising image quality, adjusting video technology to evaluate the impact of anorectal disorders upon rectal voiding, and studies comparing the sitting and decubitus positions – the latter of which is indicated in case of incontinence and premature evacuation of the barium sulphate solution.

The main role of videodefecography is not to evaluate and interpret absolute values of patient parameters for comparison with control groups (which has led to much frustration), but to provide comparative data on pelvic dynamics for individual patients. The technique's value lies in the possibility of comparing measures of pelvic dynamics during rest, maximum voluntary contraction, and evacuation. During the examination, most patients evacuate the rectal content within 15–20 s [15], but evacuation time may be affected by content consistency or uneasiness on the part of the patient. In the latter instance, the patient may be allowed to evacuate in private and return for a fluoroscopic reevaluation.

Many disorders diagnosed with videodefecography, especially small rectoceles and intussusceptions, are observed in 25–77% of asymptomatic subjects [16]. Failure to recognize such normal variations can lead to diagnostic and therapeutic exaggerations. Thus, it is of crucial importance to distinguish between videodefecographic findings and the factors causing constipation – the distinction being based on the observation of similar findings in the clinical history and the evaluation of rectal voiding time during the examination.

More recently, dynamic anorectal ultrasonography [17, 18] and magnetic resonance imaging (MRI) [19, 20] have been used in evaluating these disorders, with satisfactory results. Dynamic anorectal ultrasonography may be performed with different types of transducers. Barther et al. [17] used a linear transrectal transducer, whereas Beer-Gabel et al. [21] employed a transperineal transducer with intrarectal and intravaginal gel, in both cases with results similar to those generated by defecography. More recently, dynamic ultrasonography techniques have been developed using two- and three-dimensional imaging for diagnosing functional changes in the pelvic floor [19, 22]. The ultrasonographic technique presents the advantage of evaluating anatomical integrity and sphincter lesions simultaneously. It is quick to perform, well tolerated, produces high-resolution images, and does not expose patients to radiation.

With the introduction of open-configuration MRI, image acquisition in the vertical or even sitting position is now possible and provides a global view and analysis of the musculature, pelvic viscera, anorectal angle, PR muscle function, and pelvic-floor descent.

With this technique, the rectal wall is seen more clearly, making intussusception and rectocele evaluation more reliable, and the concurrent evaluation of the structures surrounding the rectum and anal canal help evaluate patients with perineal descent and enterocele [23]. Dynamic magnetic resonance (DMR) has been found to be equivalent to conventional defecography in all aspects tested [24, 25]. The advantage of the method is to simultaneously show sphincter function and global motility of the pelvic floor while avoiding radiation exposure, constituting a significant aid in the surgical and therapeutic planning and decision making [26].

References

1. O'Kelly TJ, Mortensen NJ (1992) Test of anorectal function (editorial). Br J Surg 79:988–989
2. Taraska JM (1994) Tort reform. In: Taraska, JM. Legal guide for physicians. Matthew Bender, New York, pp 1–64
3. Walldén L (1952) Defecation block in cases of deep rectogenital pouch. A surgical, roentgenological and embryological study with special reference to morphological conditions. Acta Chir Scand 165:1–122
4. Finlay JG, Bartolo DCC., Bartram CI et al (1988) Symposium: Proctography. Int J Colorectal Dis 3:67–89
5. Mahieu P, Pringet J, Bodart (1984) Defecography: contribution to the diagnosis of defecation disorders. Gastrointest Radiol 9:253–261
6. Halligan S, Megee, Bartran CI (1994) Qualification of evacuation proctography. Dis Colon Rectum 37:(1)151–154
7. Burhennè HJ (1964) Intestinal evacuation study: a new roentgenologic technique. Radiol Clin North Am 33:79–84
8. Mahieu P, Pringot J, Bodart P et al (1984) Defecography: I. Description of a new procedure and results in normal patients. Gastrointest Radiol 9:247–251
9. Wexner SD, Jorge JMN (1994) Colorectal physiological tests: Use or abuse of technology? Eur J Surg 160:167–174
10. Agachan F , Pfeifer J, Wexner SD (1996) Defecography and proctography. Results of 744 patients. Dis Colon Rectum 39(8):899–905
11. Freimauis MG, Wald A, Carvana B, Bauman DH (1991) Evacuation proctography in normal volunteers. Invest Radiol 26(6):581–585
12. Harvey CJ, Halligan S, Bartram CL et al (1999) Evacuation proctography: a prospective study of diagnostic and therapeutic effects. Radiology 211(1):223–237
13. Altringer WE, Saclarides TJ, Dominguez JM et al (1995) Four-contrast defecography: pelvic "flooroscopy". Dis Colon Rectum 38(7):685–689
14. Kelvin FM, Maglinte DD, Homback JA et al (1992) Pelvic prolapse: assessment with evacuation proctography (defecography): Radiology 184(2):547–551
15. Turnbull GH, Bartram RW Jr, Lennard-Jones JE (1988) Radiologic studies of rectal evacuation in adults with idiopathic constipation. Dis Colon Rectum 31:190–197
16. Bartram CL, Turnbull GK, Lennard-Jones JE (1988) Evaluation proctography: an investigation of rectal expulsion in 20 subjects without defecatory disturbance. Gastrointest Radiol 13:72–80
17. Barthed M, Portier F, Heynies L et al (2003) Dynamic anal endosonography may challenge defecography

for assessing dynamic anorectal disorders: results of a prospective pilot study. Endoscopy 32(4):300–305

18. Van Outryve SM, Van Outryve MJ, De Writer BY, Pelckmans PA (2002) Is anorectal endosonography valuable in dyschezia? Gut 51(5):695–700

19. Murad-Regadas SM, Regadas FSP, Rodrigues LV et al (2008) A novel three-dimensional dynamic anorectal ultrasonography technique (Echodefecography) to assess obstructed defecation comparison with defecography. Surg Endoscopy 22(4):974-979

20. Kelvin FM, Maglinte DD, Hale DS et al (2000) Female pelvic organ prolapse: a comparison of triphasic dynamic MR imaging and triphasic fluoroscopic cystocoloproctography. AJR Am J Roentgenol 174:81–88

21. Beer-Gabel M, Teshler M, Barzilai N et al (2002) Dynamic trans-perineal ultrasound (DPT-US) – a new method for diagnosis of pelvic-floor disorders: technical details and preliminary results. Dis Colon Rectum 45:239–248

22. Regadas SMM, Regadas FSP, Rodrigues LV et al (2006) A novel procedure to assess anismus using three-dimensional dynamic ultrasonography. Colorect Dis 9(2):159–165

23. Beer-Gabel M, Teshler M, Barzilai N et al (2002) Dynamic transperineal ultrasound in the diagnosis of pelvic floor disorders: pilot study. Dis Colon Rectum 45:239–245, discussion 245–248

24. Schafik A (2001) Magnetic pudendal neurostimulation: a novel method for measuring pudendal nerve terminal motor latency. Clin Neurophysial 112:1049–1052

25. Kumar S, Rao SSC (2003) Diagnostic test in fecal Incontinence. Current Gastroenterol Rep 5:406–413

26. Diamant NE, Kamm MA, Wald A, Whitehead WE (1999) AGA technical review on anorectal testing techniques. Gastroenterology 116:735–760

CHAPTER 20

Dynamic Transperineal Ultrasonography

Andrew P. Zbar, Marc Beer-Gabel

Abstract

In assessing patients who present as the final common pathway with the symptom complex of evacuatory dysfunction, there is general recognition that the vast majority of them have a multiplicity of pelvic-floor and perineal soft-tissue abnormalities across compartments. A dynamic imaging modality is required to define the real-time integration of these anomalies and to highlight their significance in each case, particularly when there is clinical or radiographic evidence of a dominant pathology and where corrective surgery is contemplated. Dynamic transperineal ultrasound (DTP-US) is a simple, radiation-free, inexpensive, and learnable technique that highlights pathology in each pelvic compartment and the interplay between compartments during straining and simulated bolus defecation. Another significant advantage of the technique is its ability to demonstrate tissues that lie well beyond the focal distance of an endoanal probe. Studies on selected patient subgroups with complex evacuatory difficulty are awaited that compare DTP-US with its counterpart, dynamic magnetic resonance (MR) imaging. We suggest that using DTP-US for real-time assessment of pelvic-floor function is best performed by the clinician managing the case or in close collaboration with the radiologist for the best potential clinical outcome. Consideration should be given to its formal accreditation by coloproctologists, gastroenterologists, radiologists, gynecologists, and biofeedback therapists.

Introduction

Transperineal ultrasonography (TP-US) is not particularly new as a technique for assessing perineal structures, being first described for use in assessing the bladder neck in patients presenting with urinary stress incontinence [1]. It may be used in both static and dynamic (DTP-US) modes. The latter exploits the real-time capability of ultrasound to assess the component parts of the anterior, middle, and posterior pelvic compartments to define their interaction during straining and simulated defecation in patients who present to specialized pelvic-floor clinics with the principal symptom of evacuatory difficulty [2]. This original TP-US technique was either a combination of perineal sonography or transintroital (as distinct from transvaginal) sonography [3, 4] and has the advantage of being widely available for adapted transducer heads with the facility for real-time determination of sagittal images by probe rotation. Application of simple transperineal sonography for assessing the anal region was suggested by Pittman et al. in 1990 [5] at a time when anal endosonography was redefining the effect on the anal sphincter of complicated vaginal delivery [6, 7]. As a result of this work, Beer-Gabel et al. in Israel [8], Kleinübing in Brazil [9], Roche et al. in Switzerland [10], and Piloni in Italy [11] independently in effect "rediscovered" this method for assessing the posterior perineum and pelvic floor, showing that images could be obtained axially that rivaled those provided by conventional endosonography. In this respect, it was

M. Pescatori, F.S.P. Regadas, S.M. Murad Regadas, A.P. Zbar (eds.), *Imaging Atlas of the Pelvic Floor and Anorectal Diseases*. ISBN 978-88-470-0808-3. © Springer-Verlag Italia 2008

recognized that the images obtained with transvaginal endosonography were of low quality for assessing the anterior external anal sphincter (EAS) and the perineal body in patients presenting with fecal incontinence [12–14].

Quite apart from the validation of TP-US static images in assessing anal sphincter disruption, where transperineal images somewhat better delineate the outer borders of the atrophic EAS compared with the standard endosonographic view [15], it was realized that its real-time capability and sagittal transducer shift could provide a dynamic image of the interaction of pelvic floor and perineal structures during provocative maneuvers, such as simulated defecation, as well as in patients who present to pelvic multidisciplinary clinics with severe evacuatory dysfunction [16]. It has been increasingly recognized that functional difficulties in defecation are extremely common [17–19], particularly following pelvic gynecologic surgery [20, 21] and perineal procedures. [22]. It is known that >90% of these patients present with multicompartmental disease of the pelvic floor, even when there may be a dominant clinical feature such as rectocele [23, 24]. Lately, Dietz and colleagues have exploited the benefits of three-dimensional reconstructed translabial ultrasound in depicting the pelvic floor and perineal soft tissues when assessing the effects of vaginal delivery [25] and examining the alteration of levator-plate structure [26, 27]. Traditionally, such patients have been studied by a somewhat extended technique of defecating cine proctography [28], which may require instillation of contrast into the bladder, vagina, and even the peritoneal cavity for the specific diagnosis of enteroceles [29, 30]. The technique causes unnecessary exposure to radiation and has relatively poor patient compliance and acceptance [31]. This approach has been complemented by dynamic MR imaging, which has been extensively validated in patients with defecation difficulty [32, 33] and which has shown a high sensitivity for detecting enteroceles missed by proctography [34]. This modality, although particularly sensitive and interpretation friendly is, however, often restricted in its availability (and necessary expertise) for specific examination of the pelvic floor and has not yet been validated against DTP-US in these specialized patients [35].

This chapter outlines the technical aspects, necessary experience, and recommendations for the use of clinician-led DTP-US in patients presenting with the symptom a complex of evacuatory difficulty, discussing its advantages, indications, pitfalls, and limitations.

Technique

The technique for using DTP-US has been previously outlined [36] but is reiterated here. The principles for performing DTP-US are simple (although its interpretation can be quite difficult and has a somewhat steep learning curve). The technique utilizes standard ultrasound probes to determine the disposition of the perineal and pelvic-floor soft-tissues of the posterior, middle, and anterior compartments by a scout sweep of the basic bony and soft-tissue landmarks. These include the pubic symphysis, the urethrovesical junction, the vaginal vault, the puborectalis sling and levator floor, and the anal sphincter anlage. No specific preparation is required for the examination, although in patients with evacuatory dysfunction, it is advisable to perform the procedure with oral contrast to assess the likelihood of an enterocele. The procedure is videotaped for retrograde and orthograde scrolling of dynamic images if these are performed. Static images may be used for specific measurements. The examination begins with static TP-US. The probe of a basic ultrasound, either a 7.5- or 10-MHz curvilinear or customized transducer C4-7 and C8-12 and a linear 5-10 transducer (HDI 3000; Advanced Technology Laboratories Bothell, WA, Australia), is lightly placed against the perineal body (with the patient in the left lateral position) in front of the anus in a transverse disposition. This allows axial anal structures to be outlined, including the anal mucosa and submucosa and the internal anal sphincter (IAS) and EAS and provides images that are comparable with those obtained using an endoluminal probe. A latex condom is used to protect the transducer head.

The sphincter layers delineated naturally have the same echogenic characteristics as images obtained with endoanal ultrasonography, although there is relatively poor delineation of the perineal body. The anal mucosa and submucosa are more demonstrable where Duplex sonography defines blood flow in patients with hemorrhoids and rectal mucosal prolapse, although there is as yet no specific classification system that correlates with clinical or endoscopic grades. Initial evidence from transvaginal sonography shows that there is some correlation between clinical endoscopic grade of hemorrhoids and measurement of the submucosal area between the lumen and the inner border of the IAS as detected when the anal canal is left undisturbed [37]. A standard TP-US static axial view of the anal sphincter is shown in Figure 1.

Rotation of the probe through 180° defines a sagittal view of the anal canal and anorectal junction (ARJ) that shows the hypoechoic IAS and the hyperechoic puborectalis (PR) muscle in profile. The former is a specific landmark of the examination and appears as a double dark strip on either side of the anal canal, with the latter as a bright cone behind the air-filled rectum as the anal canal shifts direction. This view, also displaying the bright hyperechoic elliptical bundle of the PR muscle in relief, is shown in Figure 2. This shift in direction permits the calculation of ARJ movement during forcible straining or simulated evacuation, and allows measurement of the anorectal angle (ARA) during these provocative maneuvers, both of which have been shown to correlate closely with these parameters as measured during conventional defecography [36, 38]. In this comparison, measurements were made of the ARA and

descent of the ARJ based on a blinded comparison by two observers of the change in direction of the lumen on both defecography and DTP-US. The ARJ tended to lie at a higher position on DTP-US but to descend more during defecography [8].

Further sagittal examination shows the brilliantly hyperechoic pubis. The transducer is worked backward by downward angulation against the perineum to locate the hypoechoic, partially filled bladder and the urethrovesical junction (Fig. 3). The position and movement of this junction is dependent upon the filling status of the bladder [39]. The middle compartment is identified by focusing on the contrast-filled vagina, with broad assessment of the depth and contents (if any) located in the rectogen-

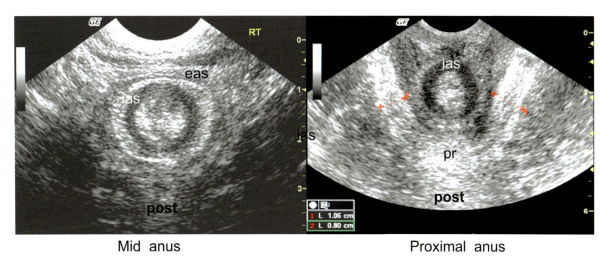

Mid anus   Proximal anus

Fig. 1. Rostral movement of the probe provides different levels of an axial view of the internal (hypoechoic) and external (hyperechoic) anal sphincters and puborectalis sling, which rival those obtained with endoanal sonography. *eas* external anal sphincter, *ias* internal anal sphincter, *pr* puborectalis muscle

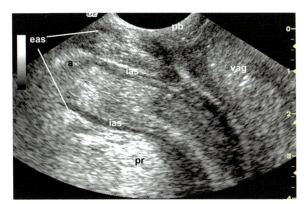

Fig. 2 Sagittal view of the rotated probe showing the hypoechoic internal anal sphincter and the hyperechoic external anal sphincter in relief, along with the vaginal lumen and the rectovaginal septal area. *a* anus, *eas* external anal sphincter, *ias* internal anal sphincter, *pr* puborectalis muscle, *pb* perineal body, *vag* vagina

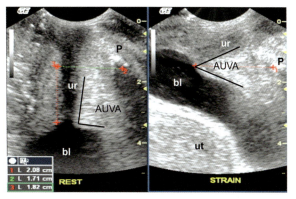

Fig. 3. Axial and sagittal views of the bladder neck with measurable urethrovesical descent on straining. On straining, closure of the anterior urethrovesical angle (*AUVA*) from 90° at rest to 45° during straining, with descent of the bladder neck (2.08 cm in this case) is evident. *bl* bladder, *P* pubis, *ur* urethra, *ut* uterus

ital septum. This area is critical for diagnosing both enterocele and peritoneocele and is abnormal in its dimensions in patients with rectocele [24, 40]. An example of an emptying rectocele with associated intrarectal rectoanal intussusception on sagittal DTP-US is shown in Fig. 4.

It is recognized that although left-lateral DTP-US images provide standardization for image comparison, simulated defecation in this position is non-physiological [41, 42]. In this respect, others advocate the use of open-architecture MR imaging technology (not widely available) for comparison with dynamic MR imaging where conditions that appear at the end of defecation, such as rectal prolapse, rectoanal intussusception, and extreme perineal descent, may be more readily diagnosed [43]. Recently, this approach has been adopted for DTP-US by Piloni and Spazzafumo for "squatting" conduct of evacuation sonography with squeeze, strain, and evacuation maneuvers [44]. Overall, these measurements were made by our group for initial validation of the technique; however, we recognize they offer little spe-

cific clinical value. [45]. Bland-Altman comparisons by our group of patients at rest and during maximal straining [38, 46] show that the ARA between the two techniques is nearly identical (defecography value in degrees minus DTP-US value), with a higher ARA on straining using proctography ($123.3° \pm 4$ for proctography vs. $116.4° \pm 3.32$ for DTP-US). At rest, the limits of agreement ranged from $-65°$ to $+26°$ and during straining from $-36°$ to $+62°$, with more proctographic than ultrasonographic outliers.

The instillation of small volumes (≤ 50 ml) of acoustic contrast gel (more recently, we use saline) into both the rectum and the vagina permits better definition of these structures and allows dynamic representation of the pelvic structures during straining. It permits adequate diagnosis of rectocele, rectoanal intussusception, and mucosal (or full-thickness) rectal prolapse in patients who present with evacuatory difficulty. Claims that overdistension of either the vagina (in particular) or rectum may diminish the capacity for rectocele diagnosis – the so-called "crowded pelvis syndrome" [47] – have not proved evident.

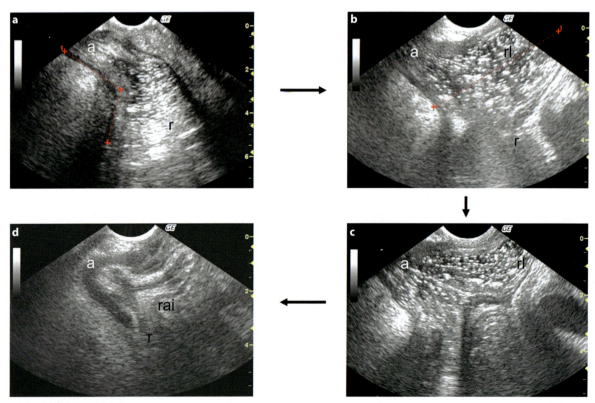

Fig. 4 a-d. Sagittal dynamic view of rectal evacuation with an emptying rectocele and associated rectoanal intussusception. **a** The rectum is filled with 60 cc of contrast. The patient is resting in the left lateral position. **b** The patient starts to strain. There is a small rectocele (*rl*). **c** While the patient is bearing down, the rectocele is emptying. There is a mucosal prolapse of the anterior rectal wall, which is pushed downward. **d** At the end of the Valsalva maneuver, there is no more contrast in the rectum. Rectoanal intussusception is clearly seen as an intrarectal invagination. *a* anus, *r* rectum, *rl* rectocele, *rai* rectoanal intussusception

In our experience varying the volume of intravaginal contrast, on blinded examination, has not altered the incidence of rectocele diagnosis where DTP-US in comparison with defecating proctography generally shows more diagnoses per patient with the former technique [36].

Clinical Indications and Recommendations

One of the inherent advantages of DTP-US is its ability to display the interrelationship between the pelvic viscera and soft tissues in real time without complex algorithms or irradiation, which has proven to be of specific use in younger patients and even in children. This dynamic interplay is crucial for a three-dimensional understanding of the altered anatomy of the region and provides assistance in operative decision making regarding rectocele and/or enterocele repair, the role of attendant sphincteroplasty/levatorplasty, and the place or sacrocolpopexy [48]. It is also more likely to provide an understanding in complex cases for treatment failure and provide a medicolegal record of the clinical status of the patient, which can provide valuable consensus in multidisciplinary management meetings [49, 50]. Another intrinsic advantage of this technique utilizes the acoustic merits of the procedure. DTP-US is able to examine tissues that lie beyond the focal distance of any endoanal probe (either ultrasonographic or MR) and that have their origin above the puborectalis sling, where coupling of an endoluminal probe is typically poor. This can be of value in assessing patients with complex recurrent fistulas and impaired function and allows definition of supralevator disease where perineal surgery may compromise healthy sphincter musculature [51, 52]. As with all other forms of ultrasound, however, there is limited capacity for distinguishing scar tissue from recrudescent sepsis.

This technique proves invaluable in difficult cases presenting with evacuatory problems because of its capacity to demonstrate diagnostic sensitivity for multiple pelvic-floor pathologies. Many such patients have been multiply referred, highlighting the importance of a multidisciplinary response to these problems [53, 54] where traditionally more complex approaches toward investigation in patients with suboptimal postoperative outcomes may be predicted [22, 55]. In this setting, DTP-US also suggests those patients more readily assisted by an initial biofeedback approach [56, 57].

The specific advantage of DTP-US lies in the objective delineation of rectocele and in decision making regarding surgical repair when rectocele is deemed to be the dominant clinical finding in patients who present with incomplete evacuation and the need for perineal or transvaginal manipulation [58]. Here, measurement may be made of the rectocele depth by projection on static TP-US images of the anterior rectal wall, showing high correlation with defecographic measurements [36]. However, it is recognized that emptying capacity does not specifically correlate with functional outcome after rectocele repair, regardless of how that repair is attempted [59, 60]. In this regard, larger nonemptying rectoceles do appear to be associated with more symptoms than smaller ones that tend to empty on defecography [61, 62]. Figure 3a shows the preoperative appearance of a rectocele in sagittal-mode DTP-US in which a subjective interpretation may be made regarding emptying capacity during forcible straining and evacuation. This dynamic sonography is useful in equating the contribution the rectocele makes to the overall pelvic floor dysfunction and may be semiquantified for postoperative comparison with clinical outcome after operative repair (Fig. 3b).

Preoperative diagnosis of a coincident enterocele will significantly change the surgical approach [63] where diagnosis of an enterocele is a more common finding in patients posthysterectomy, particularly when initial culdosuspension of the vaginal vault has not been performed [48, 64]. Although the relationship and pathophysiology of posthysterectomy constipation and defecation difficulty is complex and at present poorly understood, there is an association between subsequent vaginal-vault prolapse, enterocele, and rectocele because of failure to obliterate the peritoneal cul-de-sac of the pouch of Douglas and to suspend the vaginal apex [65]. These concomitant disorders in rectocele patients undergoing surgery have been shown to adversely affect functional outcome if they are not surgically addressed. They also diminish the reported efficiency after surgery of satisfactory rectal evacuation, and the need for assisted defecation by perineal or vaginal pressure and manipulation [66, 67].

In our previous study [36], more enteroceles were diagnosed in patients who had proven rectoceles using DTP-US when compared with defecography and who presented with objectively scored evacuatory difficulty exceeding 6 months in duration (<1 bowel movement ever 4 days or longer, or if ≥25% of bowel movements were accompanied by excessive straining). There was also a higher multiplicity of diagnosed pathologies of clinical importance using DTP-US, particularly in the posthysterectomy patient.

Figure 4 shows the DTP-US appearance of rectoanal intussusception, which may be ultrasonographically graded in accordance with the clinical grade depending on the extent of descent toward the anal canal. This typically appears as a bright echogenic buffer on straining, occupying the anal canal in the absence of contrast evacuation, an appearance similar to rectal internal mucosal prolapse (RIMP). The DTP-US grading of RIMP also appears to correlate with its clinical endoscopic grade [66, 68]. At present, DTP-US, although accurate in diagnosing both of these conditions, has not been prospectively validated as part of the treatment algorithm in terms of its impact on surgical management based on preoperative ultrasonographic grade. There is much prospective work that needs to be performed comparing DTP-US with standard modalities in a range of pelvic-floor disorders, including uterovaginal prolapse [69], rectal prolapse, and reported evacuatory "block", as well as in the morphological effects on the pelvic floor of vaginal and abdominal hysterectomy [21].

There are several pitfalls of the DTP-US technique in coloproctologic practice. It is time consuming, mildly embarrassing for some patients because of the close proximity of the examiner, somewhat messy on occasion, and has a substantial learning curve, requiring between 20 and 40 min to perform depending on one's level of expertise. Although no accreditation programs are established, it is likely that a minimum of 100 examinations are required to make the clinician relatively proficient in this examination. What is clear is that there is an increasing onus on coloproctologists to understand, interpret, and perform the available range of anal and perineal ultrasonography techniques in patients with complex anorectal disorders and to correlate these findings with operative indications and with postoperative functional outcomes. Such a view provides motivation for surgeons to become actively involved in the performance and accreditation of all forms of anorectal sonography, with the need for close cooperation between radiologists and colorectal surgeons in the credentialing and training of this important modality as part of their wider colorectal apprenticeship.

As stated, the position adopted for the performance of DTP-US is nonphysiological for most disorders, which appear at the end of defecation. Also, the proximity of the operator's hand and the probe, even with technique modifications [44], may create some patient reticence to strain adequately on request and limit the diagnostic capacity of the technique, as occurs in some scrutinized patients during proctography. Moreover, its use in men or obese women is frequently impaired because of the sheer bulk of the buttocks and the inability to properly position the probe on the perineum [70].

In summary, the ready availability of ultrasound, its lack of irradiation, and it portability and repeatability make DTP-US an exciting novel technique for use in selected patients where the indications and contraindications of the procedure are still being determined in those presenting with evacuation difficulty. It provides dynamic multiplanar imaging capacity for a multidisciplinary approach toward pelvic-floor disorders and confirms the clinical impression of rectocele, enterocele, cystourethrocele, and genital descensus. In this context, it complements the clinical examination and is selectively used to provide specific data not readily obtainable with other methodologies [71].

References

1. Schaer GN, Koechli OR, Scheussler B, Haller U (1995) Perineal ultrasound for evaluating the bladder neck in urinary stress incontinence. Obstet Gynecol 85:220–224
2. Beer-Gabel M, Frudinger A, Zbar A (2005) Dynamic transperineal ultrasound and transvaginal sonography. In: Wexner SD, Zbar AP, Pescatori M (eds) Complex anorectal disorders: investigation and management. Springer, London, pp 246–258
3. Quinn MJ, Beynon J, Mortensen NJ, Smith PJ (1988) Transvaginal endosonography: a new method to study the anatomy of the lower urinary tract in urinary stress incontinence. Br J Urol 62:414–418
4. Koebl H, Bernaschek G, Dentinger J (1990) Assessment of female urinary incontinence by introital sonography. J Clin Ultrasound 18:370–374
5. Pittman JS, Benson JT, Sumners JE (1990) Physiological evaluation of the anorectum: a new ultrasound technique. Dis Colon Rectum 33:277–284
6. Sultan AH, Nicholls RJ, Kamm MA et al (1993) Anal endosonography and correlation with in vitro and in vivo anatomy. Br J Surg 80:508–511
7. Sultan AH, Kamm MA, Hudson CN et al (1993) Anal sphincter disruption during vaginal delivery. N Engl J Med 329:1905–1911
8. Beer-Gabel M, Teshler M, Barzilai N et al (2002) Dynamic trans-perineal ultrasound (DTP-US) in the diagnosis of pelvic floor disorders: a pilot study. Dis Colon Rectum 45:239–248
9. Kleinübing H Jr, Janini JF, Malafaia O et al (2000) Transperineal ultrasonography: new method to image

the anorectal region. Dis Colon Rectum 43:1572–1574

10. Roche B, Fransioli A, Deleaval J, Marti MC (2001) Comparison of transanal and external perineal ultrasonography. Eur Radiol 11:1165–1170

11. Piloni V (2001) Dynamic imaging of the pelvic floor with transperineal sonography. Techn Coloproct 5:103–105

12. Sultan AH, Loder PB, Bartram CI et al (1994) Vaginal endosonography: new approach to image the undisturbed anal sphincter. Dis Colon Rectum 37:1296–1299

13. Frudinger A, Bartram CI, Kamm MA (1997) Transvaginal versus anal endosonography for detecting damage to the anal sphincter. AJR Am J Roentgenol 168:1435–1438

14. Frudinger A, Zbar AP (2005) Transvaginal endosonography in the assessment of the anorectal sphincter. In: Wexner SD, Zbar AP, Pescatori M (eds) Complex anorectal disorders: investigation and management. Springer, London, 258–262

15. Sarnelli G, Bosio C, Ciccarelli G et al (2000) Sonographic anatomy of the posterior perineum: technique and methodology. Ital J Coloproct 2:39–43

16. Beer-Gabel M, Zbar AP (2002) Dynamic transperineal ultrasonography (DTP-US) in patients presenting with obstructed defecation. Techniques in coloproctology 6:141

17. Thompson WG, Longsteth GF, Drossman DA et al (2000) Functional bowel disorders and functional abdominal pain. In: Drossman DA, Corazziari E, Talley NJ (eds) Functional gastrointestinal disorders. Degnon, Mclean, pp 351–432

18. Gonzalez-Argente FX, Jain A, Nogueras JJ et al (2001) Prevalence and severity of urinary incontinence and pelvic genital prolapse in females with anal incontinence or rectal prolapse. Dis Colon Rectum 44:920–926

19. Meschia M, Buonaguidi A, Pifarotti P et al (2002) Prevalence of anal incontinence in women with symptoms of urinary incontinence and genital prolapse. Obstet Gynecol 4:719–723

20. Vierhout ME, Schreuder HW, Veen HF (1993) Severe slow transit constipation following radical hysterectomy. Gynecol Oncol 51:401–403

21. Kelly JL, O'Riordain DS, Jones E et al (1998) The effect of hysterectomy on ano-rectal physiology. Int J Colorect Dis 13:116–118

22. Paraiso MF, Weber AM, Walters MD et al (2001) Anatomic and functional outcome after posterior colporrhaphy. J Pelvic Surg 7:335–339

23. Rotholtz NA, Efron JE, Weiss EG et al (2002) Anal manometric predictors of significant rectocele in constipated patients. Techn Coloproctol 6:73–77

24. Zbar AP, Lienemann A, Fritsch H et al (2003) Rectocele: pathogenesis and surgical management. Int J Colorect Dis 18:369–384

25. Dietz HP, Steensma AB, Hastings R (2003) Three-dimensional ultrasound imaging of the pelvic floor: the effect of parturition on paravaginal support structures. Ultrasound Obstet Gynecol 21:589–595

26. Dietz HP (2004) Levator function before and after childbirth. Aust N Z Obstet Gynaecol 44:19–23

27. Dietz HP, Shek C, Clarke B (2005) Biometry of the pubovisceral muscle and levator hiatus by three-dimensional pelvic floor ultrasound. Ultrasound Obstet Gynecol 25:580–585

28. Shorvon PJ, McHugh S, Diamant NE et al (1989) Defecography in normal volunteers: results and implications. Gut 30:1737–1749

29. Bremmer S (1988) Peritoneocele: a radiologic study with defaeco-peritoneography. Acta Radiol 413 (Suppl):1–33

30. LeSaffer PA. Defecography – update 1994. The model of expulsion, digital subtraction cysto-colpo-entero-defecography and the perineal support device. Belgium, AZT Aalst Belgium Story-Scientia Ghent

31. Goei R, Kemerink G (1990) Radiation dose in defecography. Radiology 176:137–139

32. Lienemann A, Anthuber C, Baron A et al (1997) Dynamic MR colpocystorectography assessing pelvic floor descent. Eur Radiol 7:1309–1317

33. Mortele KJ, Fairhurst J (2007) Dynamic MR defecography of the posterior compartment. Indications, techniques and MRI features. Eur J Radiol 61:462–472

34. Lienemann A, Anthuber C, Baron A, Reiser M (2000) Diagnosing enteroceles using dynamic magnetic resonance imaging. Dis Colon Rectum 43:205–213

35. Kruger J, Heap X, Dietz HP (2007) OC259: a comparison of magnetic resonance imaging and 4D ultrasound in the assessment of the levator hiatus. Ultrasound Obstet Gynecol 30:A447

36. Beer-Gabel M, Teshler M, Schechtman E, Zbar AP (2004) Dynamic transperineal ultrasound vs. defecography in patients with evacuatory difficulty: a pilot study. Int J Colorect Dis 19:60–67

37. Nicholls MJ, Dunham R, O'Herlihy S et al (2006) Measurement of the anal cushions by transvaginal ultrasonography. Dis Colon Rectum 49:1410–1413

38. Zbar AP, Beer-Gabel M (2006) Clinical dynamic transperineal ultrasonography in proctologic practice: the case for its use in patients presenting with evacuatory difficulty. In: Romano G, di Falco G (eds) Benign anorectal diseases, Springer, Milan, pp 17–27

39. Dietz HP, Wilson PD (1999) The influence of bladder volume on the position and mobility of the urethrovesical junction. Int Urogynecol J Pelvic Floor Dysfunct 10:3–6

40. Aigner F, Zbar AP, Ludwikowski B et al (2004) The rectogenital septum: morphology, function and clinical relevance. Dis Colon Rectum 47:131–140

41. Jorge JM, Ger GC, Gonzales I, Wexner SD (1994) Patient position during cinedefecography: influence on perineal descent and other measurements. Dis Colon Rectum 37:927–931

42. Dietz HP, Clarke B (2001) The influence of posture on perineal ultrasound imaging parameters. Int Urogynecol J Pelvic Floor Dysfunct 12:104–106

43. Schoenenberger AW, Debatin JF, Guldenschuh I et al (1998) Dynamic MR defecography with a superconducting MR system. Radiology 206:641–646

44. Piloni V, Spazzafumo L (2005) Evacuation sonography. Techn Coloproctol 9:119–125; comment 126
45. Felt-Bersma RJ, Luth WJ, Janssen JJ, Meuwissen SG (1990) Defecography in patients with anorectal disorders: Which findings are clinically relevant? Dis Colon Rectum 33:277–284
46. Bland JM, Altman DG (1986) Statistical methods for assessing agreement between the two methods of clinical measurement. Lancet 1:307–310
47. Kelvin FM, Maglinte DD (1997) Dynamic cystoproctography of female pelvic floor defects and their inter-relationships. AJR Am J Roentgenol 369:769–774
48. Backer MH (1992) Success with sacrospinous suspension of the prolapsed vaginal vault. Surg Gynecol Obstet 175:419–420
49. van Dam JH, Hop WC, Schouten WR (2000) Analysis of patients with poor outcome after rectocele repair. Dis Colon Rectum 43:1556–1560
50. Beck DE (2005) Medicolegal aspects of coloproctological practice. In: Wexner SD, Zbar AP, Pescatori M (eds) Complex anorectal disorders: investigation and management. Springer, London, pp 767–778
51. Zbar AP (2006) Static and dynamic transperineal sonography in benign proctology. In: Pescatori M, Bartram CI, Zbar AP (eds) Atlas of clinical endosonography: 2D and 3D anal, vaginal and dynamic perineal ultrasonography of benign anorectal diseases. Springer, London, pp 84–112
52. Zbar AP, Oyetunji RO, Gill R (2006) Transperineal versus hydrogen peroxide-enhanced endoanal ultrasonography in never operated and recurrent cryptogenic fistula-in-ano: a pilot study. Tech Coloproctol 10:297–302
53. Puccini F, Rottoli ML, Bologna A et al (1998) Pelvic floor dyssynergia and bimodal rehabilitation: results of combined pelviperineal kinesitherapy and biofeedback training. Int J Colorect Dis 13:124–130
54. Brusciano L, Limongelli P, del Genio G et al (2007) Useful parameters helping proctologists to identify patients with defecatory disorders that may be treated with pelvic floor rehabilitation. Techn Coloproctol 11:45–50
55. Kelvin FM, Maglinte D, Hale DS, Benson JT (2000) Female organ prolapse: a comparison of triphasic MR imaging and triphasic fluoroscopic cystocolpoproctography. AJR Am J Roentgenol 174:81–88
56. McKee RF, McEnroe L, Anderson JH, Finlay IG (1999) Identification of patients likely to benefit from biofeedback for outlet obstruction constipation. Br J Surg 86:355–359
57. Zbar AP (2005) The role of functional evaluation before anorectal surgery. Società Italiana di Chirurgia ColoRettale (SICCR) 9:74–83. www.siccr.org. Cited 23 Mar 2008
58. Ayabaca SM, Zbar AP, Pescatori M (2002) Anal continence after rectocele repair. Dis Colon Rectum 45:63–69
59. Ting KH, Mangel E, Eibl-Eibesfeldt B, Muller-Lissner SA (1992) Is the volume retained after defecation a valuable parameter at defecography? Dis Colon Rectum 35:762–768
60. Halligan S, Bartram CI (1995) Is barium trapping in rectoceles significant? Dis Colon Rectum 38:764–768
61. Heslop JH (1987) Piles and rectoceles. Aust N Z J Surg 57:935–938
62. Karlbom U, Graf W, Nilsson S, Pahlman L (1996) Does surgical repair of a rectocele improve rectal emptying? Dis Colon Rectum 39:1296–1302
63. Kahn MA, Stanton SL (1998) Techniques of rectocele repair and their effects on bowel function. Int Urogynecol J 9:37–47
64. Cruiskshank SH (1991) Sacrospinous fixation – should this be performed at the time of vaginal hysterectomy? Am J Obstet Gynecol 164:1072–1076
65. McCall ML (1997) Posterior culdoplasty: surgical correction of enterocele during vaginal hysterectomy. A preliminary report. Obstet Gynecol 10:596–602
66. Pescatori M, Boffi F, Russo A, Zbar AP (2005) Complications and recurrence after excision of rectal internal mucosal prolapse for obstructed defecation. Int J Colorectal Dis 7:107–108
67. Saclarides TJ, Brubaker L (2005) Evacuatory dysfunction following gynecologic surgery. In: Wexner SD, Zbar AP, Pescatori, M (eds) Complex anorectal disorders: investigation and management. Springer, London, pp 532–545
68. Pescatori M, Quandamcarlo C (1999) A new grading of rectal internal mucosal prolapse and its correlation with diagnosis and treatment. Int J Colorect Dis 14:245–249
69. Bump RC, Mattiasson A, Bo K et al (1996) The standardization of terminology of female pelvic organ prolapse and pelvic floor dysfunction. Am J Obstet Gynecol 175:10–17
70. Kapoor DS, Davila GW, Rosenthal RJ, Ghoneim GM (2004) Pelvic floor dysfunction in morbidly obese women: pilot study. Obes Res 12:1104–1107
71. Brusciano L, Limongelli P, Pescatori M et al (2007) Ultrasonographic patterns in patients with obstructed defecation. Int J Colorect Dis 22:969–977

CHAPTER 21

Two-dimensional Introital Sonography in Patterns of Anorectal Prolapse in Women

Vittorio Piloni, Liana Spazzafumo

Abstract

The anal cross-sectional area on 2D introital ultra-sonography (IUS) represents a new sensitive index capable of providing both superior anatomic details and clear depiction of anorectal prolapse in women. The parameter is calculated at rest and on straining by outlining the inner and the outer margin of the hypoechoic internal anal sphincter (IAS) and measuring the included area at the level of the middle anal canal in the axial plane. Average values of the inner area (1.08 ± 0.25 cm^2 vs 3.02 ± 0.73 cm^2), as well as the inner-to-outer ratio (49.6 ± 8.2 % vs 81.3 ± 2.9 %) and percentage increase on straining ($\Delta -0.007$ vs $+0.42$) have been found by us to differ significantly ($p < 0.01$) in control groups ($n = 10$) and patients with rectal prolapse ($n = 20$). Further differentiation is made possible at sonography between those patients with rectal prolapse and obstructed defecation as their main presenting symptom from those with staining episodes and/or fecal incontinence by noting whether or not the integrity of the anal sphincter is preserved. Thanks to rapid advances in technology and recent refinements in interpretation, IUS can be considered, especially in young female patients, the best imaging modality to start with in assessing rectal prolapse in a safe and noninvasive manner.

Introduction

Clinical assessment of women with anorectal symptoms is sometimes difficult, necessitating further evaluation with imaging techniques. Dynamic contrast radiography, either in its simplest [1, 2] or more extended ver-

sion [3, 4], provides excellent information on luminal abnormalities occurring within the anal canal and adjacent organs. However, it is invasive (radiation burden) and not widely accepted by patients. Recent advances in ultrasound (US) imaging has dramatically improved evaluation of the female anorectal junction, clarifying findings at physical examination and providing accurate road maps for surgeons in specific cases. Ultrasonography of the pelvic floor has assumed a central role in the diagnostic workup of pelvic prolapse syndromes, obstructive defecation, and fecal incontinence. It has been proposed as the first-line imaging approach for proper diagnosis and management, as it helps to discriminate patients with anatomical abnormalities who are likely to benefit from surgery (Fig. 1)

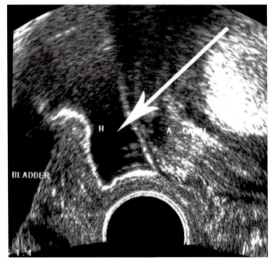

Fig. 1. Introital sonography, sagittal view. Extensive fluid accumulation (*arrow*) is seen in the deep rectovaginal pouch of a 52-year-old woman with obstructed defecation who had had a total hysterectomy 5 years earlier

M. Pescatori, F.S.P. Regadas, S.M. Murad Regadas, A.P. Zbar (eds.), *Imaging Atlas of the Pelvic Floor and Anorectal Diseases*. ISBN 978-88-470-0808-3. © Springer-Verlag Italia 2008

and those requiring conservative treatment. Despite considerable variation among centers, high-resolution transvaginal US and transperineal US are considered reliable techniques for diagnosing and characterizing anorectal abnormalities in a number of clinical applications, including inflammatory and functional coloproctological diseases [5–15]. The procedure is quite easy to perform and relatively easy to interpret.

In this chapter, we discuss and illustrate the potential of this noninvasive technique using high-resolution introital ultrasonography (IUS) to demonstrate the anatomical details of the anal canal in the cross-sectional plane in women with and without anorectal prolapse.

Imaging Technique

Sonographic examination is performed with a broadband 5- to 9-MHz curved array for transvaginal scanning. The probe is placed approximately 1–2 cm in the vaginal introitus. Gray-scale images are obtained in both sagittal and coronal planes for properly centering the region of interest (ROI) before turning the probe in the axial plane. The procedure we follow has been described in a previous report [16]. In particular, the patient is asked to reach the imaging department with her bladder half filled by natural urine. She is then placed in the Sims position, and 60 ml of hypoechoic contrast (the same as that used for evacuation proctography) are administered through a rectal tube to enhance rectal visualization. Thereafter, the patient is turned supine with her knees bent and feet flat on the table. Despite a greater distortion of image anatomy, we prefer using a 5- to 7.5-MHz endocavitary probe for the following two reasons: (1) the head of the transducer can be placed closer to the ROI to provide superior axial and lateral resolution of the pelvic anatomy, and (2) with the head of the transducer placed at the introital region, scanning through an arc of 195° is possible in the sagittal plane, even during evacuation of the intrarectal contrast.

The transducer is connected to a portable US scanner equipped with advanced software, freeze-frame, and postprocessing and recording facilities (General Electric Medical Systems, Logiq Book, Milwaukee, WI, USA), allowing delayed examination of moving images. Prevention of cross contamination between patients is achieved by using a disposable cover (latex condom or the finger of a surgical glove) over the tip of the probe. Following a preliminary transabdominal inspection of the urogenital hiatus size and shape (Fig. 2), examination of the ROI, i.e., the anorectum, includes the systematic combination of longitudinal

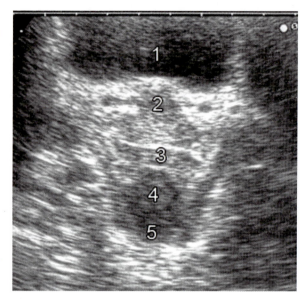

Fig. 2. Preliminary transabdominal scout sonography of the pelvis showing normal urogenital hiatus. Axial view: *1* bladder, *2* urethra, *3* vagina embedded in the endopelvic fascia, *4* anal canal, *5* puborectalis sling

with transversely oriented scans to localize the anatomical structures accurately and to provide 3D measurements during rest, squeeze, and straining maneuvers by the patient before emptying the rectum.

To obtain quantitative data from sonograms, the following anatomic landmarks and measurements are noted:

- Anal canal length: According to Sandridge et al. [9], this is measured on sagittal scans with caliper placed at the anal verge and the anorectal junction. The latter is assumed to be located where the gut lumen turns down over the puborectalis (PR) muscle. The same anatomical landmark is used to measure the diameter of the anus from the outside borders of the muscularis propria.
- Internal (IAS) and external (EAS) anal sphincters: These are measured in their short axis at either the 3, 6, or 9 o'clock position from the cross section of the anal canal at a point where it is seen to assume a perfect ring shape. The reported mean thickness is 5 mm ± 1.3, range 3–7 mm (EAS); and 3 mm ± 0.9, range 2–5 mm (IAS).
- Thickness of the PR muscle: This is measured on axial scans in the midpoint of its lateral portion, where the muscle diverges from the anal canal. The same anatomic landmark is also used to draw a line tangential to the lateral aspect of the muscle on both sides to allow measurement of the angle formed in between, which is referred to as the PR angle. Mean values reported are 5 mm ± 1.04, range 2.5–7 mm (thickness) and 40° ± 8.8 (angle).

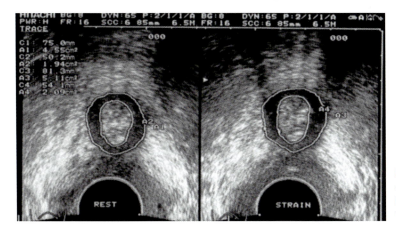

Fig. 3. Method for measurement by manual tracing of anal cross-sectional area at rest and on straining, taking the inner and outer borders, respectively, of the internal anal sphincter as reference. Reprinted from [19]

Table 1. External (A1) and internal[a] (A2) anal cross-sectional area (cm^2) at sonography by two repeated measurements (1st and 2nd) at rest and on straining in ten asymptomatic women

Case	Rest					Strain			
	A1		A2			A1		A2	
	1st	2nd	1st	2nd		1st	2nd	1st	2nd
1	3.20	3.00	1.74	1.83		2.87	2.98	1.72	1.75
2	2.40	2.35	1.21	1.30		2.21	2.27	1.10	1.17
3	1.75	1.80	0.92	1.01		1.39	1.42	0.74	0.78
4	2.41	2.38	1.06	1.02		2.57	2.60	1.17	1.12
5	1.84	1.90	0.96	0.92		1.54	1.58	0.98	1.01
6	2.15	2.20	1.01	1.05		2.23	2.18	1.08	1.11
7	2.31	2.28	1.11	1.06		2.10	2.04	1.04	0.98
8	2.75	2.69	1.03	1.08		2.80	2.73	0.95	1.03
9	1.90	1.86	0.84	0.90		2.10	2.08	1.01	1.05
10	2.30	2.28	1.03	0.98		2.38	2.31	1.05	1.08

[a] Relative to the outer and inner border, respectively, of the internal anal sphincter

Table 2. Average values of external (A1) and internal (A2) and paired t test of anal cross-sectional area in ten asymptomatic women without rectal prolapse

	Mean ± SD	Confidence interval of Δ	Paired t test	Significance
A1				
Rest	2.30 (0.43)	−0.027 − 0.081	1.132	NS
Strain	2.21 (0.48)	−0.049 - 0.049	0.00	NS
A2				
Rest	1.09 (0.24)	−0.068 - 0.020	−1.22	NS
Strain	1.08 (0.25)	−0.095 - 0.131	0.35	NS

SD standard deviation, *NS* not significant

- Anal cross-sectional area: This is calculated at rest and on straining by outlining the inner and outer margins of the smooth IAS muscle and measuring the included area at the level of the middle anal canal in the axial plane (Fig. 3). Test–retest analysis of this parameter (see Tables 1 and 2) has shown it to be both reliable and accurate. In addition, it seems to have sufficient discriminatory capacity to allow distinction between patients with and without anorectal prolapse (inner to outer ratio and increase on straining 81.3 ± 2.9% vs 49.6 ± 8.2%, $p < 0.01$ and $\Delta 0.42$ vs $\Delta -0.007$, $p < 0.01$, respectively).

Image analysis

To reduce difficulties in interpretation and to eliminate discrepancies with radiographs and MR sagittal images of the pelvis with regard to the side of the pictures, sonograms are standardized to display the caudal side of the patient's body at the lower edge of the screen, the cranial portion at the top, the dorsal portion on the right, and the ventral portion on the left. To obtain this positioning, the upside-down facility is activated so that the transducer is seen at the bottom and the image is always generated from below upward. On all other planes, i.e., axial and coronal, the right and left sides are designated following the convention used for routine imaging, in which the left side of the monitor corresponds to the right side of the patient and vice versa.

Rectal Prolapse: Definition and Imaging on Sonography

Traditionally, dynamic contrast radiography (evacuation proctography) provides a baseline to which other, more recent, modalities can be compared for investigating intraluminal anorectal abnormalities, and criteria for diagnosing rectal prolapse derived from proctographic examinations are generally applicable to either US or MR imaging. In its classic description [1, 2], mucous prolapse is defined as a rectal wall infolding of <3-mm thick confined to the anterior or posterior margin, which does not show a tendency to migrate distally on straining. Conversely, a circumferential infolding of the rectal wall ≥3 mm that descends toward the anal canal is defined as intussusception, which is termed intrarectal when it remains within the rectum and intra-anal if its apex penetrates the anal canal. Morphological features of intussusception to be determined include thickness, depth of descent, and the point of inversion from the anal verge. In addition, intussusception can be graded by using a three-point scale depending on the involved rectal-wall appearance at the end of evacuation, as follows: grade 1 intussusception is a 3- to 5-mm thick intraluminal filling defect that presumably has a mucosal component only; grade 2 intussusception is 5- to 10-mm thick and includes both the mucosal and mural components; grade 3 or full-thickness intussusception is assumed if the prolapsed folds are thicker than 10 mm, penetrate the anal canal, and appear to impede the expulsion of rectal content. A complete external rectal prolapse is diagnosed when the entire thickness of the rectal wall is extruded

through the anal canal, It is termed *reducible* when it disappears at the end of evacuation either spontaneously or by voluntary squeezing the pelvic floor musculature. It is called *unreducible* if it can be reduced only with the hands. Finally, a rectocele appears as any rectal protrusion anterior to a line extending upward through the anal canal. Its depth, either at rest or on straining, should be measured as the shortest distance from the deepest margin of where it actually reaches the anterior rectal wall and the expected line mentioned above. Rectocele [17] is graded as small if it measures <2-cm deep, moderate if it measures from 2 to 4 cm, and large if it measures ≥4 cm.

A distinct advantage of sonography over contrast radiography is its ability to depict the cross-sectional anatomy of the anal canal in fine detail, including that of the mucosa-submucosa complex and the IAS and EAS. Obtaining information on both these structures is unanimously considered an essential part of anorectal prolapse syndrome, with important therapeutical implications. In asymptomatic patients, via the introital route, the undisturbed anatomy of the anal canal is always displayed on axial scans (identification rate 100%) as follows: The virtual lumen of the anal canal is wrapped up by the hypoechoic mucosa that reproduce the "X-like" shape of a clover. Directly outside the mucosa, two to three triangular-shaped images of intermediate echogenicity that represent the submucosa are found. The IAS is the innermost muscular structure and is the continuation of the circular part of the rectal mucosa wall. It is clearly seen as a symmetric 3-mm-thick, hypoechoic ring encircling completely the submucosa. Outside the IAS is the mixed echogenic intersphincteric space. Within this space is the relatively hypoechoic longitudinal muscle, which is a continuation of the longitudinal part of the rectal muscular wall. The intersphincteric space is bordered by the relatively echoic EAS (Fig. 4). The intensively hyperechoic PR muscle is the most peripheral structure of the upper part of the sphincter. The upper part of the anal sphincter complex is connected to the levator ani muscle. In mucous prolapse, a focal deformity becomes visible that affects one or more of the arms of the X-shaped hypoechoic mucosa, leading to the appearance of a cudgel (Fig. 5). This has been found by us to correspond to the intraluminal filling defect of contrast radiography and is described as grade 1 intussusception, which has a mucosal component only. On the other hand, a circumferential infolding of the rectal wall that descends and penetrates the anal canal with its apex (intra-anal intussusception) shows a different pattern as follows: Taking the hypoechoic IAS as reference, the cross-

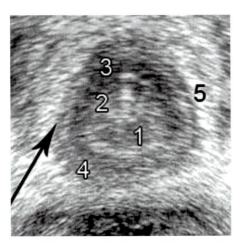

Fig. 4. Normal short-axis (axial) echotexture of the anal canal: *1* mucosa, *2* submucosa, *3* internal anal sphincter, *4* intersphincteric space with the longitudinal muscle (*arrow*), *5* external anal sphincter

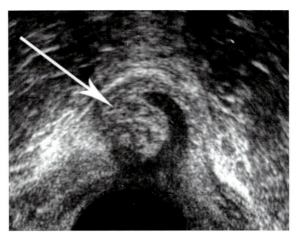

Fig. 5. Mucous prolapse. Disruption of the normal mucosa–submucosa pattern (*arrow*) on straining

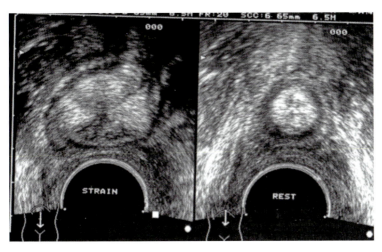

Fig. 6. Full-thickness external rectal prolapse on straining (*left panel*) is seen to disappear spontaneously when the effort is discontinued (*right panel*) in a 18-year-old woman with obstructed defecation who subsequently underwent surgical repair. Note the significant (>50%) inner to outer area ratio and increase on straining

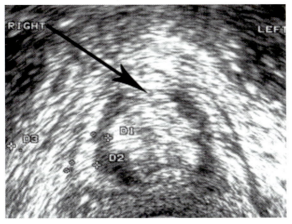

Fig. 7. Intra-anal intussusception in a 38-year-old woman with obstructed defecation and episodes of anal leakage following birth trauma. Note the internal anal sphincter derangement and attenuation (*arrow*)

sectional area of the anal canal measured on straining from the inner border of the sphincter is seen to enlarge (Fig. 6) until it overcomes by 50% that measured from its outer border. When present, a full-thickness prolapse involving both the mucosal and mural components can also be assumed (which corresponds to grades 2 and 3 intussusception at radiography), which is seen to impinge on the anal lumen and obstruct defecation. Conversely, complete external rectal prolapse with associated fecal incontinence is diagnosed when the entire thickness of the rectal wall is extruded through the anal canal and appears encircled by concentric rings of an attenuated or disrupted IAS (Fig. 7). This discriminating capability by sonography is highly suggestive. It encourages further investigation considering that for patients with rectal prolapse and obstructed defecation as their primary symptom, only approximately 40% improve following surgery, whereas continence improves to some degree in up to 75% for those with incontinence as their main symptom.

It might be argued, however, that just stressing the perineum, though giving useful information, is of limited value for detecting the most important abnormalities affecting the posterior compartment, such as trapping in a rectocele and enterocele, that occur only when the rectum is stressed maximally by evacuation. Thus, transperineal sonography may have to include rectal voiding to become a valuable study in coloproctology. Not by chance, a special technique has been developed by us that is capable of providing details of the anorectal anatomy during evacuation of semisolid barium sulphate suspension. Characteristically, this substance appears radiopaque at contrast radiography and, unlike acoustic gel, hydrogen peroxide, or tap water, is homogeneously anechoic at sonography, thus enhancing optimal visualization of inner anorectal layers. For the emptying phase, patients are scanned in the squatting position with their knees flexed and thighs abducted sufficiently to allow placement of the transducer in a sagittal orientation between the labia majora after having positioned a pad on the floor of the diagnosis room. Major drawbacks of this technique are that it is: (1) somewhat difficult for the sonographer, who sits in front of the patient, to keep the probe fixed in place during the process of evacuation; (2) potential risk of wrong assessment due to shift of the anatomic plane during strain resulting in measurement of sections different from those intended. In fact, determining a rectal base position during evacuation with respect to the starting position used by evacuation sonography has not been proven by us [16] to be sufficiently accurate and reproducible to match dynamic contrast radiography in cases of rectal prolapse. On the other hand, the examination is capable of showing soft-tissue details not seen on defecograph-ic sequences, including a curvilinear hyperechoic structure that extends from the posterior border of the gut lumen to the anterior anorectal junction on sagittal dynamic images, which has been suggested to represent the locked valve mechanism initially proposed by Phillips and Edwards [18]. This structure, which becomes visible only at sonography, thanks to the anechoic contrast medium injected intrarectally, lies as a flap over the upper end of the anal canal, effectively occluding it. At the beginning of defecation, a downward bulge is seen to occur in the linear stripe, which is followed by opening of the anorectum into a funnel shape. It is possible to suggest that any impairment in the mechanism for breaking the seal of the valve may lead to outlet obstruction, strain at defecation, and eventually to rectal prolapse.

Conclusion

Whereas dynamic radiography (proctography) is commonly considered superior to US in evaluating the presence and extent of abnormalities affecting the gut lumen, it has limited value in demonstrating anatomic derangements of extraluminal structures, including in particular the anal sphincters, fat recesses, muscles, and fascia. Perineal sonography, on the other hand, has limited value during the emptying phase and is highly operator dependent but is safe, inexpensive, and well tolerated by the patient. Its main value in patients with obstructed defecation and anorectal prolapse consists of giving objective evidence of relationships between pelvic organs and concomitant anal-sphincter derangements, which, in turn, allows better therapeutic decisions.

Acknowledgements

The authors are especially indebted to Dr. Ebe Tartufo for her assistance in formatting the manuscript.

References

1. Ekberg O, Mahieu PHG, Bartram CI et al (1990) Defecography: dynamic radiological imaging in proctology. Gastroenterol Int 3:63–69
2. Kelvin FM, Maglinte DDT, Benson JT (1994) Evacuation proctography (defecography): an aid to the investigation of pelvic floor disorders. Obstet Gynecol 83:307–314
3. Hock D, Lombard R, Jehaes C et al (1993) Colpocystodefecography. Dis Colon Rectum 36:1015–1021
4. Kelvin FM, Maglinte DDT, Benson JT et al (1994) Dynamic cystoproctography: a technique for assessing disorders of the pelvic floor in women. AJR Am J Roentgenol 163:368–370
5. Piloni V, Spazzafumo L (2007) Sonography of the female pelvic floor: clinical indications and techniques. Pelviperineology 26:59–65
6. Rubens DJ, Strang JG, Bogineni-Misra S et al (1988) Transperineal sonography of the rectum: anatomy and pathology revealed by sonography compared with

CT and MR imaging. AJR Am J Roentgenol 170:637–642

7. Chang TS, Bohm-Velez M, Mendelson EB (1993) Nongynecological applications of transvaginal sonography AJR Am J Roentgenol 160:87–93

8. Sultan AH, Loder PB, Bartram CI et al (1994) Vaginal endosonography: new approach to image the undisturbed anal sphincter. Dis Colon Rectum 37:1296–1299

9. Sandridge DA, Thorp JM (1995) Vaginal endosonography in the assessment of the anorectum. Obstet Gynecol 86:1007–1009

10. Halligan S, Northover J, Bartram CI (1996) Vaginal endosonography to diagnose enterocele. Br J Radiol 69:996–999

11. Alexander AA, Liu JB, Merton DA et al (1997) Fecal incontinence: transvaginal US evaluation of anatomic causes Radiology 199:529–532

12. Peschers UM, DeLancey JO, Schaer GN et al (1997) Exoanal ultrasound of the anal sphincter: normal anatomy and sphincter defects. Br J Obstet Gynaecol 104 (9):999–1003

13. Stewart LR, Wilson SR (1999) Transvaginal sonography of the anal sphincter: reliable or not? AJR Am J Roentgenol 173 (1):179–185

14. Piloni V (2001) Dynamic imaging of pelvic floor with transperineal sonography. Tech Coloproctol 5:103–105

15. Beer-Gabel M, Zbar AP (2002) Dynamic transperineal ultrasound in patients presenting with obstructed evacuation Tech Coloproctol 6:141

16. Piloni V, Spazzafumo L (2005) Evacuation sonography. Tech Coloproctol 9:119–126

17. Kelvin FM. Maglinte DDT, Hale DS et al (2000) Female pelvic organ prolapse: a comparison of triphasic dynamic MR imaging and triphasic fluoroscopic cystocolpoproctography. AJR Am J Roentgenol 174: 81–88

18. Phillips SF, Edwards DAW (1965) Some aspect of anal continence and defecation. Gut 6:396–406

19. Piloni VL, Bazzocchi A, Golfieri R (2007) Functional imaging in rectal prolapse. In: Altomare DF, Pucciani F (eds) Rectal prolapse. Springer-Verlag Italia, pp 21-32

CHAPTER 22

Dynamic Two- and Three-dimensional Ultrasonography: Echodefecography

Sthela M. Murad Regadas, F. Sérgio P. Regadas

Abstract

Here we describe a novel dynamic ultrasonography technique – echodefecography – using a 360° two- and three- dimensional transducer with automatic scanning to assess patients with obstructed defecation. The technique is useful to evaluate evacuation disturbances affecting the posterior compartment (anorectocele, intussusception, prolapse, and anismus) and the middle compartment (enterocele). Echodefecography may be used as an alternative method to assess patients with obstructive defecation syndrome, as it has been shown to detect the same anorectal dysfunctions identified by defecography.

Introduction

Techniques using dynamic anorectal ultrasonography (DA-US) using transperineal US [1, 2], endorectal 2D endoprobe [3], transrectal approaches by filling the rectal lumen with water [4], or US gel with a 3D endoprobe [5–7] have been described to assess patients with obstructed defecation (OD). Such dynamic evaluations require viewing the entire pelvis and the anorectal segment longitudinally. Thus, as the conventional 360° axial transducer cannot produce 3D images, it is of limited use. Murad Regadas et al. [5–7] developed the echodefecography technique using a 360° 2D and 3D transducer (model 2050) with automatic scanning, frequencies in the range of 10–16 MHz, and a focal distance of 2.8–6.2 cm. The transducer is kept in the position of initial image acquisition and follows the movement of the pelvic floor muscles during straining. These techniques are useful to evaluate evacuation distur-

bances affecting the posterior compartment (anorectocele, intussusception, prolapse, and anismus) and the middle compartment (enterocele).

Echodefecography Technique

The patient is submitted to rectal enema 2 h before the exam and is duly informed about the procedure, including the need for alternating between rest and straining over a 20-s period. The result of the exam depends on the degree of cooperation obtained from the patient. The transducer is introduced into the rectum and positioned at 6–7 cm from the anal margin. Four automatic scans are performed to identify anatomical and functional changes induced by straining. The images are evaluated in the axial and longitudinal planes and, if necessary, in the diagonal plane. Each scan takes 50 s and may be repeated if necessary. The examination takes 10–15 min on the average.

Scan One

The transducer is positioned 6 cm from the anal margin. The lower rectum, anorectal junction, and anal canal are then scanned with the patient at rest. The anatomical configuration of the anal canal is checked for muscle injury, even in asymptomatic patients (occult lesions).

Scan Two

The transducer is positioned 6 cm from the anal margin. The patient alternates between rest and strain-

M. Pescatori, F.S.P. Regadas, S.M. Murad Regadas, A.P. Zbar (eds.), *Imaging Atlas of the Pelvic Floor and Anorectal Diseases*. ISBN 978-88-470-0808-3. © Springer-Verlag Italia 2008

ing during the same scan. Scanning starts with the patient at rest for 15 s while images of the lower rectum are acquired. The patient is then asked to strain for 20 s while the scanner captures dynamic images of the lower rectum, anorectal junction, upper anal canal, and proximal part of the mid anal canal. Finally, the patient rests for 15 s while the lower and distal part of the mid anal canal are scanned.

This scan evaluates the movements of the puborectalis (PR) muscle during the evacuatory effort, identifying normal relaxation or paradoxical contraction (anismus).

Scan Three

The transducer is positioned 7 cm from the anal margin during a sequence of rest and straining similar to that described for scan two. However, scanning is initiated more proximally to check for rectal invagination. Findings are confirmed in the following scan.

Scan Four

After injecting 120–180 ml of US gel into the rectal ampulla, the transducer is positioned 7 cm from the anal margin, and the scanning sequence described above is followed. If straining is not maintained properly for 20 s or if the transducer is not positioned centrally in the rectum, scanning may have to be repeated, including reapplication of gel as needed. During scanning, the intrarectal gel distends the rectal walls, making it possible to view the layers and inducing voiding desire as in defecation. All anatomical structures of the anal canal, anorectal junction, and pelvic floor may be viewed, and anatomical and functional changes associated with voiding may be demonstrated and quantified while confirming findings from the previous scan. It is important to make sure the patient is effectively straining despite the presence of the intrarectal transducer and despite being in the left lateral position. Straining may be confirmed by observing evacuatory efforts on the transducer, by eliminating the intrarectal gel, and by changes in the position of anatomical structures.

Image Interpretation

Static and dynamic images acquired during the four scanning procedures described above are analyzed. The position of the anatomical structures involved during the evacuatory effort is compared for the rest-

ing and straining positions (dynamic images), and measurements are taken by drawing lines and angles. Images are analyzed according to evacuatory dysfunction.

Anismus

Anismus may be evaluated in either 2D or 3D mode.

Two-dimensional Mode

The transducer is positioned at the PR level. The angle, which is measured during both rest and straining, is produced by drawing two diagonal lines at the 3 and 9 o'clock positions of the internal circumference of the transducer and making them converge at the 6 o'clock position of the internal border of the PR muscle [8].

Normal findings: The angle is relatively closed due to PR muscle relaxation during straining, increasing the distance between the transducer and the PR muscle (Fig. 1).

Diagnosis of anismus: The angle is wider due to the paradoxical contraction of the voluntary anal muscles during the evacuatory effort, decreasing the distance between the transducer and the PR muscle (Fig. 2).

Three-dimensional Mode (Sagittal Plane)

An angle is formed by the convergence of a 1.5-cm line drawn parallel to the internal border of the PR muscle and a vertical line drawn perpendicular to the axis of the anal canal. The angle is measured during rest (scan one) and straining (scan two) [6] (Fig. 3).

- Normal findings: The distance between the transducer and the PR muscle is increased during straining, widening the angle due to relaxation of the PR muscle and the external anal sphincter (EAS) [6] (Fig. 3).
- Diagnosis of anismus: The distance between the transducer and the PR muscle is reduced during straining, narrowing the angle due to the paradoxical contraction of the striated anal muscles [6] (Fig. 4).

The angle measures are inverted in the axial (2D) and longitudinal (3D) projection due to the references established, but they are easy to interpret, as both projections evaluate the movements of the PR muscle during straining. The advantage of the 3D projection is that movement of the PR muscle and the EAS may

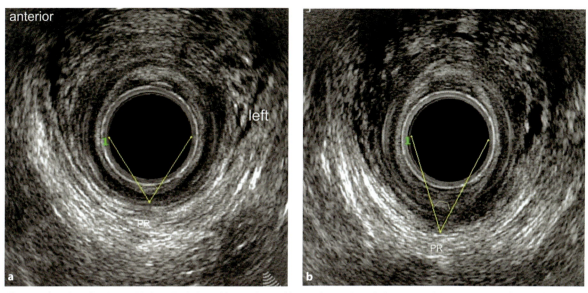

Fig. 1 a, b. Normal patient, axial plane. Angle formed by *two diagonal lines* at the 3 and 9 o'clock positions of the internal circumference of the endoprobe, converging at the 6 o'clock position of the internal border of the puborectalis (*PR*) muscle. **a** Resting. **b** Evacuatory effort. Reduced angle

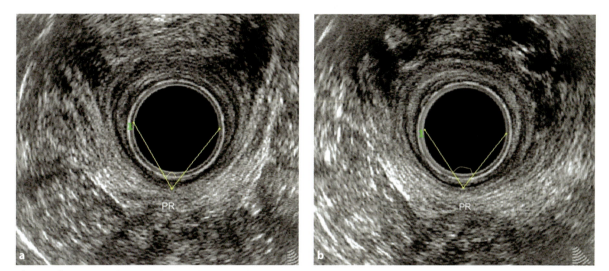

Fig. 2 a, b. Patient with anismus (2D image), **a** Resting. **b** Evacuatory effort. Increased angle. *PR* puborectalis muscle

be evaluated in their entire longitudinal extension. Despite the movement, the high spatial resolution of the image makes it possible to observe the beginning and end of straining without distortion, in addition to other changes of interest.

Anorectocele

Anorectocele may be identified in scan four. The vagina is the anatomical structure of reference. Movements of the posterior wall of the vagina, the anterior wall of the lower rectum, the anorectal junction, and the upper anal canal are evaluated. The effect of straining is demonstrated by comparing the distance between two parallel lines drawn on the projection of the posterior wall of the vagina during rest and straining. In normal women, the vagina is displaced downward and backward and presses against the anterior wall of the lower rectum, the anorectal junction, and the upper anal canal during straining. At rest, the vagina remains at the same level or slightly posterior to its original position on the projection of the lower rectum [5, 7, 8] (Fig. 5).

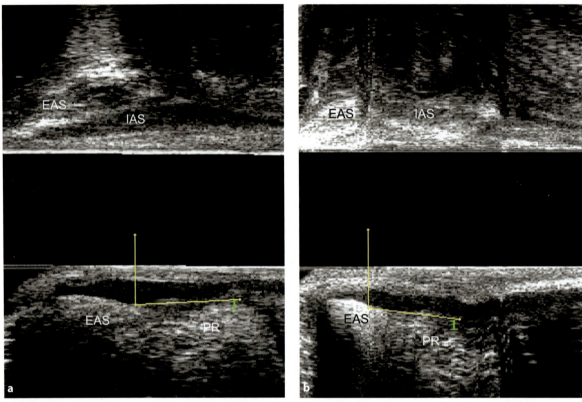

Fig. 3 a, b. Normal patient, mid sagittal plane. Angle formed by the confluence of a line traced parallel with the internal edge of the puborectalis (*PR*) muscle (*line 1*) and another vertical line according to the anal canal axis. **a** Resting. **b** Straining. Increased angle. *EAS* external anal sphincter, *IAS* internal anal sphincter

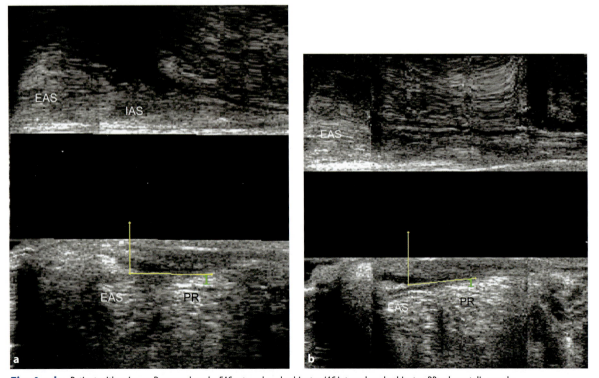

Fig. 4 a, b. Patient with anismus. Decreased angle. *EAS* external anal sphincter, *IAS* internal anal sphincter, *PR* puborectalis muscle

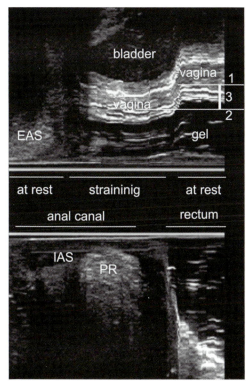

Fig. 5. Normal patient. *Line 1*: parallel with the vaginal wall at rest. *Line 2*: parallel with the vaginal wall during straining. *Line 3*: distance between lines 1 and 2 (*arrow*). *EAS* external anal sphincter, *IAS* internal anal sphincter, *PR* puborectalis muscle

Diagnosis of Anorectocele

During straining when the pressure rises in the lower rectum and the anal canal, the vagina is pressed forward by the anterior wall of the lower rectum, anorectal junction, and the upper anal canal. Based on echodefecographic images [9], Regadas et al. [10] demonstrated that the herniation starts probably on the anterior wall of the anorectal junction and upper anal canal and then involves the lower rectum as it enlarges. Therefore, the term anorectocele was proposed. The site of largest herniation is on the upper anal canal (Fig. 6). Anorectocele is demonstrated and quantified by measuring the distance between two horizontal lines drawn in parallel with the posterior vagina wall, one at the point where straining starts (when the posterior vaginal wall displaces the anterior wall of the lower rectum downward and backward) and one at the point of maximum distension of the anterior wall of the anorectal junction and upper anal canal (herniation into the vagina) (Fig. 6). If the anorectocele is very large, the focal distance of the transducer may have to be increased up to 6.2 cm to allow viewing the entire herniation. At this focal distance, the image is preserved without distortion, and the anatomical structures are clearly visualized. The echodefeco-

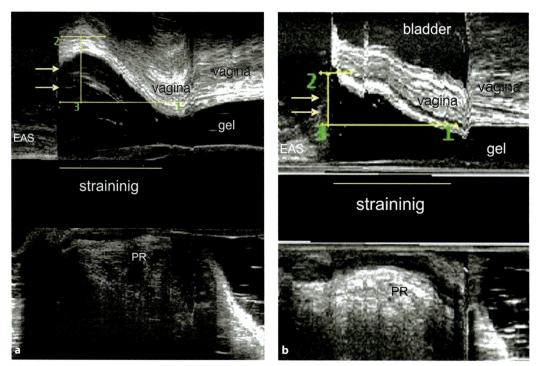

Fig. 6 a, b. Patient with anorectocele grade III, mid sagittal plane. *Line 1*: parallel with the vaginal wall during initial straining. *Line 2*: parallel with the vaginal wall at maximal herniation point. *Line 3*: distance between lines 1 and 2 (anorectocele size) (*arrows*). *EAS* external anal sphincter, *PR* puborectalis muscle

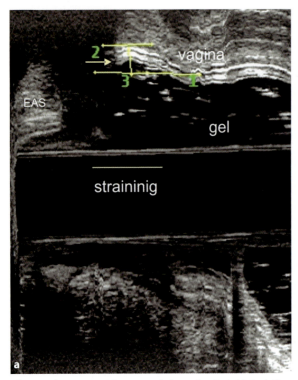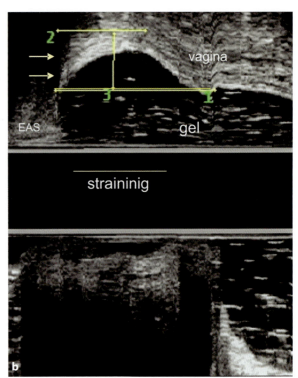

Fig. 7 a, b. Patient with anorectocele (*arrows*). **a** Grade I. **b** Grade II

graphic classification, which is based on a comparison with cinedefecography, establishes that herniations measuring 0.2–0.6 cm (average 0.5 cm) correspond to stage I anorectocele (Fig. 7a), 0.7–1.3 cm (average 1.0 cm) to stage II anorectocele (Fig. 7b), and >1.3 cm to stage III anorectocele [6–8] (Figs. 6 and 8c).

Intussusception

Intussusception is easily identified when two parallel muscle layers are visualized in the axial and longitudinal planes during straining without intrarectal gel (scan three) (Fig. 8a). When intrarectal gel is employed (scan four), the two muscle layers are seen projecting into the rectal lumen (Fig. 8b, c). Cases of minor intussusception are characterized by small displacements with practically parallel muscle layers (Fig. 9), but in more severe cases, muscle layers are displaced much further and appear perpendicular to each other (Figs. 10–12). Associating the diagonal plane can improve visualization significantly (Figs. 10b and 12c). Intussusception is easily identified even when it occurs at the level of the anorectocele (Figs. 8–12).

Anal Prolapse

Anal prolapse is a thickening of the subepithelial tissue of the anal canal, observed between the transducer and the internal anal sphincter (IAS). It can be measured in the axial and longitudinal planes and evaluated during both rest and straining [5, 8] (scans one and two) (Fig. 13).

Enterocele

The intestinal loops are usually visualized on the projection of the anterior quadrant of the mid to lower rectum close to the bladder and the uterus, even during straining. Enterocele is identified by the presence of intestinal loops on the projection of the lower rectum and upper anal canal at the level of the PR muscle and is easily observed in the axial and longitudinal planes (scans two, three and four) (Figs. 14 and 15).

Perineal Descent

Perineal descent is diagnosed and quantified with a single scan showing displacement of the pelvic floor

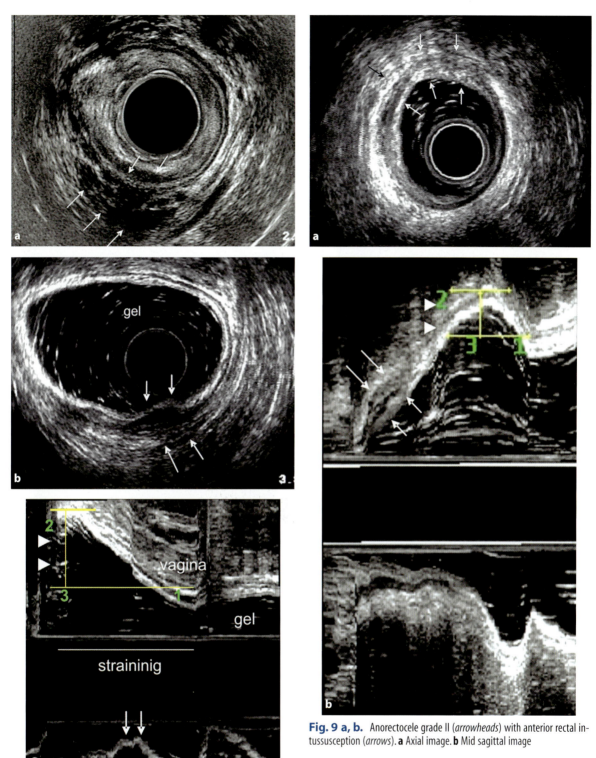

Fig. 8 a-c. Patient with anorectocele grade III (*arrowheads*) with posterior rectal intussusception (*arrows*). **a** Axial image without gel. **b** Axial image with gel. **c** Mid sagittal image with gel

Fig. 9 a, b. Anorectocele grade II (*arrowheads*) with anterior rectal intussusception (*arrows*). **a** Axial image. **b** Mid sagittal image

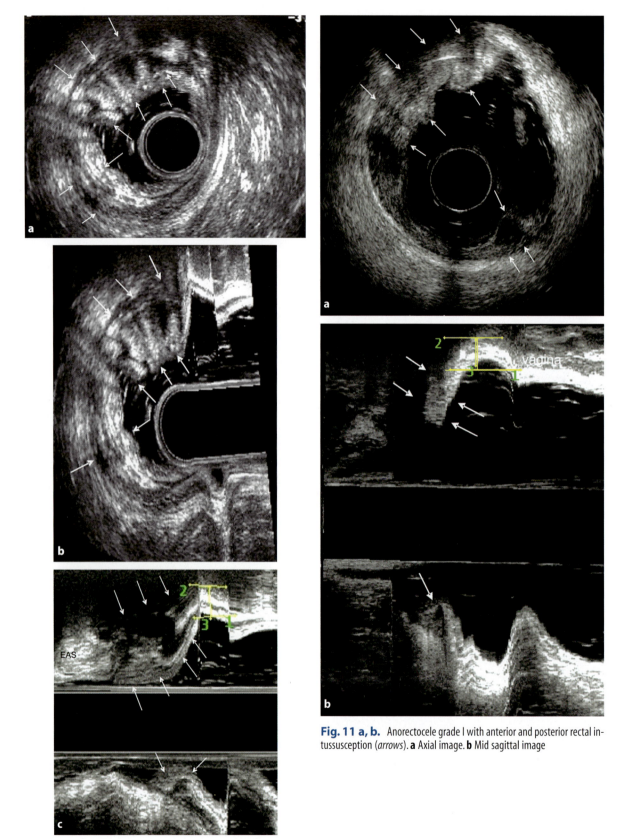

Fig. 11 a, b. Anorectocele grade I with anterior and posterior rectal intussusception (*arrows*). **a** Axial image. **b** Mid sagittal image

Fig. 10 a-c. Anorectocele grade II with hemicircumferential rectal intussusception (*arrows*). **a** Axial image. **b** Axial and sagittal image with diagonal plane. **c** Mid sagittal image. *EAS* external anal sphincter

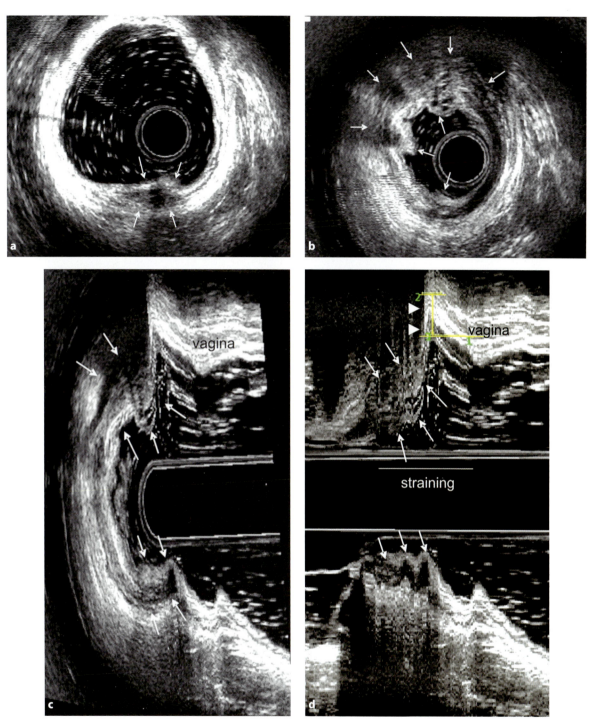

Fig. 12 a-d. Anorectocele grade II (*arrowheads*) with circumferential rectal intussusception (*arrows*). **a**, **b** Axial image. **c** Axial and sagittal image with diagonal plane. **d** Mid sagittal image

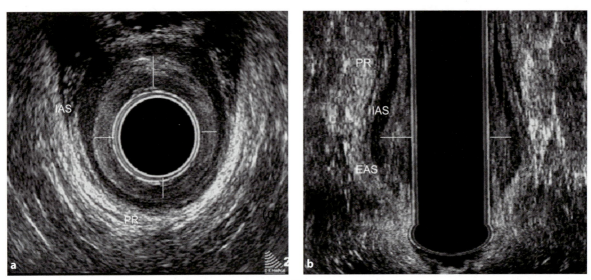

Fig. 13 a, b. Mucosa prolapse (*lines*). **a** Axial image. **b** Coronal image. *EAS* external anal sphincter, *IAS* internal anal sphincter, *PR* puborectalis muscle

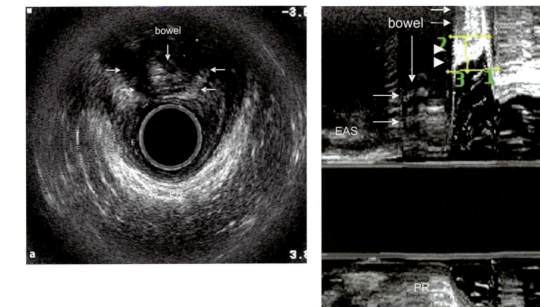

Fig. 14 a, b. Enterocele (*arrows*) with anorectocele grade II (*arrowheads*). **a** Axial image without gel. **b** Mid sagittal image with gel. *EAS* external anal sphincter, *PR* puborectalis muscle

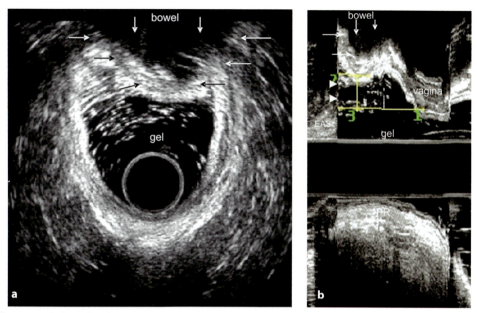

Fig. 15 a, b. Enterocele (*arrows*) with anorectocele grade II (*arrowheads*). **a** Axial image with gel. **b** Mid sagittal image with gel. *EAS* external anal sphincter

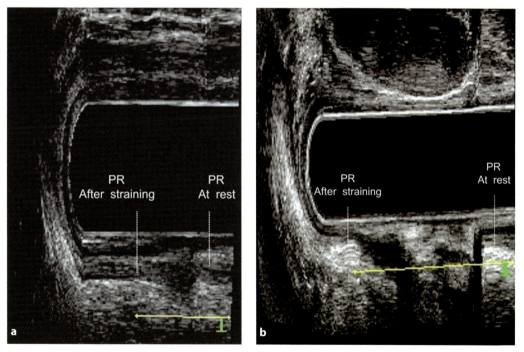

Fig. 16 a, b. **a** Normal patient, mid sagittal plane. **b** Patient with perineal descent. Increased distance between both positions of the puborectalis (*PR*) muscle

muscles between resting and straining. The transducer is positioned proximally to the PR muscle. The PR muscle is initially scanned at rest (3 s), then during straining. Unlike in the previous scanning procedures, the transducer does not follow the descending muscles of the pelvic floor but remains in the same position until the PR muscle becomes visible distally, then the scan is stopped. Straining time is directly proportional to the distance of perineal descent. The perineal descent length is quantified by measuring the distance between the position of the proximal border of the PR muscle at rest and at the point it is identified again after being displaced due to the evacuatory effort (Fig. 16).

Conclusion

Dynamic US scanning is a helpful tool in evaluating patients with obstructed defecation, as it clearly shows the anatomical structures and mechanisms involved in defecation. It also demonstrates the anorectal anatomical integrity and detects sphincter injury with high spatial resolution. It is quick, inexpensive, well tolerated by patients, and requires no radiation exposure.

References

1. Beer-Gabel M, Teshler M, Barzilai N et al (2002) Dynamic trans-perineal ultrasound (DTP-US) – a new method for diagnosis of pelvic floor disorders: technical details and preliminary results. Dis Colon Rectum 45:239–248
2. Beer-Gabel M, Teshler M, Schechtman E, Zbar AP (2004) Dynamic transperineal ultrasound vs. defecography in patients with evacuatory difficulty: a pilot study. Int J Colorectal Dis 19:60–67
3. Brusciano L, Limongelli P, Pescatori M et al (2007) Ultrasonographic patterns in patients with obstructed defaecation. Int J Colorectal Dis 22:969–977
4. Barthet M, Portier F, Heyries L (2000) Dynamic anal endosonography may challenge defecography for assessing dynamic anorectal disorders: results of a prospective pilot study. Endoscopy 32(4):300–305
5. Murad Regadas SM, Regadas FSP, Rodrigues LV et al (2006) A novel procedure to assess anismus using three-dimensional dynamic ultrasonography. Colorectal Dis 9:159–165
6. Murad Regadas SM, Regadas FSP, Rodrigues LV et al (2006) Ecodefecografia tridimensional dinâmica nova técnica para avaliação da síndrome da defecação obstruída (SDO) rev bras. Coloproctol 26(2):168–177
7. Murad Regadas SM, Regadas FSP, Rodrigues LV et al (2008) A novel three-dimensional dynamic anorectal ultrasonography technique (echodefecography) to assess obstructed defecation, a comparison with defecograhy. Surg Endoscopy 22:974-979
8. Murad Regadas SMM, Regadas FSP, Lima DMR (2006) Ultra-sonografia anorretal dinâmica novas técnicas In: Regadas FSP, Murad Regadas SMM (eds) Distúrbios funcionais do assoalho pélvico atlas de ultra-sonografia anorretal bi e tri-dimensional. Editora RevinterRio de Janeirop, pp 79–94
9. F. Sergio P. Regadas, Sthela M et al (2007) Anal canal anatomy shown by three-dimensional anorectal ultrasonography. Surg Endoscopy 21(12):2207–2211
10. Regadas FSP, Murad Regadas SM, Wexner SD et al (2006) Anorectal three-dimensional endosonography and anal manometry in assessing anterior rectocele in women. A new pathogenesis concept and the basic surgical principle. Colorectal Dis 9:80–85

Commentary

Mario Pescatori

The experience of the Regadas group in this field has progressively increased over recent years. US defecography (US-DFG) is expected to become an essential part of the anorectal physiology testing in specialized centers due to its advantages over conventional defecography, which are clearly stated in the conclusions of this chapter.

1. Anismus, which according to Bouchoucha et al. [1] is part of a multiorgan disorder (i.e., psychoneurological-gastrointestinal-urogenital), may be easily identified with US-DFG. As suggested for anal manometry, however, the diagnosis of anismus is perhaps better based on three consecutive attempts of straining and three positive finding of either nonrelaxing or paradoxical contracting puborectalis (PR) muscle. It should be noted that the presence of nurses and doctors might affect the normal behavior of the patients being tested by inducing tension in their pelvic floor muscles. To overcome such artefacts, the 24-h ambulant electromyogram using thin loop wires attached to the PR muscle – like a halter for the heart – allows measurement of the PR muscle's motor activity with the patient at home, in a more favorable psychological environment, and has been found to be helpful in distinguishing true anismus from artefacts.

2. Enterocele was one of the hot topics of the past decade. At least two important papers from the Schouten group [2, 3] showed that mesh obliteration of the pelvic outlet is likely to improve symptoms such as pelvic tension and perineal discomfort but is unlikely to effectively manage obstructed defecation, the reason being that only the "central" abnormality is dealt with. Instead, US-DFG might allow the clinician to achieve a simultaneous diagnosis of enterocele, anorectocele, and rectal intussusception, thus allowing a multifactorial correction of associated disorders. One of the advantages of US-DFG vs. DFG alone is that it also allows detection of the descent of the bowel loop, whereas the latter only depicts the wide opening of the rectovaginal space, without giving direct visualization of the visceral descensus. We developed a novel combined approach for enterorectocele and rectal prolapse and intussusception that consists of a modified pouch of Douglas, omentoplasty associated with either levatorplasty or endoanal rectocele repair (Pescatori, unpublished studies). US-DFG might support the preoperative assessment of such a complex condition. Another useful test is dynamic magnetic resonance imaging (MRI), which, unfortunately, is much more expensive and less well tolerated by the patient.

3. Solitary rectal ulcer syndrome, particularly in its pseudopolypoid version, might benefit from the application of US-DFG, as it may well detect both pseudopolyps inside the hypoechoic ring of the rectal smooth muscle and IAS hypertrophy as a possible consequence of an overactive IAS. This technique has been described at St. Mark's Hospital [4] for contrasting the above occurring neuromuscular dysfunction.

Last but not least, if we take in account appropriate treatment choice, both surgical and rehabilitative, the unexpected finding of an anteriorly interrupted EAS, possibly caused by obstetric injuries in multiparous women as reported by Brusciano et al. [5], might induce the clinician to perform an anterior sphincteroplasty or at least exclude an endoanal procedure, which might worsen sphincter function and cause fecal incontinence.

References

1. Bouchoucha M, Devroede G, Arsac M (2004) Anismus: a marker of multi-site functional disorder? Int J Colorect Dis 19:374-379
2. Gosselink MJ, van Dam JH, Huisman WM, Schouten WR (1999) Treatment of enterocele by obliteration of the pelvic inlet. Dis Colon Rectum 42.940–944
3. Oom DM, van Dijl VR, Gosselink MP, Schouten WR (2007) Enterocele repair by abdominal obliteration of the pelvic inlet: long-term outcome on obstructed defaecation and symptoms of pelvic discomfort. Colorect Dis 9:845–580
4. Halligan S, Sultan AH, Rottenberg G, Bartram CI (1995) Endosonography of the anal sphincter in solitary rectal ulcer syndrome. Int J Colorect Dis 10:79–82
5. Brusciano L, Limongelli P, Pescatori M et al (2007) Ultrasonographic pattern in patients with outlet obstruction. Int J Colorect Dis 22:969–977

CHAPTER 23

Dynamic Magnetic Resonance Defecography

Alice Brandão

Abstract

Defecography by magnetic resonance imaging is an accurate method for evaluating morphology and function of the anorectal and pelvic muscles and organs. The dynamics of the pelvic floor may be evaluated in multiple compartments in high-resolution images and video mode, and the diseases affecting the evacuation mechanism may be identified.

Introduction

Unlike earlier forms of imaging, such as conventional defecography, magnetic resonance imaging (MRI) makes it possible to view the pelvic floor in its entirety and in multiple compartments, both at rest and dynamically, thus providing information essential for surgical planning and choice of treatment approach. The technique has been shown to be equivalent to conventional defecography in all respects [1, 2] and has not only confirmed findings of simpler tests, such as proctography, but is capable of detecting unsuspected abnormalities in two thirds of cases [2].

Using MRI, the opening of the anal canal and the anorectal angle may be evaluated during sphincter contraction and evacuation, and the elimination of endorectal contrast may be quantified. The rectal walls may also be clearly observed, and disorders such as intussusception and rectocele may be identified. The global evaluation of the pelvic floor makes it possible to view the descent of the anterior, mid, and posterior compartments. Furthermore, the structure of the anal sphincters, with emphasis on the internal anal sphincter (IAS), may be examined simultaneously with the addition of an endorectal or endoanal coil [3, 4] (Fig. 1). Compared with conventional defecography, MRI may be limited by restricted access to health care services, high cost, and lack of studies comparing asymptomatic to abnormal individuals [5].

MRI is available in open-configuration systems that acquire images with the patient in the sitting or vertical position. Because of the easy access and high spatial and temporal resolution afforded by the technique, MRI findings in a closed magnetic field are discussed in this chapter, and the technique, details of pelvic floor anatomy, and the most commonly observed anatomical and functional abnormalities are described [6-8].

MRI Technique

The three compartments of the pelvic floor should be identified before and after administration of rectal contrast medium with no need for further opacification of the vagina or bladder, as the soft tissues provide an excellent contrast during MRI acquisition (Fig. 2). The examination is divided into three steps:

1. Analysis of the pelvic floor structures at rest without endorectal contrast in T2-weighted high-resolution sequences in the axial, sagittal, and coronal planes: In these images, it is possible to analyze the components of the levator ani muscle; the levator hiatus; the position of the pelvic organs, vagina, and urethra; the presence of lesions associated with uterine leiomyoma, which can accentuate symptoms; and the solitary rectal ulcer, which can be associated with intussusception (Fig. 3).

2. Dynamic video evaluation in the sagittal and coronal planes: In the sagittal plane, the exami-

M. Pescatori, F.S.P. Regadas, S.M. Murad Regadas, A.P. Zbar (eds.), *Imaging Atlas of the Pelvic Floor and Anorectal Diseases*.
ISBN 978-88-470-0808-3. © Springer-Verlag Italia 2008

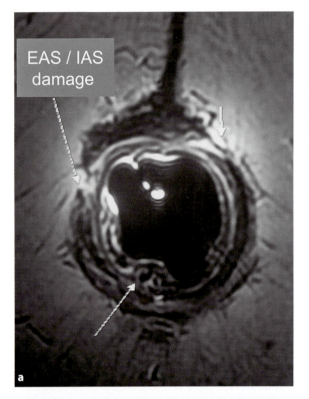

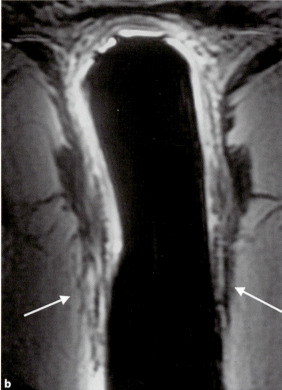

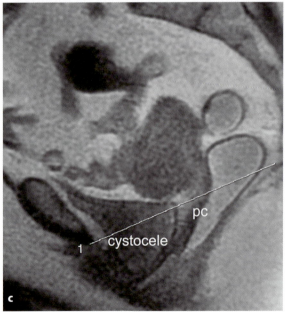

Fig. 1 a-c. Endorectal coil. Patient with complete descending perineum syndrome. Sphincter fragmentation. **a** Axial plane. **b** Coronal plane. **c** Dynamic resonance showing cystocele, ureterocele, and descending perineum according to the pubococcygeal (*pc*) line. *EAS* external anal sphincter, *IAS* internal anal sphincter

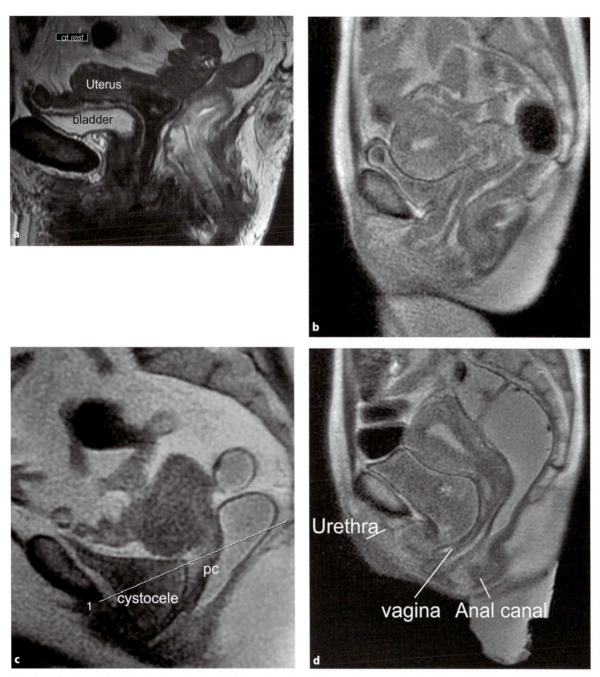

Fig. 2 a-d. Sagittal plane. Identification of urethra, bladder, vagina, uterus, rectum, and anal canal. **a** Pelvic floor at rest. **b** Valsalva maneuver. **c** Sphincter contraction. **d** Defecation

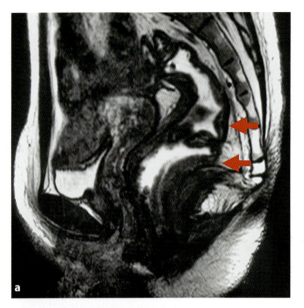
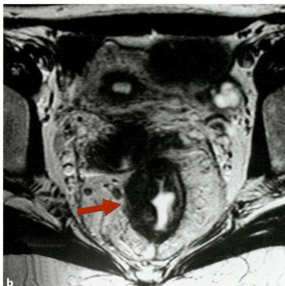
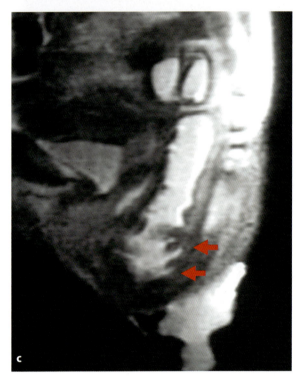

Fig. 3 a-c. Solitary rectal ulcer. **a** Sagittal plane. **b** Axial plane: rectal wall is thickened (*arrows*). **c** Dynamic resonance: anorectal intussusception (*arrows*)

nation is performed during Valsalva maneuver to determine the severity of the pelvic floor injury. In the coronal plane, mobility of the iliococcygeal component of the levator ani muscle is assessed as a reflex of unilateral or bilateral muscle bulging during increased intra-abdominal pressure (Valsalva maneuver) (Fig. 4).

3. Evacuation after the introduction of endorectal contrast medium (gel). The dynamic study is performed while the patient is lying down with bent knees during sphincter contraction and evacuation. Images showing intussusception are acquired in video mode in the sagittal plane and sometimes in the axial plane (Figs. 5 and 6).

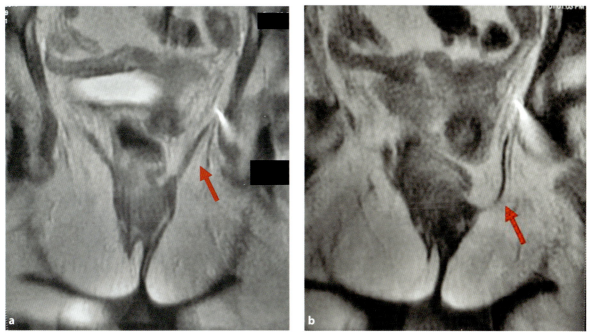

Fig. 4 a, b. Coronal plane. Levator ani muscle at rest (*arrow*) (**a**). Coronal plane: Valsalva maneuver; iliococcygeus muscle injury, with protrusion on the left side (*arrow*) (**b**)

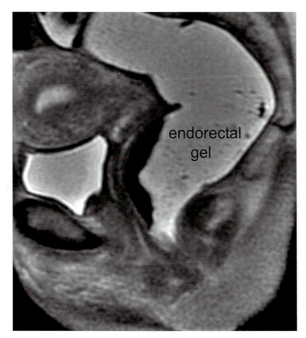

Fig. 5. Sagittal plane. Dynamic resonance with endorectal contrast gel.

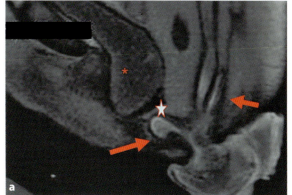

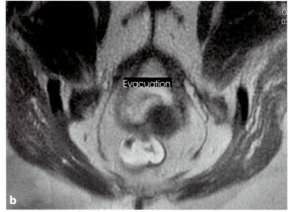

Fig. 6 a, b. Dynamic resonance demonstrating a patient with descending perineum syndrome. Cystocele and colpocele (*red star*), enterocele (*white star*) and intussusception (*arrows*). **a** Sagittal plane. **b** Coronal plane

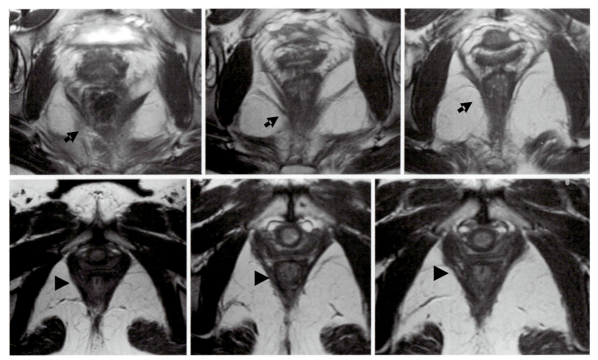

Fig. 7. Axial plane. T2-weighted imaging demonstrating normal anatomy of levator ani muscle. Iliococcygeus muscle (*arrow*) and puborectalis are well visualized (*arrowhead*)

Types of Intrarectal Contrast Medium

The bowel is prepared with a glycerine suppository or a clyster with fleet enema. Intrarectal contrast gel is introduced until the patient reports a sensation of fullness and voiding urge or until using 250 ml.

Monitoring the Examination

The examination is easily monitored using a rapid sequence of 1-s MRI scans for approximately 90 s. The variation between images acquired during rest, sphincter contraction, and evacuation helps determine the severity of abnormalities of the muscle support.

Interpretation

Levator Ani Muscles

The levator ani muscles, especially the puborectal bundle, may be viewed in the axial plane, whereas the iliococcygeal muscle is easily identified in the coronal plane. Analysis should focus on muscle mor-

phology and thickness and on signal strength [9, 10]. In the axial plane, the healthy levator ani sling should be evenly thick throughout, and the signal should be low and homogenous in T2-weighted images [11] (Fig. 7).

On the other hand, levator ani muscle injury is characterized by asymmetric or diffuse reduction in thickness with or without fat infiltration of the muscle fibers. Fat infiltration appears as high signal intensity in the muscle fibers on T1- and T2-weighted sequences [9-11] (Fig. 8).

In more severe cases, the puborectalis (PR) muscle may have become detached from the pubis, and the proximal extremity may appear retracted and irregular. Concurrently, the vagina and sometimes the urethra may have been diverted toward the injury [9, 12] (Fig. 9). In very severe lesions, the distance between the PR fibers and the levator hiatus appears increased in the axial plane. In women with an intact pelvic floor, the length should be 4.5 cm [11] (Fig. 8).

In images acquired in the coronal plane, the healthy iliococcygeal muscle appears intact with smooth ascending outlines. However, when the muscle is injured, the lower fibers tend to bulge during Valsalva maneuver [11, 13] (Fig. 4).

The levator plate remains parallel to the pubococcygeal line at rest and during Valsalva straining

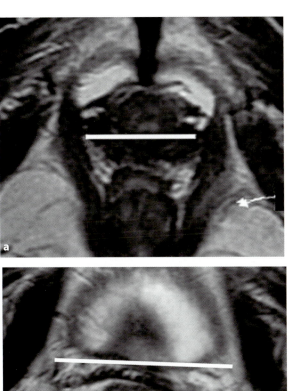

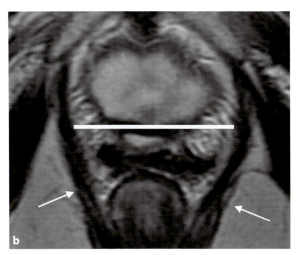

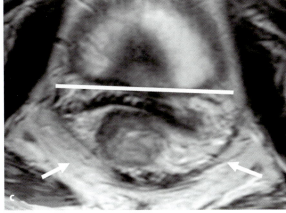

Fig. 8 a-c. Axial plane. Levator ani muscle. **a** Fat infiltration on left puborectalis muscle (*arrow*) with normal levator hiatus (<4.5cm) (*horizontal line*). **b, c** Advanced fat infiltration, specially on c, where it is not possible to identify muscle fiber (*arrows*); the levator hiatus is increased (*line*)

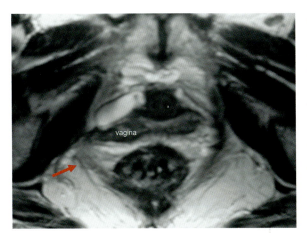

Fig. 9. Axial plane. Puborectalis muscle without pubic insertion (*arrow*) and its proximal extremity is retracted and irregular. Vagina is also dislodged to the injured muscle side (*right*)

in normal women. Increased caudal inclination indicates loss of posterior muscle support (iliococcygeal bundle) and may be identified even at rest (sagittal plane) [13] (Figs. 10 and 11).

Evaluation of the Pubococcygeal Line

The pubococcygeal line extends from the lower border of the pubic symphysis to the last coccygeal joint. It is drawn electronically and represents the level of the pelvic floor [13, 14] (Fig. 12). The distance between the pubococcygeal line and the bladder, cervix, and anorectal junction should be measured on images obtained during rest, Valsalva maneuver, and evacuation [5] (Fig. 13), whereas the anorectal

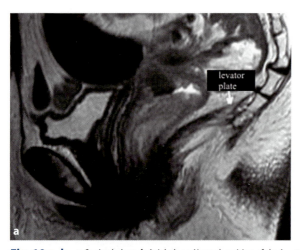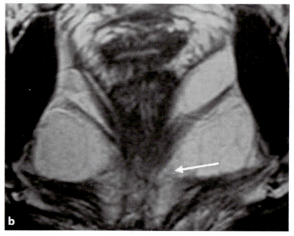

Fig. 10 a, b. a Sagittal plane. **b** Axial plane. Normal position of the levator plate (*arrow*)

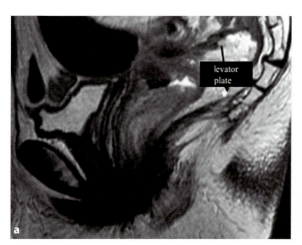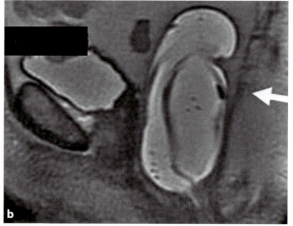

Fig. 11 a, b. Sagittal plane. **a** Normal position of the levator plate (*arrow*). **b** Sagittal plane; at rest: descending perineum syndrome and fecal incontinence. Levator plate abnormally positioned (vertical) (*arrow*)

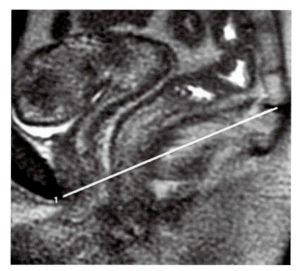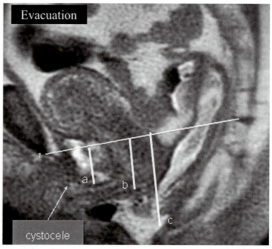

Fig. 12. T2 sagittal plane. Pubococcygeal line (*line*) extends from the inferior border of the pubic symphysis to the apex of the coccyx and represents the inferior limit of the pelvic floor

Fig. 13. (Dynamic resonance) demonstrates the distance from the pubococcygeal line (*line 1*) to the bladder (*line a*), cervix (*line b*), and anorectal junction (*line c*) during the evacuatory effort. Excessive descent of these organs in relation to the pc line. Urethra is positioned horizontally due to cystocele (*arrow*)

junction is defined by the PR muscle. In women with normal continence, the bladder, the vaginal vault, and the anorectal junction remain above the pubococcygeal line [13]. During Valsalva maneuver, the pelvic organs may move very slightly, but if the organ descends from 1 to 2 cm below the pubococcygeal line, the pelvic floor has likely been weakened. If the prolapse exceeds 2 cm, then surgery may be indicated [13] (Figs. 13 and 14).

Anterior Compartment

In sagittal images acquired during pelvic floor contraction, the healthy urethra remains slightly anterior to the base of the bladder. The loss of urethral integrity intrinsic to the sphincter and the anterior fascial support of the bladder lead to urethral hypermobility, as observed when comparing the organ's position during rest, Valsalva maneuver, and evacuation (Fig. 15).

In cystocele and stress-induced incontinence, the levator ani muscle and the pubocervical fascia are injured, making the posterior bladder wall descend below the pubococcygeal line and thereby displacing the anterior vaginal wall. Depending on severity, the injury may be identified at rest or during Valsalva maneuver and evacuation [12] (Fig. 16).

MRI scans performed during Valsalva maneuver show how much the bladder has moved in relation to the pubococcygeal line. Cystocele may be small (<3 cm), medium (3-6 cm), or large (>6 cm) [5, 15, 16].

Middle Compartment

The normal vagina is H-shaped, indicating adequate lateral fascial support [17] (Fig. 17). When normal support is lost, the vagina becomes longer and sometimes asymmetrical, depending on which side of the levator ani muscle has been most severely injured [8, 12] (Fig. 18). A downward displacement (uterocele or uterine prolapse) is also observed and may be classified as mild (<3 cm), moderate (3-6 cm), or severe (>6 cm) [16] (Fig. 19).

Enterocele is the protrusion of the peritoneum between the rectum and the vagina, with the descent of the pouch of Douglas into the rectovaginal space due to disruption of the fascia of the rectovaginal septum. A pouch is formed that may contain fat or be accompanied by the small bowel (enterocele) and/or the sigmoid (sigmoidocele). Enterocele may be identified at rest and by accentuating the dynamic images acquired in the sagittal plane during evacuation, when the sig-

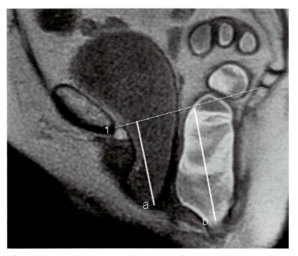

Fig. 14. Post hysterectomy. The distance from the pubococcygeal line (*line 1*) to the bladder (*line a*) and anorectal junction (*line b*) is longer than 2 cm during the evacuatory effort. It is compatible with multicompartmental defect

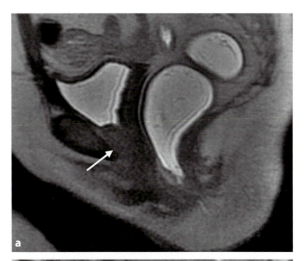

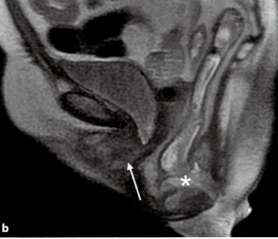

Fig. 15 a, b. Loss of urethra integrity with hypermobility comparing the **a** resting position with the **b** evacuatory effort. Rectoanal intussusception (*)

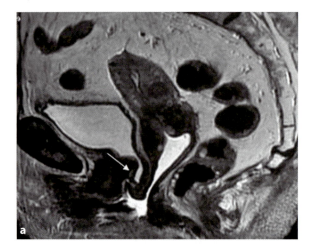

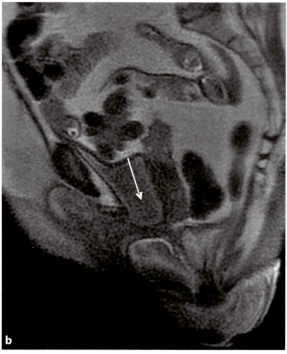

Fig. 16 a, b. Cystocele visualized in the at-rest position. **a** Protruding through vagina. **b** During the evacuatory effort (*arrows*)

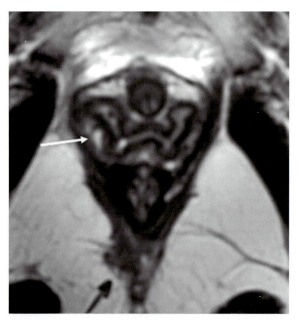

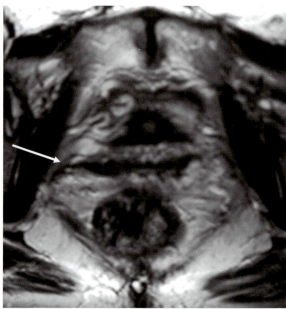

Fig. 17. T2-weighted axial plane. Normal vagina. "H" shape (*white arrow*), suggesting normal lateral fascial support. Supralevator fistulous tract (*black arrow*)

Fig. 18. T2-weighted axial plane. Vagina is straightened (arrow) due to lack of fascial support

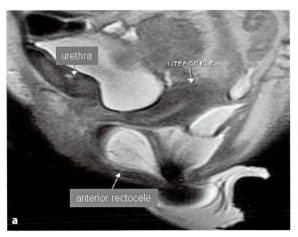

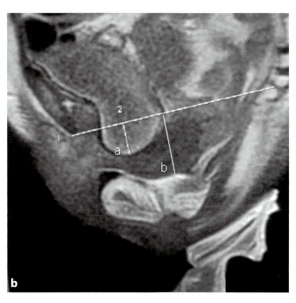

Fig. 19 a, b. Sagittal plane. Descending perineum syndrome (multi-compartmental). **a** Uterus prolapse and anterior rectocele identified during evacuatory effort (*arrows*). **b** Measurement of the cystocele (*line a*) and uterus prolapse (*line b*) in relation to pubococcygeal line (*line 1*)

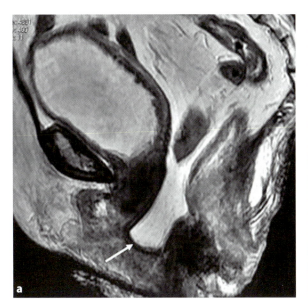

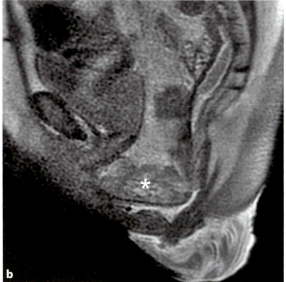

Fig. 20 a, b. Enterocele. **a** At rest (*arrow*). **b** Increased size during the evacuatory effort (*)

moid or small bowel loops may be seen invading the space between the rectum and the vagina [18] (Fig. 20).

Posterior Compartment

Observations at rest: The outline of the anterior wall is observed in order to identify small rectoceles, view the position of the anorectal junction in relation to the pubococcygeal line, and evaluate the levator plate.

Measurements during evacuation: The anorectal angle, the length and degree of the anal canal opening, the position of the anorectal junction in relation to the pubococcygeal line (perineal descent), the degree of rectal voiding, and the duration and number of contractions required to eliminate the rectal contrast should be quantified. The existence of voluntary loss of endorectal gel during rest and sphincter contraction should also be observed.

Anorectal Angle

The anorectal angle is measured from the midline of the anal canal to a tangent of the posterior rectal wall. At rest, the angle is 95° on average (range 70-134°), although it rarely exceeds 120° in healthy individuals [19] (Fig. 21). The anorectal angle normally decreases during sphincter contraction and increases during evacuation due to the contraction and relaxation, respectively, of the PR muscle [20].

Anal Canal Length

The average length of the anal canal at rest is 16 mm (range 6-26 mm) in women and 22 mm (range 10-38 mm) in young men. During sphincter contraction, the length of the anal canal is slightly reduced to an average 14 mm (range 6-20 mm) in young women and 17 mm (range 9-27 mm) in young men (Fig. 22).

Perineal Descent

The perineum is considered to have prolapsed or descended when it extends more than 2 cm below the pubococcygeal line during evacuation. This is commonly observed in patients with chronic intestinal constipation and in multiparous women [21] (Fig. 23). Perineal descent may be mild (<3 cm), moderate (3-6 cm), or severe (>6 cm) [5].

Types of Disorders

Rectocele

Rectocele is an anterior protrusion in the rectal wall. An anterior rectal protrusion in relation to a line drawn upward from the anterior wall of the anal canal to the anterior rectal wall may be defined as a rec-

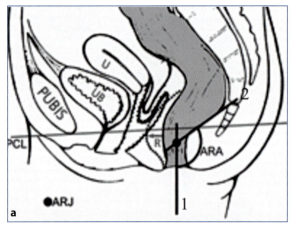

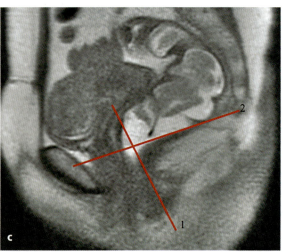

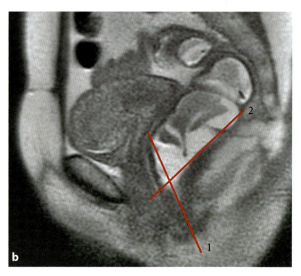

Fig. 21 a-c. The anorectal angle is measured between the axis of the anal canal and posterior rectal wall. **a** Schematic representation (line 1- anal canal line 2- posterior rectal wall). *UB* bladder, *PCL* pubococcygeal line, *ARA* anorectal angle, *ARJ* anorectal junction. **b** At rest (*line 1* anal canal, *line 2* posterior rectal wall). **c** Straining (*line 1* anal canal, *line 2* posterior rectal wall)

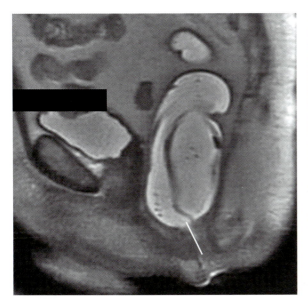

Fig. 22. Sagittal plane. Anal canal length at rest (*white line*)

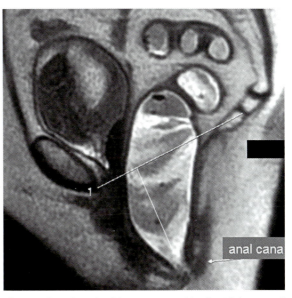

Fig. 23. Excessive perineal descent, at rest position. *Line 1* Pubococcygeal, *line 2* Anal canal

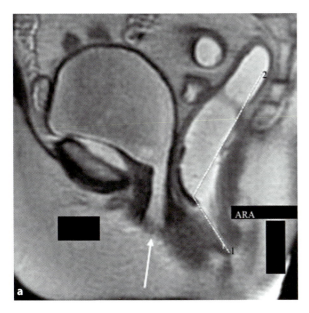

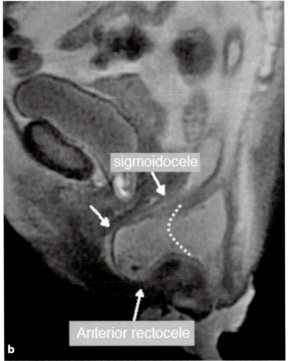

Fig. 24 a, b. Rectocele. **a** Small anterior rectal wall herniation (*arrow*). **b** Larger rectocele with enterocele and sigmoidocele (*arrows*)

tocele. Rectoceles <2.0 cm are common in asymptomatic women but are clinically unimportant [8 22] (Fig. 24). Anterior rectoceles are classified according to the size of the protrusion [5]:
- Degree 0: no rectocele is visible
- Degree 1 (small): rectocele <2.0 cm

- Degree 2 (moderate) rectocele between 2.0 cm and 4.0 cm
- Degree 3 (severe): rectocele >4.0 cm

Complete or partial voiding of the rectocele and the need for manual voiding should also be observed (Fig. 25).

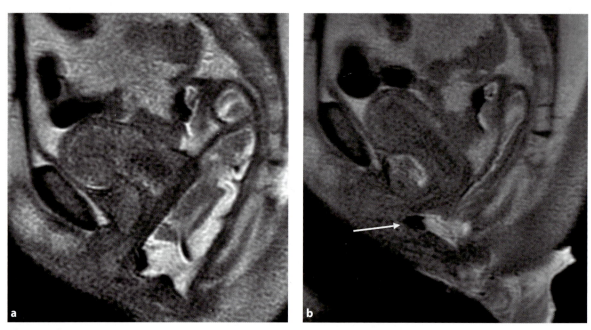

Fig. 25 a, b. Endorectal gel is evacuated during straining. **a** Initial evacuatory effort. **b** After maximal straining Rectocele (*arrow*)

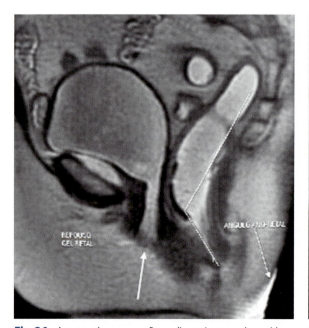

Fig. 26. At rest posthysterectomy. Descending perineum syndrome. A large cystocele is identified (*arrow*). *Line 1* anal canal, *line 2* posterior rectal wall, *ARA* anorectal junction

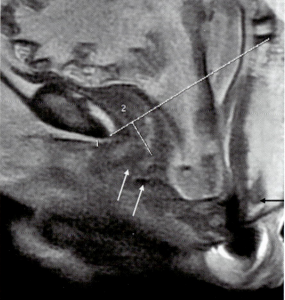

Fig. 27. Straining posthysterectomy. Increased descending perineum on the three compartments, identifying cystocele, colpocele (*white arrow*), and excessive anorectal junction descent (*black arrow*)

Descending Pelvic Floor Syndrome

In this syndrome, pelvic floor muscle tone is highly reduced. The diagnosis is usually based on clinical symptoms, electrophysiological tests, and image findings, especially MRI [5, 23]. The descent of the rectum, bladder, and vagina in relation to the pubo-coccygeal line, covering one, two, or all three compartments, is defined as pathological. The examination is performed at rest and during Valsalva maneuver and evacuation. The pelvic floor is likely to be more severely compromised when abnormalities are observed both at rest and during evacuatory effort (Figs. 26 and 27).

Spastic Pelvic Floor Syndrome

At rest, the PR muscle tractions the rectum anteriorly to maintain the anorectal angle (the angle between the posterior border of the distal rectum and the center of the anal canal). In spastic pelvic floor syndrome, the PR muscle is not relaxed physiologically during defecation but remains hypertonic throughout the entire evacuation [21, 24]. MRI T2-weighted sagittal images show how the PR muscle fails to relax during evacuation either because the anorectal angle does not increase as it should early in the evacuation process or because paradoxical contraction of the muscle reduces the angle. As a result, the patient makes a considerable effort to evacuate [5, 18] (Figs. 28 and 29).

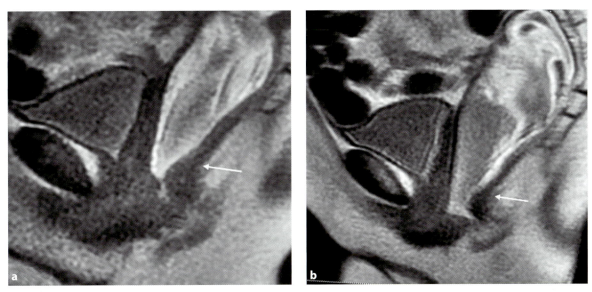

Fig. 28 a, b. Paradoxical puborectalis (PR) muscle contraction syndrome (anismus) (*arrows*). **a** At rest. **b** Straining.)The PR muscle does not relax during the evacuatory effort, keeping the same anorectal angle and suggesting anismus

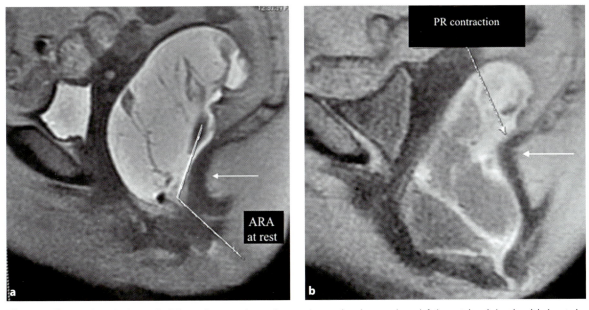

Fig. 29 a, b. Paradoxical puborectalis (PR) muscle contraction syndrome. **a** Anorectal angle at rest (*arrow*). **b** Anorectal angle is reduced during straining (*arrow*) due to paradoxical PR contraction

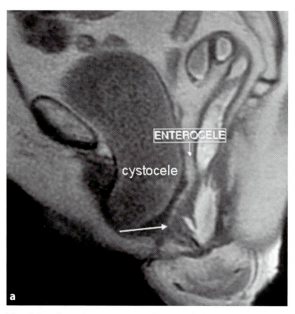 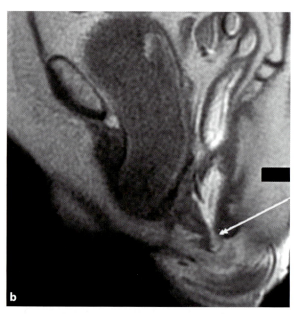

Fig. 30 a, b. a Asymptomatic small rectoanal intussusception (*arrow*) associated to cystocele and enterocele. **b** Anal mucosa prolapse (*arrow*)

Intussusception and Rectal Prolapse

Invaginations of the rectal wall and mucous membrane toward the anal canal are referred to as intussusceptions. The invagination includes the mucous membrane and may be accompanied by parietal components [18]. As in rectocele, invagination starts in the rectal wall and extends toward the anorectal junction. It is relatively commonly observed in otherwise asymptomatic patients. If the intussusception reaches the anal canal, the patient may experience a sensation of incomplete voiding due to obstruction [24] (Fig. 30). Intussusception is classified according to the degree of rectal exteriorization at the end of evacuation [5]:

– Degree 0: No intussusception
– Degree 1: Intussusception is intrarectal, with minimal involvement of the rectal wall or circumferential involvement restricted to the rectum (Fig. 30)
– Degree 2: Intussusception is restricted to the inside of the anal canal
– Degree 3: Intussusception reaches beyond the anal canal and exteriorizes through the anus (Fig. 31).

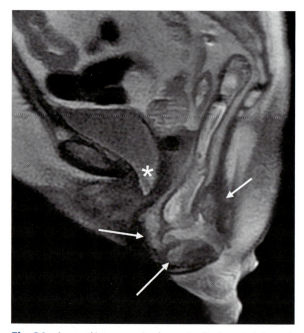

Fig. 31.   Anorectal intussusception, better visualized anteriorly (*arrows*), and a cystocele (*)

Enterocele

Enterocele is a herniation of the lower peritoneal pouch along the anterior rectal wall, in the posterior pouch of Douglas, and in the rectus recess. A wide rectovaginal fossa is formed that may contain omen-

tal and mesenteric fat, small bowel, or sigmoid [18]. Defecography with MRI easily identifies enterocele and its related components, showing prolapse of the small bowel and sigmoid (Fig. 20) into the space between the vagina and the anterior rectal wall and the sliding apart of these two organs. Enterocele is classified into three types [5]:

- Degree 0: No enterocele
- Degree 1: Herniation as far as the distal third of the vagina
- Degree 2: Herniation as far as the perineum
- Degree 3: Herniation extending beyond the anal canal.

If asymptomatic, and enteroceles are not detected prior to pelvic floor corrective surgery, they may evolve with increasingly visible symptoms and eventually require surgical correction [18].

Conclusion

Defecography with MRI provides accurate evaluation of the morphology and function of the anorectal and pelvic muscles and organs involved in pelvic floor dynamics. Imaging in the sagittal plane makes it possible to completely evaluate the anal canal and the position of the anorectal junction, vaginal vault, and bladder base in relation to the pubococcygeal line and thereby detect any pelvic organ descent. With high-resolution imaging, it is also possible to define the anatomy and functioning of the levator ani muscle, one of the most important components of the pelvic floor.

The spatial and temporal resolution is high enough to view the relevant morphological structures and dynamics of the pelvic floor, demonstrating the major pathologies affecting the defecation mechanism. Classification of findings into mild, moderate, and severe degrees is a direct and reproducible method of describing, staging, and quantifying visceral pelvic prolapse.

References

1. Shafik A (2001) Magnetic pudendal neurostimulation: a novel method for measuring pudendal nerve terminal motor latency. Clin Neurophysiol 112:1049–1052
2. Kumar S, Rao SSC (2003) Diagnostic test in fecal incontinence. Current Gastroenterol Rep 5:406–413
3. Rociu E, Stoker J, Eijkemans MJ et al (1999) Fecal incontinence: endoanal US versus endoanal MR imaging. Radiology 212:453–458
4. Malouf AJ, Halligan S, Williams AB et al (2001) Prospective assessment of interobserver agreement for endoanal MRI in fecal incontinence. Abdom Imaging 26:76–78
5. Hetzer F, Andreisek G, Tsagari C et al (2006) MR defecography in patients with fecal incontinence: imaging findings and their effect on surgical management. Radiology 240:449–457
6. Bertschinger KM, Hetzer FH, Roos JE et al (2002) Dynamic MR imaging of the pelvic floor performed with patent sitting in an open-magnet unit versus with patient supine in a closed-magnet unit. Radiology 223:501–508
7. Lienemann A, Anthuber C, Baron A et al (1997) Dynamic MR colpocystorectography assessing pelvic floor descent. Eur Radiol 7:1309–1317
8. Bertschinger KM, Hetzer FH, Roos JE, Hilfiker PR (2002) Dynamic MR imaging of the pelvic floor performed with patient sitting in an open-magnet unit versus with patient supine in a closed-magnet unit. Radiology 223:501–508
9. Bezerra MRL, Soares FFA, Fainthch S et al (2001) Identificação das estruturas músculo-ligamentares do assoalho pélvico feminino na ressonância magnética. Riod Bras 34(6):312–319
10. Jaap S, Halligan S, Bartram CI (2001) Pelvic floor imaging. Radiology 218:621–641
11. Fielding RF, Dumanli H, Schreyer AG et al (2000) MR-based three-dimensional modeling of the normal pelvic floor in women. Quantification of muscle mass. AJR Am J Roentgenol 174:657–660
12. Rodrigues, CJ, Fagundes Neto HO, Lucon M et al (2001) Alterações no sistema de fibras elásticas da fáscia endopélvica de paciente jovem com prolapso uterino. Rev Bras Ginec Obstet 23(1):234–239
13. Fielding JR (2002) Practical MR imaging of female pelvic floor weakness. Radiographics 22:295–304
14. Underweger M, Marincek B, Gottstein-Aalame N (1998) Ultrafast MR imaging of the pelvic floor. AJR Am J Roentgenol 176:959–963
15. Comiter CV, Vasavada SP, Barbaric ZL et al (1999) Grading pelvic prolapse and pelvic floor relaxation using dynamic magnetic resonance imaging. Urology 54:454–457
16. Kelvin FM, Maglinte DD, Hale DS, Benson JT (2000) Female pelvic organ prolapse: a comparison of triphasic dynamic MR imaging and triphasic fluoroscopic cystocolpoproctography. AJR Am J Roentgenol 174:81–88
17. Yang A, Mostwin JL, Rosenshein NB, Zerhouni EA (1991) Pelvic floor descend in women: dynamic evaluation with fast MR imaging and cinematic display. Radiology 179:25–33
18. Ross JE, Weishaupt D, Wildermuth S et al (2002) Experience of 4 years with open MR defecography: pictorial review of anorectal anatomy and disease. Radiographics 22:817–832
19. Stoker J, Rociu E, Zwarborn AW et al (1999) JS. Endoluminal MR imaging of the rectum and anus: technique, applications, and pitfalls. RadioGraphics 19:383–398
20. Ferrante SL, Perry RE, Schreiman JS et al (1991) The reproducibility of measuring the anorectal angle in defecography. Dis Colon Rectum 34:51–55

21. Karasick S, Karasick D, Karasick SR (1993) Functional disorders of the anus and rectum: findings on defecography. AJR Am J Roentgenol 160:777–782
22. Yoshioka K, Matsui Y, Yamada O et al (1991) Physiologic and anatomic assessment of patients with rectocele. Dis Colon Rectum 34:704–708
23. ltringer WE, Saclarides TJ, Dominguez JM et al (1995) Four contrast defecography: pelvic "floor-oscopy". Dis Colon Rectum 38:969–973
24. Shorvon PJ, McHugh S, Diamant NE et al (1989) Defecography in normal volunteers: results and implications. Gut 30:1737–1749

Subject Index

Printed in June 2008